PHARMACOLOGY – RESEARCH, SAFETY TESTING AND REGULATION SERIES

MULTIPLE DRUG RESISTANCE

PHARMACOLOGY – RESEARCH, SAFETY TESTING AND REGULATION SERIES

Antibiotic Resistance: Causes and Risk Factors, Mechanisms and Alternatives
Adriel R. Bonilla and Kaden P. Muniz (Editors)
2009. ISBN: 978-1-60741-623-4

Antibiotic Resistance: Causes and Risk Factors, Mechanisms and Alternatives
Adriel R. Bonilla and Kaden P. Muniz (Editors)
2009. ISBN: 978-1-61668-162-3 (Online Book)

Poisons: Physiologically Active Substances
S. B. Zotov and O. I. Tuzhikov
2009. ISBN: 978-1-60741-973-0

Drug Monitoring by HPLC: Recent Developments
Victoria Samanidou and Eftichia Karageorgou
2010. ISBN: 978-1-60876-183-8

Nonprescription Drugs: Considering A New Class for Behind-the-Counter Drugs
Lars P. Eliassen (Editor)
2010. ISBN: 978-1-60741-961-7

Biogenic Amines: Pharmacological, Neurochemical, and Molecular Aspects in the CNS
Tahira Farooqui and Akhlaq A. Farooqui (Editors)
2010. ISBN: 978-1-60876-625-3

Safety Efforts in Pediatric Drug Development
Conor D. Byrne (Editor)
2010 ISBN: 978-1-60741-565-7

Handbook of Drug Targeting and Monitoring
Boris Andreev and Vasily Egorov (Editors)
2010 ISBN: 978-1-60741-839-9

Biopharmaceutics and Drug Hypersensitivity
Paul Mossillo and John Pinzini (Editors)
2010 ISBN: 978-1-60741-830-6

Multiple Drug Resistance
Agoston Meszaros and Gusztav Balogh (Editors)
2010 ISBN: 978-1-60741-595-4

PHARMACOLOGY – RESEARCH, SAFETY TESTING AND REGULATION SERIES

MULTIPLE DRUG RESISTANCE

AGOSTON MESZAROS
AND
GUSZTAV BALOGH
EDITORS

Nova Biomedical Books
New York

Library of Congress Cataloging-in-Publication Data

Available upon request

ISBN: 978-1-60741-595-4

Published by Nova Science Publishers, Inc. ✦ New York

Contents

Preface		ix
Chapter I	**Profile of Genetic and Cellular Multiple Drug Resistance in a Diagnostic and Therapeutic Strategy in Acute Leukemia in Children and Adults** *Jan Styczynski and Joanna Szczepanek*	1
Chapter II	**Multidrug- Resistant *Acinetobacter baumannii* Infections: Characteristics and Treatment Options** *A. Rodríguez- Guardado, A. Blanco, F. Pérez, M. Lantero, M. Álvarez Vega, JM Torres and JA Cartón*	31
Chapter III	**Multiple Drug Resistance** *Paul D. Brown*	65
Chapter IV	**Herb-Drug Interactions and Implication in Drug Monitoring** *Ping Li and Shu-Feng Zhou*	99
Chapter V	**Cell Membranes, Cytosolic pH and Drug Transport in Cancer and MDR: Physics, Biochemistry and Molecular Biology** *Cyril Rauch, Adam Blanchard, Eleanor Wood, Eleanor Dillon, Miriam L. Wahl and Salvador Harguindey*	129
Chapter VI	**Genetic and Clinical Factors of Antibiotic Resistance in Bacteria** *Spyros D. Mentzelopoulos and Eleni E. Magira*	153
Chapter VII	**Bacteriophage Therapies and Enzybiotics: Novel Solutions to Antibiotic Resistance** *Noémie Manuelle Dorval Courchesne, Albert Parisien and Christopher Q. Lan*	167

Chapter VIII	**Nutrition and Tuberculosis** *Wing Wai Yew and Chi Chiu Leung*	**195**
Chapter IX	**Reversal of Multidrug Resistance (MDR) by the Isoquinoline Alkaloid Glaucine** *Yonggang Ma and Michael Wink*	**203**
Chapter X	**Uncommon *Acinetobacter Baumannii* Isolation from Leukemic Patients and Emerging of Tigecycline-Resistance** *Vincenzo Savini, Chiara Catavitello, Marzia Talia, Andrea Balbinot, Fabio Febbo, Assunta Manna, Arianna Pompilio, Giovanni Di Bonaventura, Raffaeele Piccolomini and Domenico D'Antonio*	**213**
Chapter XI	**Finding the Genetic Solution for Cancer in the Mechanism of Taxol Cytotoxicity** *Frank Un*	**219**
Chapter XII	**Genetic Regulation, Physiology, Assessment and Inhibition of Efflux Pumps Responsible for Multi-Drug Resistant Phenotypes of Bacterial Pathogens** *L. Amaral, S. Fanning, M. McCusker, G. Spengler, L. Rodrigues, C. Iversen, M. Martins, A. Martins, M. Viveiros and I. Couto*	**225**
Chapter XIII	**Antimicrobial Resistance: Evolutionary Roots** *Roberto Manfredi and Leonardo Calza*	**245**
Index		**251**

Preface

Multiple drug resistance is a condition enabling a disease-causing organism to resist distinct drugs or chemicals of a wide variety of structure and function targeted at eradicating the organism. Infections caused by multidrug-resistant (MDR) bacteria are an increasing problem worldwide. The interaction among several genetic host factors, distinctive anatomical and other features of the bacteria, and hygiene measures, play a paramount role in the treatment of infections caused by multidrug-resistant organisms. This important book gathers the latest research from around the world on multiple drug resistance and its clinical consequences.

Chapter I - Significant progress has been made in the therapy for pediatric acute lymphoblastic leukemia (ALL), while it was less evident in adult ALL and in acute myeloid leukemia (AML), both in children and in adults. Failure of therapy in acute leukemias is related to the presence of minimal residual disease, poor response to therapy and occurrence of relapses. Presence of cytogenetic aberrations and cellular multiple drug resistance in leukemic cells at presentation are important prognostic factors in ALL and to a lesser extent in AML. Individualized tumor response testing (ITRT) and analysis of drug resistance mechanisms performed on leukemic cells can provide valuable information in assessment of biology of the diseases and their prognosis. A genetic profile based on microarray analysis confirms correlation between cytogenetic changes in leukemic cells and drug resistance in ALL. Possibly, cytogenetic profile determines cellular drug resistance and final therapy outcome. A phenomenon of drug resistance in acute leukemias might be also explained by a concept of presence of leukemic stem cells (LSCs). LSCs are a population of rare leukemic cells exhibiting stem cell properties such as self-renewing, differentiation, tissue reconstitution and multiple drug resistance, expressing high levels of various members of ATP-Binding Cassette (ABC) transporters family (including MDR1 and BCRP). Identification of phenotype and molecular properties of LSCs will facilitate development of the best strategies to target leukemia. Knowledge on karyotype-related multiple drug resistance profile might enable the use of targeted therapy in resistant/refractory acute leukemias both in children and adults.

Chapter III - The problem of multiple drug resistance is a significant public health problem as health officials try to contain drug resistance in bacteria, fungi, viruses, including HIV and influenza, and particularly complicates the therapeutics for control and limits what is available for emerging infections. While most multiple drug resistant (MDR) pathogens were traditionally associated with nosocomial infections, including methicillin-resistant *Staphylococcus* species (MRSA and CoNS) and several MDR organisms, including penicillin-resistant *Streptococcus pneumoniae* and MRSA, have recently been isolated from community sources, and some of these have begun to cause problems in the hospital setting. Nosocomial infections affect a significant proportion of patients in intensive care units (ICUs) and are associated with substantial morbidity and mortality, and increased costs. Furthermore, the prevalence of antibiotic-resistant pathogens isolated in the ICU is usually significantly higher than in other hospital wards. This has precipitated a plethora of strategies to contain these organisms, while the scientific community struggle to keep pace with the need to devise new combinations of drugs.

In Jamaica, the traditional approach has been to assess the prevalence of multiple drug resistance among important nosocomial pathogens, primarily in the intensive care units. However, in more recent times, attention has been given to investigation of molecular resistance determinants, such as the presence of plasmids, such as *qnr* plasmids in *E. coli* and genetic elements, such as the staphylococcal cassette chromosome *mec* (SCCmec) elements in community- and hospital-acquired MRSA. This paper will assess the molecular and cellular mechanisms of bacterial resistance, some of the overlooked aspects concerning development and spread of antimicrobial resistance, the local situation in Jamaica, and implications for clinical practice.

Chapter IV - By searching the literature, it was found that a total of 32 drugs interact with herbal medicines in humans. These drugs mainly include anticoagulants (warfarin, aspirin and phenprocoumon), sedatives and antidepressants (midazolam, alprazolam and amitriptyline), oral contraceptives, anti-HIV agents (indinavir, ritonavir and saquinavir), a cardiovascular drug (digoxin), immunosuppressants (cyclosporine and tacrolimus) and anticancer drugs (imatinib and irinotecan). Most of them are substrates for cytochrome P450s (CYPs) and/or P-glycoprotein (P-gp) and many of which have narrow therapeutic indices. However, several drugs including acetaminophen, carbamazepine, mycophenolic acid, and pravastatin did not interact with herbs. Both pharmacokinetic (e.g., induction of hepatic CYPs and intestinal P-gp) and/or pharmacodynamic mechanisms (e.g., synergistic or antagonistic interaction on the same drug target) may be involved in herb-drug interactions, leading to altered drug clearance, response and toxicity. Toxicity arising from herb-drug interactions may be minor, moderate, or even fatal, depending on a number of factors associated with the patients, herbs and drugs. Predicting drug-herb interactions, timely identification of drugs that interact with herbs and therapeutic drug monitoring may minimize toxic drug-herb interactions. Predicting pharmacokinetic herb-drug interactions is likely if one follows the pharmacokinetic principles and utilizes proper models that are used for predicting drug-drug interactions. Identification of drugs that interact with herbs can be incorporated into the early stages of drug development. More studies are needed and new approaches are required to minimize toxicity arising from herb-drug interactions.

Chapter V - Pleiotropic resistance (or multidrug resistance, or MDR) to anticancer drugs in malignant diseases takes place either primarily or secondarily in the treatment of cancer. The first report suggesting that MDR could be the result of active drug extrusion was published in 1973 by Dano [1]. A few years later, P-glycoprotein (Pgp) was identified by

Juliano and Ling as a membrane protein that actively extrudes membrane embedded drugs. Biochemistry is a "science of contacts" between at least two biochemical elements (e.g. a drug and a transporter). These elements have to interact in order for a reaction to occur (e.g. drug extrusion). Taking into account that drugs do not necessarily incorporate into the membrane in the vicinity of a drug transporter, these transporters have been thought to exhibit a "vacuum cleaner" like-activity on membrane embedded drugs. Accordingly, understanding this activity is essential; as the movement of membrane embedded drugs, or otherwise, movement of the transporters must occur if extrusion is to take place. These activities should be considered as targets for anticancer drugs. Drug movement occurs by lateral diffusion (Brownian movement) in the membrane and the physical conditions required for drug extrusion by membrane transporters is known as the "2D random walk" theory. A deeper understanding is now possible, because there is enough literature enabling understanding of: (a) why the membrane is central to Pgp-mediated drug extrusion; (b) why the drug's molecular weight is an essential determinant in MDR, and; (c) why an alkaline cytosolic pH is essential in MDR.

After recalling the importance of pH in many aspects of cancer, including MDR, the authors will focus on the reason why a better understanding of the "vacuum cleaner" hypothesis is needed to clarify the subsequent processes involved in MDR. This will lead us to consider the cell membrane's mechanical properties and cytosolic pH alkalinization as important factors in the etiopathogenesis and understanding of MDR.

Chapter VI - Infectious diseases still remain an important cause of mortality. The emergence of pathogenic bacteria resistant to many antibiotics (multidrug-resistant strains) has created the need for exploring resistance to antimicrobial therapy along with the development of novel therapeutic agents. This need has become urgent, because during the last three decades, only two new classes of antibiotics with novel mechanisms of action (i.e., linezolid and daptomycin) have been introduced. Also, the overall antibiotic consumption has increased. The development of drug resistance over time limits the efficacy of antimicrobial agents and exerts a negative effect on patient outcomes.

Interaction between several genetic host factors, distinct anatomical and other features of the bacteria, and hygiene measures play a paramount role in the treatment of infections caused by multidrug-resistant organisms. The recent progress in molecular biology and bacterial genome analysis has revolutionized our understanding of the infectious diseases mechanisms. The evolution of antibiotic resistance is primarily the result of natural selection acting on variant bacterial phenotypes. Both the rigid base sequence of DNA and the more plastic expression patterns of the genes contribute to the bacterial phenotype. Several categories of antibiotic resistance genes have been identified. Examples include silent genes such as the *E. coli* AmpC gene, which when activated confers potent antibiotic resistance, the glutamate decarboxylase genes, which enable the passage through the acidic environment of the stomach, genes regulating the expression of other genes related to antibiotic resistance, genes encoding beta lactamases, etc.

Crosstransmission is frequent in pathogens causing nosocomial outbreaks. Contact precautions, compliance with universal hand hygiene measures, and maximum barrier precautions should be implemented in hospitals, and particularly, in intensive care units. Multiple drug resistance is a very complicated issue perplexed by various mechanisms that have several implications on the pathogenesis, the epidemiology, and the clinical outcome of the infections. In this article, the authors attempt to clarify the multiple and different genetic paths involved in the pathogenesis of antibiotic resistance. Furthermore, the authors describe clinical factors related to multiple drug resistance.

Chapter VII - Bacteriophages (phages) and bacterial cell wall hydrolases (BCWHs) have been recognized as promising alternative antibacterials. Phages are bacterial virsuses that kill bacteria by causing bacteriolysis. It is estimated that there are about 10^{31} phages on earth and approximately 5,100 have been identified and reported towards the end of last century, providing a vast pool of candidates for applications such as phage therapy. Phages are highly effective and specific to target bacteria. They have been generally accepted as effective antibacterials that could potentially provide safe and cost effective means for the treatment and prephylaxis of bacterial infections. BCWHs are lytic enzymes that cause bacteriolysis by hydrolyzing the peptidoglycan of bacterial cell wall. BCWHs are also called enzybiotics because they are enzymes that have antibiotic-like antibacterial activities. They are produced by amost all cellular organisms including microorganisms, plants, and animals. Virolysins (also called lysins, endolysins) are a special group of BCWHs encoded by phages but produced naturally by bacteria infected by lytic phages. They are probably the most promising enzybiotics.

Chapter VIII - Evidences are accumulating in both human and animal studies that undernutrition is associated with increased risk and severity of tuberculosis. In addition, obesity appears to protect against tuberculosis. Diabetes mellitus increases risk of tuberculosis, but poor diabetic control contributes to the bulk of such risk. In both under-nutrition and poor diabetic control, the increased risk is seen mainly in the pulmonary form of the disease, and the exact reason for relative sparing of the extrapulmonary sites remains unclear. Undernutrition has also been associated with worsened prognosis, poorer response to treatment and increased risk of relapse. Data from randomized controlled trials are scanty, as nutritional supplementation trials are often costly and difficult to implement. Micronutrients have been shown to decrease the risk of reversion of sputum culture to positivity after initial conversion, but there was no significant effect on mortality. With the putative roles of systemic inflammatory responses in tuberculosis manifestations, adjunctive corticosteroid administration treatment has been found to afford earlier and more significant body weight gain, albeit no differences in sputum bacteriological conversion and disease relapse rate. Further studies, with better study designs and serial monitoring of relevant nutritional parameters, are required to clarify the complex situation.

Chapter IX - The most important mechanism for multidrug resistance (MDR) in tumor cells is that mediated by highly expressed ABC transporters, such as P-gp and BCRP. These transporters expel various lipophilic anti-cancer drugs, which can enter cells by free diffusion. In this study, 96-well plate based assays and flow cytometry analysis were employed to screen natural products for P-gp and BCRP inhibition. The isoquinoline alkaloid glaucine inhibits P-gp and BCRP activity. Glaucine (10 μM) can enhance the cytotoxicity of doxorubicin in P-gp expressing Caco-2 and CEM ADR5000 cells 2.5 and 5.4-fold, respectively. In a BCRP overexpressing breast cancer cell line (MDA-MB-231) the cytotoxicity of mitoxantrone was increased 2.5 fold at 1 μM and that of camptothecin 2.9-

fold at 5 μM. Glaucine may be a candidate for the development of broad spectrum reversal agents.

Chapter X - *Acinetobacter baumannii* is associated with nosocomial outbreaks worldwide. Particularly, it has been known to be responsible for significant morbidity and mortality among immunosuppressed patients, mostly those admitted to intensive care units (ICU). The authors isolated only three *A. baumannii* strains over a 2-year period from leukemic patients. Two of them were found to be commensal of the upper airways, wheras the third one was collected from stool, and played an uncertain role as the cause of an enteritis episode. All of strains were found to be multidrug-resistant. Surprisingly, they also exerted tigecycline-resistance. Authors emphasize the role of multidrug-resistant *A. baumannii* as an emerging bacterium in haematologic hosts. Also, the first enteric isolation of this species is reported, althoug its role as the cause of the patient's diarrhoea remained controversial.

Chapter XI - For almost five decades, chemotherapy has played a vital role in managing cancer. With the combination of targeted therapies such as *Cetuximab* targeting EGF receptor, chemotherapy has seen even greater efficacy in clinics. Yet, the advances have been limited to prolonging the survival rather than decreasing mortality. This is largely due to the problem of drug resistance that remains unresolved. Even with the introduction of targeted therapeutics, the inherent ability of the cancer cells to mount resistance through genetic alterations eventually depreciates the therapy. It explains the nearly unchanged percentage of mortality for those with metastatic cancers amongst others. Multi-drug resistance (MDR) phenomenon is associated with the expression of ABC (ATP-binding cassette) transporters, which includes p-glycoprotein, MRP2, ABCG2, and possibly MRP3. By limiting to MDR, i.e. the drug import step, these traditional approaches have largely avoided addressing the drug induced lytic mechanism directly. This is, in part, due to our lack of knowledge concerning the molecular mechanism through which these drugs kill human cancer cells. By limiting to MDR, physicians remain incapable of countering drug resistance occurring as a result of cancer cell's interference with the steps lying further downstream in the lytic path. Instead, the authors need to develop counter-strategies based on the lytic path. In this commentary, the discovery of 'hyperploid progression-mediated death (HPMD)', a tumor specific lytic path targeting cancers mutated in tumor suppressor genes like RB or p53, is described. HPMD was discovered serendipitously while investigating the mechanism through which Taxol (widely used to treat breast cancer) induces aneuploidy in human cancer cells [*Carcinogenesis* 20, 1161-8 (99)]. The discovery of the lytic path provides a mechanistic basis for understanding how resistance to chemotherapy arise, thus providing a framework to develop counter strategies in a methodical way.

Chapter XII - The response of bacteria to a given antibiotic or other toxic agent that does not immediately kill them results in an adaptive response that secures their survival. This response may involve a number of distinct mechanisms, among which is the activation of genes that promote the appearance of transporters that extrude the agent prior to its reaching its target. These transporters extrude a large variety of chemically unrelated compounds and hence they bestow on the bacterium a multi-drug resistant (MDR) phenotype. The appearance of this MDR phenotype during therapy makes therapy problematic. Understanding the genetic and physiological properties of MDR efflux pumps is an absolute requirement if

MDR bacterial infections are to be successfully managed. There is much to learn and methods that afford the needed understanding will eventually pave the way for the successful management of an MDR bacterial infection. Therefore, the application of recently developed methods that assess the MDR bacterium at its genetic and physiological levels is the focus of this chapter. The material presented in this chapter is only the beginning for the evaluation and assessment of MDR efflux pumps.

In: Multiple Drug Resistance
Editors: A. Meszaros, G. Balogh, pp. 1-29

ISBN: 978-1-60741-595-4

Chapter I

Profile of Genetic and Cellular Multiple Drug Resistance in a Diagnostic and Therapeutic Strategy in Acute Leukemia in Children and Adults

Jan Styczynski [*] ***and Joanna Szczepanek***
Department of Pediatric Hematology and Oncology, Collegium Medicum, Nicolaus Copernicus University, Bydgoszcz, Poland

Abstract

Significant progress has been made in the therapy for pediatric acute lymphoblastic leukemia (ALL), while it was less evident in adult ALL and in acute myeloid leukemia (AML), both in children and in adults. Failure of therapy in acute leukemias is related to the presence of minimal residual disease, poor response to therapy and occurrence of relapses. Presence of cytogenetic aberrations and cellular multiple drug resistance in leukemic cells at presentation are important prognostic factors in ALL and to a lesser extent in AML. Individualized tumor response testing (ITRT) and analysis of drug resistance mechanisms performed on leukemic cells can provide valuable information in assessment of biology of the diseases and their prognosis. A genetic profile based on microarray analysis confirms correlation between cytogenetic changes in leukemic cells and drug resistance in ALL. Possibly, cytogenetic profile determines cellular drug resistance and final therapy outcome. A phenomenon of drug resistance in acute leukemias might be also explained by a concept of presence of leukemic stem cells (LSCs). LSCs are a population of rare leukemic cells exhibiting stem cell properties such as self-renewing, differentiation, tissue reconstitution and multiple drug resistance, expressing high levels of various members of ATP-Binding Cassette (ABC) transporters family (including MDR1 and BCRP). Identification of phenotype and molecular properties of LSCs will facilitate development of the best strategies to target leukemia.

[*] Coresponding author: Fax: +48 52 585 4867 E-mail: jstyczynski@cm.umk.pl.

Knowledge on karyotype-related multiple drug resistance profile might enable the use of targeted therapy in resistant/refractory acute leukemias both in children and adults.

Keywords: Acute lymphoblastic leukemia, acute myeloblastic leukemia, children, adults, drug resistance, gene expression profile, microarray, cytogenetics.

Drug Resistance and Therapy Failure in Acute Leukemia

Leukemias account for about 30% of all types of cancer in childhood and about 8% in adults. The distribution of subtypes of leukemia varies between age groups (**Table 1**). Acute lymphoblastic leukemia (ALL) is diagnosed in 3000 to 4000 persons in the United States each year; two-thirds of them are children. The current rate of cure of nearly 80 percent in pediatric patients attests to remarkable progress in the development of effective treatments for resistant subtypes of the disease. Progress has been incremental, from the introduction of combination chemotherapy and central nervous system treatment for presymptomatic leukemia to newer, intensive treatment regimens for patients at high risk for relapse. In contrast, only 30 to 40 percent of adults with ALL are cured. This discrepancy can be attributed in part to the higher frequency of adverse genetic abnormalities in the leukemic lymphoblasts of adults [1].

In spite of continuous progress in therapy of acute leukemias, relapses still occur frequently both in children and adults. Efficacy of therapy of relapsed disease is worse than at first diagnosis. Failure in the therapy is dependent on three factors: pharmacokinetic resistance, cellular drug resistance and minimal residual disease [2]. Cellular drug resistance can be defined as cellular insensitivity to drug reaching the cell. It can be classified as primary (congenital, intrinsic) or acquired (secondary), external or internal, passive or active (**Table 2**). Primary drug resistance is observed in about 10% of children with acute lymphoblastic leukemia, and recognized clinically as steroid-resistant after 7 days of prednisolone monotherapy (with one dose of intrathecal methotrexate).

Mechanisms of Cellular Drug Resistance

The most important classical drug resistance mechanism includes the presence of multidrug resistance proteins (PGP, MRP, LRP/MVP, BCRP and others), changes in drug metabolism and its detoxification, impairment in intracellular signal transduction, decrease of target enzymes (eg., topoizomerase II), increase in DNA repair, cytogenetic changes, cell cycle disregulation and resistance to apoptosis, both mitochondrial and receptor pathways [3, 4]. Multidrug resistance proteins include 48 proteins. The most important in leukemia are: ABC (ATP binding cassette) proteins, such as: PGP (Permeability Glycoprotein), encoded by MDR1 (multidrug resistance gene), MRP 1-6 (multidrug resistance-related protein), BCRP (breast cancer resistance protein). Non-ABC protein responsible for development of drug resistance includes LRP/MVP (lung-resistance related protein / major vault protein). Current classification of multidrug resistance mechanisms is shown in **Table 3** (acc. to Marie [4]).

Table 1. Frequency of ALL and other leukemias in childhood and adulthood

Characteristics	Children	Adults
Frequency of leukemia	24 / million children / year	50 / million / year
Leukemia among all cases of cancer	30%	8%
Acute : chronic leukemia ratio	95 : 5	50 : 50
ALL : AML ratio	80 : 15	10 : 40
CLL : CML ratio	0 : 5	35 : 15

ALL – acute lymphoblastic leukemia, AML – acute myeloid leukemia, CLL – chronic lymphatic leukemia, CML – chronic myeloid leukemia

Table 2. Types of cellular drug resistance

Type of drug resistance	Characteristics
Primary	Present at cancer diagnosis
Acquired	Developing during or after chemotherapy/radiotherapy. Clinically recognized as occurrence of relapsing or refractory disease.
External	Mechanisms present before drug reaches the cell
Internal	Mechanisms related to properties of cancer cell: selective to one drug, or pleiotropic – to many drugs (most frequently observed in patients)
Proximal (passive)	Deficiency to obligate target or drug activating enzyme; blocking the drug to reach its target
Distal (active)	Mechanism induced with drug exposure; modification of drug target (i.e. enzymes, DNA)

Table 3. Classification of drug resistance mechanisms

I. Before drug reaches the cell	II. On cellular target
1. Pharmacology: a. Inefficient drug metabolism b. Inefficient drug transport	1. Target modification: a. Upregulation or downregulation of target activity b. Changes in function of target
2. Intracellular transport: a. Decreased drug uptake b. Increased drug efflux	2. DNA repair: a. Increased DNA repair b. Lack of recognition of DNA changes
3. Cellular metabolism: a. Decreased drug activation b. Increased drug catabolism	3. Apoptosis and cell cycle: a. Changes in function b. Changes in regulation

Biology of Acute Lymphoblastic Leukemia in Age Groups

Comparing outcomes of various types of cancer in childhood and adulthood, the most striking differences could be found for acute lymphoblastic leukemia (ALL), which accounts for 28% of all newly diagnosed cases of cancer in childhood and 1% in adults. Two thirds of all ALL cases occur below 18 years of age [1]. With multi-agent chemotherapy, currently 80% of children but only 40% of adults reach long-term remission [5]. This outcome is related to differences in biology and cytogenetics of lymphoblasts, which are followed by differences in drug resistance profile in children and adults [6, 7]. The most striking adverse prognostic factors in adults are: the high rate of presence of BCR-ABL rearrangement, low rate of favorable cytogenetic aberrations such as hyperdiploid state or presence of TEL-AML1 rearrangement, higher frequency of T-cell and lower of common-pre-B immunophenotype, and presence of multidrug resistance proteins [7, 8]. Co-existence and induction of various drug resistance mechanisms are frequent phenomena in adults. Probably, age itself, more than any other factor, is the most important prognostically unfavorable continuous variable in ALL. This is related to various biology, cytogenetics and drug resistance in age groups. The number of prognostically unfavorable factors increases with the age of patients [5, 7, 8]. Also, ability to tolerate chemotherapy, differences in treatment protocols and rigor in adherence to protocols in children and adults are other important factors. ALL might be regarded as model disease, showing age-dependent therapeutic difficulties in oncology [9]. In spite of the differences in clinical outcome, the gene expression pattern in children and adults with ALL is very similar and is primarily dependent to immunophenotype and cytogenetic aberrations. When age groups are compared, the expression patterns of infants and adults over 40 also show a remarkable similarity [10].

Age has important prognostic impact in ALL. Prognostic factors in childhood acute lymphoblastic leukemia are shown in **Table 4**. Infants below 1 year have a dismal prognosis. Children 1-9 year have the best prognosis and then a progressive worsening in outcome is seen with an increasing age. The incidence of important genetic and immunophenotypic features varies with age. However, even when corrected for the association with other risk factors, age itself is related to induction failure, drug resistance, resolution of minimal residual disease and relapse. Although differences have been described in morphologic and immunologic characteristics and, more important, in the distribution of molecular abnormalities, no single feature among these variables appears to account for the marked differences in clinical and biologic behaviors. Compared to children, adults with ALL are more refractory to initial chemotherapy and more likely to develop resistance to ongoing treatment. Possibly, two different subsets of the disease are represented in these age groups, which are caused by different populations of pluripotent leukemic stem cells [11, 12].

Biology of Acute Myeloid Leukemia in Age Groups

Taking into account both children and adults, age is adversely related to therapy outcome in AML, and the percentage of patients with favorable cytogenetics decreases with age. On the other hand, age is positively correlated with multi-drug resistance and the proportion of patients with unfavorable cytogenetics (**Table 5**). Even within each cytogenetic risk group, treatment outcome deteriorates markedly with age. The distinct biology and clinical responses argue for age-specific assessments when evaluating therapies for AML. In childhood AML no drug is more effective in comparison to ALL, and cellular drug resistance is partially related to chromosomal abnormalities. In vitro drug resistance in childhood AML on relapse probably is not higher than at first diagnosis. With respect to age, infant AML cells are more in vitro sensitive than older AML children, while adult AML is not more in vitro resistant than childhood AML. Pediatric AML is more drug resistant than pediatric ALL. Pediatric AML is equally resistant as adult AML. Pediatric and adult AML, respectively, are probably equally drug resistant on initial diagnosis and at relapse. Probably there are no differences between cellular drug resistance in adult ALL between initial diagnosis and relapse.

Table 4. Prognostic factors in childhood acute lymphoblastic leukemia

Factor	Favorable	Unfavorable
Age	1–10 years	<1 year, >10 years
Leukocytosis	Low e.g. <50 x 10^9/L	High, e.g. ≥50 x 10^9/L
Immunophenotype	common/pre-B	pro-B, T
DNA index	Hiperdiploid ie. ≥1,16	Hypodiploid <0,95
Cytogenetics	Hyperdiploidy >50 chromosomes, t(12;21)	t(9;22), t(4;11), translocations 11q23
CNS involvement	No	Yes
Response to steroids after 7 days of therapy	Blast count (in PB) <1,0 x 10^9/L	Blast count (in PB) ≥1,0 x 10^9/L
Drug resistance *in vivo* *in vitro*	 Fast response Sensitive profile	 Late response Resistant profile
Bone marrow in 15 days	<5% blasts in BM	≥5% blasts in BM
Bone marrow in 33 days	<5% blasts in BM	≥5% blasts in BM
Minimal residual disease	≤10^{-4} leukemic cells	≥10^{-2} leukemic cells

AML is considered to be a stem cell disease. BCRP, PGP and MRPs are preferentially expressed in leukemic stem cells, making this disease drug resistant [13]. Except infants, the higher the age, the worse the outcome in AML, however cellular drug resistance in AML cells seems to be similar throughout all other age groups. Possible applications of cell culture assays include risk-group stratification, rational improvements of current treatment protocols for subgroups of patients based on specific drug resistance profiles, individualized tailored therapy, the study of cross-resistance patterns between drugs, the study of possibilities to modulate or circumvent drug resistance, the study of drug interactions, and drug screening [14, 15].

Table 5. Prognostic factors in childhood acute myeloid leukemia (AML)

Factor	Favorable	Unfavorable
Age	Infants	Older children
Secondary leukemia	Down syndrome	Myelodysplastic syndromes
Therapy-related AML	No	Yes
Leukocytosis	Low	High
Morphology	FAB M2 with Auer rods, FAB M4 Eo, FAB M3	Other FAB subtypes
Cytogenetics	t(8;21), t(15;17), inv(16), t(9;11)	Anomalies 11q23 [other than t(9;11)], monosomy 7/7q
FLT3-ITD	Absent	Internal tandem duplication
MRP3 and BCRP	Low expression	High expression
In vitro drug resistance	Sensitive profile	Resistant profile
Early response to therapy	<5% blasts in bone marrow in day 15	≥5% blasts in bone marrow in day 15
Minimal residual disease (MRD)	Low levels of MRD	High levels of MRD

Current treatment strategies of acute myeloid leukemia based on conventional cytotoxic agents provide complete remission in 60%-80% of younger patients, however, only 30%-40% are alive at 5 years [16]. As shown with adolescents with ALL, so far, there is no study suggested that young adult patients with AML have far superior outcome when treated on more intensive pediatric regimens. For elderly patients significant improvements in survival have not emerged for years [17]. Most recently, insights into the molecular pathogenesis of AML have led to the development of specific targeted therapy [18]. The new approaches are being studied alone or in combination with chemotherapy, such as immunoconiugate gemtuzumab ozogamicin, multidrug resistance inhibitors, farnesyltrasferase inhibitors, histone deacetylase and proteasome inhibitors, antiangiogenesis agents, FLT3 inhibitors, apoptosis modulators, new alkylating agent and nucleoside analogs, and immunotherapy [18].

Cytogenetics and *In Vitro* Drug Resistance in Acute Leukemia in Children and Adults

Increased in vitro cellular drug resistance is related to poor outcome in high-risk childhood ALL [19-22]. No such correlation was so far proved in pediatric AML, although a possibility of prognostic value of combined in vitro drug resistance profile to fludarabine, treosulfan and mitoxantrone or etoposide was observed [23, 24]. Since fludarabine and treosulfan are not used in first line therapy of pediatric AML, it is difficult to confirm in clinical conditions the value of this observation.

Presence of cytogenetic aberrations in leukemic cells at presentation is an important prognostic factor in acute leukemias. Translocation t(9;22) and 11q23/*MLL* rearrangement are related to poor prognosis, while hyperdiploidy ≥50 chromosomes and translocation t(12;21) are good prognosis factors in acute lymphoblastic leukemia (ALL). In acute myeloid leukemia (AML), t(8;21), t(15;17) and inv(16) have good prognosis, whereas 5/5q-, 7/7q- and complex karyotype have poor prognosis. It seems that prognostic value of cytogenetic changes is related to differences in cellular drug resistance in ALL, and to lesser extent, in AML. genetic profile based on microarray analysis confirms correlation between cytogenetic changes in leukemic cells and drug resistance in ALL. Possibly cytogenetic profile determines cellular drug resistance and final therapy outcome. Knowledge on karyotype-related drug resistance profile might enable the use of targeted therapy in resistant/refractory acute leukemias both in children and adults.

In Vitro Drug Resistance Profile in ALL Subgroups

In Vitro Drug Resistance Profile of Philadelphia Positive Acute Lymphoblastic Leukemia is Heterogeneous and Related to Age

The t(9;22)(q34;q11) translocation leading to the Philadelphia (Ph+) chromosome resulting in *BCR-ABL* gene fusion is associated with a poor prognosis in acute lymphoblastic leukemia (ALL). Both childhood and adult Ph+ precursor B-cell ALL samples display a heterogeneous in vitro resistance profile, with relatively sensitive and resistant cases. The adult Ph+ samples, however, are generally more resistant compared to matched Ph- controls. In vitro drug resistance, measured by the MTT assay, did not differ significantly between pediatric Ph+ and Ph- samples for prednisolone, dexamethasone, L-asparaginase, vincristine, anthracyclines, thiopurines, epipodophyllotoxins, and 4HOO-ifosfamide, even after matching for important prognostic features (age, white blood cell count (WBC), and immunophenotype). On the other hand, adult Ph+ALL was more resistant to prednisolone (>270-fold, P=0.030), and displayed an overall tendency to resistance when compared to matched cases of Ph- adult precursor B-cell ALL. Within Ph+ALL, in vitro prednisolone resistance increased significantly with age (P=0.006). The expression of lung resistance protein (LRP), but not P-glycoprotein (PGP) or multidrug resistance protein (MRP), was significantly higher in all Ph+ patients. The correlation of prednisolone resistance with age within the Ph+ cases might help explain the poorer prognosis of adult Ph+ALL [25, 26].

In Vitro Drug-Resistance Profile in Infant Acute Lymphoblastic Leukemia in Relation to Age, *MLL* Rearrangements and Immunophenotype

ALL in infants under 1 year is strongly associated with translocations involving 11q23 (*MLL* gene), CD10-negative B-lineage (proB) immunophenotype, and poor outcome. Infants with ALL appear to have a distinct in vitro resistance profile with the proB immunophenotype being of importance. In analysis of the relationship between age, *MLL* rearrangements, proB-lineage, and in vitro drug resistance determined using the MTT assay, in comparison to children aged over 1 year with common/preB (c/preB) ALL, the infants were highly resistant to steroids (for prednisolone (PRED) more than 580-fold, P=0.001) and

L-asparaginase (L-ASP) (12-fold, P=0.001), but more sensitive to cytarabine (AraC) (1.9-fold, P=0.001) and 2-chlorodeoxyadenosine (2-CdA) (1.7-fold, P<0.001). No differences were found for vincristine, anthracyclines, thiopurines, epipodophyllotoxines, or 4-hydroperoxy (HOO)-ifosfamide. ProB ALL of all ages had a profile similar to infant ALL when compared with the group of c/preB ALL: relatively more resistant to L-ASP and PRED (and in addition thiopurines), and more sensitive to AraC and 2-CdA. Age was not related to cellular drug resistance within the proB ALL group (<1 year, n=32, vs >/=1 year, n=19), nor within the *MLL*-rearranged ALL (<1 year, n=34, vs >/=1 year, n=8). The translocation t(4;11)(q21;q23)-positive ALL cases were more resistant to PRED (>7.4-fold, P=0.033) and 4-HOO-ifosfamide (4.4-fold, P=0.006) than those with other 11q23 abnormalities. The expression of P-glycoprotein, multidrug-resistance protein, and lung-resistance protein (LRP) was not higher in infants compared to older c/preB ALL patients, but LRP was higher in proB ALL and *MLL*-rearranged ALL of all ages. The role of MLL cannot be excluded, with the t(4;11) being of special significance, while age appears to play a smaller role [27].

TEL/AML1 Gene Fusion is Related to *In Vitro* Drug Sensitivity for L-Asparaginase in Childhood Acute Lymphoblastic Leukemia

The t(12;21) translocation resulting in *TEL/AML1* (also known as *ETV6/RUNX1*) gene fusion is present in approximately 25% of patients with precursor B-lineage pediatric ALL. Studies suggest an association with a good prognosis; however, relapse can occur. Analysis of the relation between t(12;21), and in vitro drug resistance, in childhood B-lineage ALL at diagnosis, has shown that the values of drug resistance did not differ significantly between *TEL/AML1*-positive and -negative samples for prednisolone, dexamethasone, daunorubicin, thiopurines, epipodophyllotoxins, and 4-HOO-ifosfamide. However, the *TEL/AML1*-positive patients were relatively more sensitive to L-asparaginase (ASP; 5.9-fold; P=0.029) and slightly but significantly more resistant to vincristine (1.5-fold; P=0.011) and cytarabine (1.5-fold; P=0.014). After matching for unevenly distributed patient characteristics-that is, excluding patients younger than 12 months, patients with CD10-negative immature B-lineage ALL, patients with Philadelphia chromosome, and patients who were hyperdiploid (more than 50 chromosomes) from the *TEL/AML1* negative group-the only remaining difference was a relative sensitivity for ASP in the *TEL/AML1*-positive samples (10.8-fold; P=0.012). Possibly, the presence of *TEL/AML1* gene fusion in childhood precursor B-lineage ALL does not seem to be associated with a high in vitro drug sensitivity, except for ASP, indicating that these patients could benefit from treatment schedules with significant use of this drug [28].

In another study, *ETV6/RUNX1*(+) samples were significantly more sensitive than *ETV6/RUNX1*(-) samples to doxorubicin, etoposide, amsacrine, and dexamethasone, whereas the opposite was true for cytarabine. After matching for unevenly distributed patient characteristics, that is, excluding patients with high hyperdiploidy (>51 chromosomes), t(9; 22), t(1;19), or 11q23 rearrangement, the *ETV6/RUNX1*(+) samples remained significantly more sensitive to doxorubicin (P=0.001) and etoposide (P=0.001). For the other drugs tested (amsacrine, cytarabine, dexamethasone, prednisolone, vincristine, 6-thioguanine, and 4-

hydroperoxy-cyclophosphamide), no significant difference in cellular drug sensitivity was found [29].

Translocation t(1;19) and *In Vitro* Drug Resistance

Translocation t(1;19) is related to low cellular drug resistance in childhood acute lymphoblastic leukemia [30].

DNA Hyperdiploidy and *In Vitro* Drug Resistance

DNA hyperdiploidy is a favorable prognostic factor in childhood acute lymphoblastic leukemia (ALL) characterized by increased incidence of spontaneous apoptosis in the bone marrow of hyperdiploid childhood acute lymphoblastic leukemia [31]. The favorable prognosis associated with DNA hyperdiploidy in childhood common ALL may be explained by a relative sensitivity of hyperdiploid common ALL cells to antimetabolites, especially to mercaptopurine, L-asparaginase [32], and to methotrexate [33].

Drug Resistance to Methotrexate in Therapy of ALL

Impressive gains have been made in the therapy of childhood acute lymphoblastic leukemia (ALL) in recent years such that remissions today are commonly achieved in up to 95% of patients and long term disease-free survival rates approach 70%. Methotrexate is a key component in ALL consolidation and maintenance therapies and is administered intrathecally in the prophylaxis and treatment of central nervous system leukemia. Critical determinants of methotrexate sensitivity and resistance (dihydrofolate reductase levels, methotrexate membrane transport, methotrexate polyglutamylation) have been identified in lymphoblasts from children with ALL. Heterogenous expressions of increased dihydrofolate reductase or impaired methotrexate transport can be detected in both diagnostic and relapsed ALL specimens by flow cytometry with fluorescent methotrexate analogues. Lymphoblasts from children with ALL synthesize long chain polyglutamates and correlations have been established between the accumulation of methotrexate polyglutamates in ALL blasts and characteristic patient prognostic features. Variations in methotrexate polyglutamate accumulation may reflect changes in polyglutamate synthetic or degradative enzymes, or may be secondary to changes in methotrexate influx or dihydrofolate reductase levels. Other critical elements in treatment response to methotrexate include the dose and route of methotrexate administration, its catabolism to 7-hydroxymethotrexate, and the rate of methotrexate plasma clearance. A unique relationship exists between chromosome 21 and ALL leukemogenesis, and response to treatment including methotrexate. A better understanding of the molecular bases of methotrexate response and the development of methotrexate resistance in childhood ALL should facilitate further improvements in the effectiveness of methotrexate-based chemotherapy for this disease [34-36].

In Vitro Drug Resistance Profile in AML Subgroups

Cellular Drug Resistance Profiles in Childhood Acute Myeloid Leukemia: Differences between FAB Types and Comparison with Acute Lymphoblastic Leukemia

In comparison of in vitro drug resistance between childhood ALL and AML, it has been shown that AML was significantly more resistant than ALL to the following drugs, as noted by the median resistance: glucocorticoids (greater than 85-fold), vincristine (4.4-fold), L-asparaginase (6.9-fold), anthracyclines (1.8- to 3.4-fold), mitoxantrone (2.6-fold), etoposide (4.9-fold), platinum analogues (2.4- to 3.4-fold), ifosfamide (3.5-fold), and thiotepa (3.9-fold). For cytarabine and thiopurines, the median LC50 values (the drug concentration that kills 50% of the cells) were equal. Also, busulfan, amsacrine, teniposide, and vindesine showed no significant differences, but the numbers were smaller, and the median LC50 values were 1.3- to 5.2-fold higher in AML. None of the drugs demonstrated greater cytotoxicity in AML. FAB M5 was significantly more sensitive than FAB M4 to most drugs frequently used in AML, as indicated by the following ratios of median sensitivities: the anthracyclines (2.6- to 3.2-fold), mitoxantrone (12.5-fold), etoposide (8.7-fold), and cytarabine (2.9-fold). For etoposide and cytarabine (5.4- and 3.4-fold, respectively) FAB M5 was also significantly more sensitive than FAB M1/M2. FAB M5 was equally sensitive to L-asparaginase and vincristine as ALL. Only 15% of the AML samples were "intermediately" sensitive to glucocorticoids, mainly in FAB M1/M2. The poorer prognosis of childhood AML might be related to resistance to a large number of drugs, yet within AML, FAB M5 had a distinct resistance pattern. Possible, these resistance profiles may be helpful in the rational design of further treatment protocols [37].

Cellular Drug Resistance in Childhood Acute Myeloid Leukemia is Related to Chromosomal Abnormalities

Specific cytogenetic abnormalities predict prognosis in childhood acute myeloid leukemia (AML). Patients are usually classified according to the genetic abnormalities in the leukemic cells: t(8;21), inv(16), t(15;17), t(9;11), other 11q23 translocations, abnormalities of chromosome 5/7, trisomy 8 alone, normal karyotype, single random, and multiple (defined as 2 or more) abnormalities. Analysis of in vitro drug resistance and cytogenetic abnormalities of de novo childhood AML samples has shown that samples with chromosome 5/7 abnormalities were median 3.9-fold (P=0.01) more resistant to cytarabine than other AML samples. The t(9;11) samples were more sensitive to cytarabine (median 2.9-fold, P=0.002), etoposide (13.1-fold, P=0.001), the anthracyclines (2.9- to 8.0-fold, P<0.01), and 2-chlorodeoxyadenosine (10.0-fold, P=0.002) than other AML samples. All other genetic subgroups did not show specific resistance profiles. Overall, no differences in drug resistance in samples taken at diagnosis between patients remaining in continuous complete remission (CCR) versus the refractory/relapsed patients were found. Within several genetic subgroups, however, relapsed/refractory patients were more cytarabine resistant when compared with patients remaining in CCR, but numbers were small and the results were not significant. Possibly some, but not all, cytogenetic subgroups in childhood AML display specific drug-resistance profiles [38].

Possibility of Modulation of Drug Resistance In Leukemia

Possibilities of modulation of circumvention of drug resistance include development of following possibilities: new classes of drugs with higher anti-leukemic activity, new drug combinations, targeted therapy, combination of chemotherapy and radiotherapy, specific drug administration, high-dose chemotherapy, blocking drug resistance proteins, sensitization or gene therapy. Agents modulating multidrug resistance proteins can be classified as:

1. Non-PGP-specific agents
    - calcium channel blockers: verapamil, niphedipine
    - antibiotics: erythromycin, tetracyclines, ceftriaxone
    - others: trifluoperazine, cyclosporine A, quinine, amiodaron
2. Agents PGP-specifically modulating drug resistance
    - dexverapamil, amiodarone derivatives (I generation)
    - cyclosporine D (PSC 833) (II generation)
    - valspodar, bricodar, zosuquidar (III generation)
3. Modulation of MRP: probenecid
4. Modulation of BCRP: fumitremorgin, tariquidar, ABCG2 antibodies

Clinical Aspects of Cellular Drug Resistance in ALL between Children and Adults

Individualized tumor response testing (ITRT) is a new name for all kind of ex vivo drug resistance assays. ITRT and analysis of drug resistance mechanisms performed on leukemic cells can provide valuable information in assessment of biology of the diseases and their prognosis. The lymphoblasts from adults show an increased in vitro resistance to cytotoxic drugs. The group of adult ALL samples was significantly more resistant to cytosine arabinoside, L-asparaginase, daunorubicin, dexamethasone and prednisolone. The resistance ratio was highest for prednisolone (31.7-fold) followed by dexamethasone (6.9-fold), L-asparaginase (6.1-fold), cytosine arabinoside (2.9-fold), daunorubicin (2.5-fold) and vincristine (2.2-fold). Lymphoblasts from adult patients were not more resistant to mercaptopurine, thioguanine, 4-HOO-ifosfamide, mitoxantrone and teniposide. Lymphoblasts from adults proved to be relatively resistant to drugs commonly used in therapy. This might contribute to the difference in outcome between children and adults with ALL [39]. Another factor is related to differences in cytogenetic changes in acute lymphoblastic leukemia in children and adults (**Table 6**, acc. to [40]).

Glucocorticoid resistance may be a fundamental difference between children, adolescents and adults with ALL, which may underlie different biological aspects and also explain the difference in prognosis [39]. It seems that in vitro resistance to prednisolone with respect to the age might be a continuous variable in ALL patients, except infants. The greater the age, the higher the in vitro resistance to prednisolone. This may be due to induction of various defending mechanisms, such as an activation of multidrug resistance proteins, which develops throughout the life and protect the human against xenobiotics [41, 42].

Clinical Aspects of Cellular Drug Resistance in AML between Children and Adults

With current protocols 80-90% of children with AML achieve CR and about 50-60% experience survival [7, 74]. In adult AML prognosis is less favorable with 70-80% CR rate and 40% survival [75]. One of possible factors that might contribute to differences in therapy outcome can be related to differences in distribution of the most frequent primary chromosomal aberrations in childhood and adult AML (**Table 7**) [43-46]. Elderly patients (>60 years) are reported to carry an even poorer prognosis, either due to intrinsic drug resistance or the inability to withstand intensive therapy. In the comparison of in vitro drug resistance in childhood and adult AML, no significant differences were found for cytarabine, etoposide, vincristine, prednisolone, idarubicin, mitoxantrone, 6-thioguanine, amsacrin, doxorubicin, L-asparaginase and busulfan, while only for daunorubicin, cells of adult AML patients were median 1.2-fold more resistant than those from children, but this difference is presumably not clinically relevant. Within adult group, no differences were found in drug resistance between patients >60 years and <60 years, suggesting that elderly patients are not intrinsically resistant but perhaps treated less intensive. Thus, the difference in outcome between childhood and adult AML can not be explained by clinically significant differences in an in vitro drug resistance measured with the MTT assay and therefore might reflect other differences like pharmacokinetics (Zwaan et al., Blood 1998; 92:198b, abstract 3843).

Comparison of Drug Resistance in Different Types of Leukemia in Children and Adults

Pediatric AML is more resistant than pediatric ALL [43-45]. Pediatric AML is equally resistant as adult AML. Pediatric and adult AML, respectively, are probably equally drug resistant on initial diagnosis and at relapse [70, 76]. There are some discrepancies in results comparing cellular drug resistance in adult ALL between initial diagnosis and relapse [45, 76], however it seems that probably there are no differences [76].

In the comparative study of adults with ALL, AML and B-lineage CLL (chronic lymphocytic leukemia), B-CLL cells were found to be more sensitive than cells from both AML and ALL to cytarabine, cladribine, fludarabine, doxorubicin, idarubicin, vincristine and cyclophosphamide. No difference in cellular drug resistance was found between B-CLL and ALL cells for prednisolone, whereas AML cells were more resistant. However, B-CLL cells acquired cellular drug resistance during therapy, as cells obtained from patients who had received previous chemotherapy were more resistant to almost all tested drugs as compared to cells from treatment-naive patients [76].

Table 6. Cytogenetic changes in acute lymphoblastic leukemia in children and adults

Cytogenetic subgroups	Fusion transcript	Children	Adults
Normal karyotype		22%	23%
B-lineage ALL			
Hypodiploidy≤ 45 chromosomów		1%	2%
Hyperdiploidy≥ 50 chromosomów		25%	7%
t(12;21)	*TEL-AML1*	22%	2%
t(8;14), t(8;22), t(2;8)	*MYC*	2%	4%
t(1;19)	*E2A-PBX1*	5%	3%
t(9;22)	*BCR-ABL*	3%	25-40%
t(4;11), t(11;19), t(9;11)	*MLL* rearrangements	8%	10%
T-lineage ALL			
1p32	*TAL1*	7%	12%
5q35	*HOX11L2*	2.5%	1%
19p13	*LYL1*	1.5%	2,5%
10q24	*HOX11*	0.7%	8%
t(11;19)(q23;p13.1)	*MLL-ENL*	0.3%	0.5%

Table 7. Frequency distribution of the most frequent primary chromosomal aberrations in childhood and adult AML

Cytogenetic aberrations	Fusion transcript	Children	Adult s
No changes	(-)	23%	45%
t(8;21)(q22;q22)	*AML1-ETO*	15%	6%
t(15;17)(q21;q12)	*PML-RARα*	8%	8%
inv(16)(p13q22) lub t(16;16)(p13;q22)	*CBFβ-MYH11*	10%	5%
t(9;11)(p21-22;q23)	*MLL-AF9*	6%	2%
trisomia 8	(-)	3%	9%
-5/5q-	?	1%	7%
-7/7q-	?	4%	8%
11q23 rearangements	*MLL;v*	6%	5%
t(6;9)(p23;q34)	*DEK-CAN*	1%	1%
others		23%	4%

v = variable (MLL partner)

Profile of Genetic and Cellular Multiple Drug Resistance in a Diagnostic and Therapeutic Strategy in acute Leukemia in Children and Adults

Accurate and rapid diagnosis, prognostication and monitoring of the acute leukemias: acute lymphoblastic leukemia (ALL) and acute myeloid leukemia (AML) are essential for development of curative chemotherapy. Currently laboratory methods are based on analysis of level of cell morphology, immunophenotype, cytogenetic, protein and gene expression profiles of cancer cells [47-50]. A major challenge for the treatment of adults and children with acute leukemia is to improve and refine diagnostic and risk classification schemes.

It is not possible to investigate a large number of genes using traditional methods. Microarrays are such technology which promises to monitor many biological samples at the whole genome or transcriptome scale on a single chip [51]. This technique is becoming increasingly useful in molecular biology and in medicine. Microarrays have potential to analyze the expression level of thousands genes in a single reaction in quickly and efficient manner. Arrays technologies are as tools to identify genes whose expression correlates with predict risk of relapse, tailor treatment intensity and monitor response to therapy [49]. Recent studies have demonstrated the ability to stratify acute leukemias on the basis of gene expression patterns. Such analysis can provide new insights into the biologic and molecular mechanisms of drug response and facilitate the development of more effective treatment schemes.

Principles of Microarray Technology

A typical array platform is a series of many microscopic spots of DNA, cDNA or oligonucleotides that are used as probes attached to a solid support (glass slides, silicon chips or nylon membrane) [51, 52]. Each array contains thousands of different probe sequences arranged in a defined matrix. Most widely used microarrays can be categorized into two groups: (1) robotically spotted cDNA microarrays and (2) microarrays produced by synthesizing the oligonucleotides probe directly on the supporting substrate [52, 53].

A microarray study is multi-step process involves steps like: probe design, array fabrication, RNA extraction and labeling, hybridization, scanning and data analysis (Figure 1) [54]. The RNA samples are obtained from analyzed tissue (interest and reference) and are reverse transcribed into cDNA. In the next step they are assigned to different dye labels [52, 53, 55]. Array spots are hybridized with a cDNA (microarray) or cRNA (GeneChip) sample (called target) under high-stringency conditions. Following hybridization, the microarray is washed to remove unbound and non-specific material. The presence or absence of a DNA or RNA of interest is visualized using a fluorogenic or chemiluminescent detectors. Detected probe-target hybridization is quantified to determine relative abundance of nucleic acid sequences in the sample. The intensity of the signals from probe-target interaction can be used to estimate whether the expression of a particular genes is upregulated, downregulated, unchanged or absent [52, 53, 56].

A B

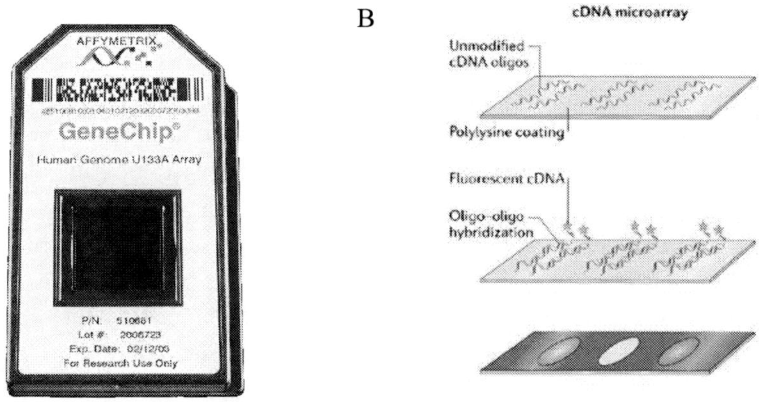

Figure 1. A - One of the most widely used chips in the study of gene expression profiles in acute leukemias GeneChip® Human Genome U133A array (http://www.affymetrix.com), B - Scheme of interaction on DNA microarray chip (http://www.nature.com).

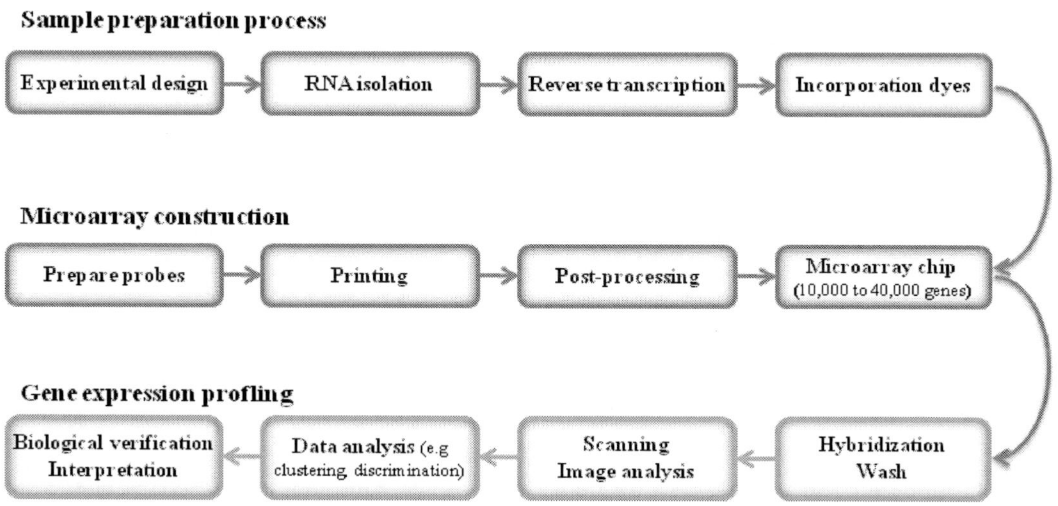

Figure 2. A microarray experiment

Microarrays are the most popular technique for gene expression profiling (GEP) [54, 57]. The main purpose of GEP is to finding groups of genes with similar expression patterns and groups of samples with similarly expressed genes. Many experiments measure an entire genome simultaneously, so expression of each gene present in a particular cell may be estimated. Analysis of genes expression involves measuring the relative amount of mRNA expressed in two or more experimental conditions. Changes in levels of a particular transcripts suggest a pathological condition.

Application of Microarray

There are two primary molecular biology applications for an array experiment: identification of sequence (gene/gene mutation) and determination of genes activity (expression profiling) [57]. Microarrays are used especially to measure changes in expression level. With the help of microarray technology, a measurement of the activity of thousands of genes simultaneously can be performed [58]. In this way it is possible to create a better picture of cellular function. Gene expression profiles can be used in: (a) gene discovery, (b) biochemical pathways elucidation, (c) disease diagnosis, (d) drug discovery - pharmacogenomics, and (e) toxicological research - toxicogenomics. This method has been used to examine gene expression profiles of various hematologic and nonhematologic tumors.

In studies of acute leukemias, the researchers are able to correlate the expression of over 30,000 genes with a number of specific leukemic features including hematopoietic lineage, immunophenotype and cytogenetics. Microarrays are useful in diagnosis, classify, monitor response to treatment response to chemotherapy, minimal residual disease (MRD) and clinical outcomes such as metastasis, recurrence, survival or second malignancies [48, 49, 59-63]. Gene expression profiling can be helpful in addition to conventional techniques. Microarray technology could improve the current procedures for diagnosis and risk assessment in acute leukemias [49, 64].

Prediction of Outcome Based on Expression Signatures

One of the most useful applications of this methodology is to define gene sets that predict outcome. Treatment of childhood ALL is based on the concept of tailoring the intensity of therapy to groups of patient's risk of relapse. Recently, genome wide studies were started in which patients are stratified according to gene expression profiling. Based on the expression profiles of the leukemic blasts it is possible to predict the relapse for T-ALL and hyperdiploid B-precursor ALL [63], *TEL-AML1*, *MLL*-rearranged and cases that lacked cytogenetic changes. The study performed by Carrol et al. [64] suggest that gene expression profiling can be helpful in prediction of slow early response for patients with precursor B-ALL. They were not able to correlate specific genes signature with rapid early response, what may suggest the existence of a variety of molecular mechanisms operate within individual cases to response to chemotherapy. Cario et al. [65] identified a characteristic gene expression profile which distinguished patients without minimal residual disease at end induction and following week 12 from those with detectable MRD at week 12 (group high risk of treatment failure). The signature was characterized by low expression of genes controlling cell cycle progression and apoptosis. Many chemotherapeutic drugs are cell cycle phase-dependent, what may contribute to lower sensitivity of leukemic cells to commonly used chemotherapeutic agents in high-risk patients. Teuffel et al. [66] observed low expression of ribosomal proteins in pediatric ALL with an unfavorable outcome. Bullinger et al. [59] determined alteration in gene expression levels from 116 adults with AML. They have shown that 133-gene model can accurately predict overall survival including the intermediate risk group. Yagi et al. [67]

used microarray for identification set of 35 genes related with poor prognosis in childhood ALL.

Drug Resistance in Leukemia Microarray Studies

Microarray technology holds great promise in identify indicator genes respond to drug exposure, discover novel gene interactions, complex regulatory networks and cross-communication between different pathways during various anticancer agent [52]. Definition of mRNA signatures can be used to estimate how the cancer cells react to a particular drug and distinguish between drug-resistant and drug-sensitive ALL cells. This method is helpful in defining whether resistance to chemotherapy can be represented by change in transcriptomic profiles and which genes are involved in drug resistance [68]. Expression signatures were able to identify patients that were eventually at risk to fail with conventional therapy. By investigating the differences in gene activity between untreated and treated tumor cells, or between blasts at relapse and at new diagnosis, it will be possible to understand how different therapies affect tumors and ability to develop more effective and less toxic treatment [64].

Several microarray studies of untreated and pre-treated acute leukemias have demonstrated that gene expression patterns can predict antileukemic drug response (Tables 8 and 9). One of the most important array experiment of the leukemic blasts is the study performed by Holleman et al. [22]. They identified a characteristic transcriptomic patterns which distinguished ALL samples taken from pediatric patients with leukemic cells either sensitive or resistant to four widely used antileukemic agents: prednisolone (PRD), vincristine (VCR), asparaginase (ASP) or daunorubicin (DNR). The expression of 172 human gene probe sets which correlated with resistant profile was shown to discriminate primary childhood ALL cells. Discriminating genes belonged to numerous functional groups, while no single gene was linked to resistance of four tested agent. Out of the 124 genes correlating with response to treatment, 121 have not previously been linked with resistance to investigated drugs [22]. The same research group identified also gene expression signatures that distinguish ALL cells with multiple drug resistance profile [69]. Only 15% of identifying genes were common in both experiments. The level of expression for all common genes was concordant between the single and cross-resistance analyses. In the next GEP study, focusing on 70 apoptosis genes Holleman et al. [70] identified BCL2L13, which was related both to L-asparaginase resistance and treatment outcome, independent from known prognostic factors in 2 independent cohorts of children with B-lineage ALL.

Sorich et al. [71] identified genes related with sensitivity or resistance of ALL cells to methotrexate. They found a large number of genes that differed in their expression level and selected highly significant 50 genes. Patients with GEP indicating a good methotrexate (MTX) response had significantly better five-year disease-free survival in comparison with profiles indicating a poor response. Researchers demonstrated that these 50 genes which expression was related to MTX response are specific to MTX only. Genes/gene expression patterns discriminating drug resistance in ALL are drug specific. Stams et al. [73] proved that overexpression of asparagine synthetase did not correlate to L-asparaginase resistance in pediatric ALL with t(12;21)(p12;q22) chromosomal translocation. The signature was characterized by 5-fold higher expression of this enzyme in the *TEL-AML1* positive ALL patients compared with *TEL-AML1* negative ALL patients. Patients without presence of translocation *TEL-AML1* had 3.5-fold higher expression level of asparagine synthetase. There were no significant differences in drug resistance between *TEL-AML1*-positive and -negative ALL cells. As shown by transcriptomic data, resistance to etoposide may be associated with alteration in expression level 3 genes: *NR2C1, MPST, SRP46* [76]. When Beesley et al. [74] compared gene expression signature to chromosomal analysis data, they found potential 'hot-spots' (e.g. translocations involving 19p13) for change of gene expression level in genes related with therapy failure. Aberrations at the molecular level were correlated with upregulation of genes at locus 19p13. Yeoh et al. [63] identified set of 7 genes, that were selectively expressed in cells from pediatric patients with T-ALL at high risk for relapse with an accuracy of 97%. 20 ranked genes for hyperdiploidy >50 chromosomes, were identified as statistically significant predictors of relapse, with accuracy of 100%.

Currently, little clinical useful information based on GEP in adult AML is available [77]. With respect to adult ALL, Chiaretti et al. [75, 78] carried out genomewide studies and compared the gene expression patterns of patients who relapsed and those who responded to induction chemotherapy. They have found only one gene (interleukin 8), that was overexpressed in refractory T-ALL cells and a set of 30 genes that were highly expressed in lymphoblast from patients who achieved complete remission. The authors defined a 3-gene model (including *AHNAK, CD2, TTK*), that was predictive for duration of remission. Low expression of genes associated with cell cycle progression was correlated with refractory to treatment [78]. Chiaretti et al. [75] focused on gene expression profile in the high-risk group. They identified set of genes that governed their response to the antileukemic therapy. The gene patterns was characterized by overexpression of genes involved in the phosphatidylinositol pathway and gene mediated in the metabolism, like asparagine synthetase. Virtaneva et al. [79] analyzed gene expression profiles in 2 groups of adult patients with acute myeloid leukemia: AML with normal cytogenetics versus AML trisomy 8 (+8). They observed significant differences in expression level for genes involved in controlled cell death. In the cohort AML+8, patients who demonstrated resistance to cytarabine-based chemotherapy, several apoptotic genes (e.g. *BAD, BCL2* and *CRADD*) were downregulated. Inhibition of normal pathway of cell death could be the reason of resistance to cytarabine. The studies of AML by Valk et al. [80] and Bullinger et al. [60] demonstrated that a newly identified gene expression profile could help in associations between genetic alteration that predict a poor outcome and mechanisms of response to chemotherapy.

Analysis of gene expression signatures, both pediatric and adult patients with T-ALL, indicate that different genes are associated with outcome in these patients [63, 78]. Even between six genetic subtype of pediatric ALL, researchers could not identify a common expression profile that predict drug resistance [63]. Genome wide expression information suggest existence of different genetic mechanisms of resistance to anticancer therapy. The ability to predict the treatment response based on GEP is a promising approach to study targeted therapies and also for development the novel drug [53].

Table 8. Applications of gene expression profiles in study of in vitro drug activity and response to treatment in acute leukemias

Tested drugs/ Analyzed mechanisms	Results	Number of discriminating genes	Functional classification of discriminating genes	Ref.
Methotrexate (MTX)	Significant differences in GEP between patients who responded well to MTX to those who responded poorly.	50 highly significant genes	DNA synthesis, its components, repair of DNA and cell proliferation.	[71]
Prednisolone (PRD) *Vincristine (VCR)* *L-Asparaginase (ASP)* *Daunorubicin (DNR)*	Identification of sets of differentially expressed genes in sensitive or resistant B-lineage childhood ALL. It have been demonstrated that the gene expression signature is related to the outcome of treatment.	42 probe sets/33 genes and 3 cDNA clones 59 probe sets/40 genes and 14 cDNA clones 54 probe sets/35 genes and 10 cDNA clones 22 probe sets/20 genes and 2 cDNA clones	cell communication, nucleic acid metabolism, carbohydrate metabolism, cell proliferation cell communication, development, nucleic acid metabolism, protein metabolism cell communication, protein metabolism, physiological process cell communication, nucleic acid metabolism, protein metabolism, transport, cell growth and maintenance	[22]
Multiple drug resistance *(1) crossresistance to PRD, VCR, ASP, DNR* *(2) resistance to ASP and VCR*	Determination of the multiple drug resistance of ALL cells to four antileukemic drugs. No single gene was associated with resistance to all four agents.	45 genes 139 genes	nucleic acid metabolism, including transcription (most genes), RNA and DNA processing, and DNA repair, transport protein biosynthesis (ribosomal proteins, translation elongation factor-related genes)	[69]
Prednisolone (PRD) *L-Asparaginase (ASP)*	Identification of genes associated with drug resistance among 70 key apoptosis genes.	4 probe sets/2 genes 3 probe sets/3 genes	genes for PRD sensitivity: *MCL1*, *DAPK1* genes for ASP resistance: *BCL2L13*, *HRK*, *TNF*	[70]
Prednisolone	Identification of genes related with response for prednisolone treatment and determination of glucocorticoid resistance	57 probe sets/51 genes	apoptosis, metabolism, proliferation	[72]
L-asparaginase	High expression of asparagine synthetase was correlated with poor prognosis only in *TEL-AML1*–negative B-lineage ALL.			[73]

GEP - gene expression profiling

Table 9. Applications of gene expression profiles in study of mechanisms of drug resistance and response to treatment in acute leukemia

Analyzed factors	Results	Number of discriminating genes	Functional classification of discriminating genes	Ref.
General mechanisms involved in therapy failure	Analysis demonstrate existing common mechanism of relapse in pre-B ALL and T-ALL childhood leukemia		oncogenesis, drug resistance and metastasis and not related to classical multidrug-resistance pathways	[74]
Identification of GEP correlated with therapy-induced AML	Developing a model to a secondary AML prediction for the *TEL-AML1* subtype (with 100% accuracy).	20 top ranked genes	genes: *RSU1*, *MSH3*, *NAB1*, tyrosine kinase	[63]
Identification of genes highly expressed in relapsed adult patients	A set of genes involved in therapy failure leukemia blasts from patients without known molecular abnormalities was found.	87 probe sets/83 genes	cell communication, cytoskeleton organization, membrane antigens, resistance to chemotherapy and DNA metabolism	[75]
Determination of genetic risk factors for secondary myeloid leukemia in diagnostic ALL cells from children treated on protocols that included topoisomerase II inhibitors and alkylating agents	The authors defined a gene expression pattern that was significantly related to risk of treatment-related myeloid leukemia	68 probe sets/63 genes	transcription factor, transcription-related oncogenes, cyclins, histone, genes linked to apoptosis	[76]

GEP - gene expression profiling

Analysis of Gene Expression Profiles in Relapsed ALL

Gene expression profiles could possibly be able to identify patients who will eventually experience relapse. Several papers related to the diagnostic application of microarrays to identify gene expression patterns that are significantly associated with relapse have recently been published. Bhojwani et al. [81] analyzed the differentially expressed genes. They observed a striking pattern of genes involved in cell cycle regulation, DNA repair and apoptosis between patients at diagnosis and early relapse. However, no common pattern of changes was observed for patients with late relapse. Yeoh et al. [63] reported that gene expression profiles predictive of relapse could only be defined for individual leukemic subtypes, such as T-cell ALL or B-precursor with hyperdiploidy ≥50 chromosomes. GEP that correlated with therapy outcome, were also identified for *TEL-AML1*, *MLL*-rearranged patients and cases without cytogenetic changes. Andersson et al. [82] described two novel subgroups among patients without characteristic cytogenetic aberrations or with a normal karyotype. First group identified basis of gene expression signature for patients remaining in complete remission. Second one recognized a few patients who eventually relapsed. On the other hand, Willenbrock et al. [48] suggested that it is possible to predict relapse independently of ALL immunophenotype, separately for pre-B and T-ALL.

Carroll et al. [64] were able to differentiate patients who were at clinical remission (CR) for more than 4 years, when compared to cases that experienced a relapse within the first 3 year, based on the level of expression of 47 probe set. These set of genes has significant prognostic value, independent on clinical covariates (e.g. gender, age, and WBC count). Most of these genes were involved in signal transduction. They have performed microarray analyses on leukemic cells from a large group of patients who experienced their first bone marrow relapse and were treated in the trial COG AALL01P2 for relapsed ALL. Microarray analysis has helped to identify large set of genes that were differentially expressed in early and late relapses. The majority of these genes were involved in cell proliferation, DNA repair and cell survival. These genes had a high level of expression in the early relapse group. Further investigations of paired diagnosis-relapse samples revealed genes and pathways that may be potential targets at relapse cohort, including survivin, topoisomerase 2A and cyclin B1.

Staal et al. [83] compared the gene expression of blasts of patients with precursor-B ALL, who relapsed during therapy or after completion of treatment. Only 6 genes which were involved in cell proliferation and cell survival (*SH3 BP5, TOSO, Smad3, CD79a (Mb1), RAS GRP2 and WAS F1*), were significantly upregulated at relapse. These genes are not accepted yet as a diagnostic or progression markers and represent potential new markers for such applications and are potential drug targets. Similar results achieved Beesley et al., [74] using gene expression profiles to discriminate leukemic samples between diagnosis and relapse in each lineage, indicating the existence of common mechanisms of relapse. Analyzing the differentially expressed genes, they observed a striking pattern of genes involved in oncogenesis, drug resistance and metastasis (e.g. *BSG, GRP58, LAMP, PBX2, FUS, GTF2F1, RoXaN, PIP5K1A*), but not related to classical multidrug-resistance pathways. Willenbrock et al. [48] focused their study on prediction of therapy failure. They achieved 87% sensitivity and 69% specificity for prediction of relapse.

In most cases, gene expression profiles that have been associated with relapse have to be verified on independent population of patients. Conflicting results arise because of differences in patient populations, the kind of analysis platforms and the treatment given.

Conclusion

Currently, clinicians are trying to correlate conventional clinical variables and genes in the common model to improve assessment of cancer prognosis. Gene expression profiling may become an important diagnostic test and research tool for the future laboratory. Microarrays allow a parallel, time- and cost-saving analysis and offer important insights into the molecular pathways and interactions present in leukemia, which would not have been explored using traditional methods. Gene expression profiling has the potential to individualize diagnosis and cancer cure and monitor efficacy of treatment strategy. Nowadays, translating large data sets obtained from microarray study into therapeutic advances and preparing generally accepted diagnostic standards still remain a major challenge. However, in the future it will be possible to design treatment targeted directly to specific types of cancer cells.

Acknowledgments

This study was partially supported by grant MNiSW N407 078 32/2964.

References

[1] Pui, CH; Relling, MV; Downing, JR. Acute lymphoblastic leukemia. *N Engl J Med*, 2004, 350, 1535-1548.

[2] Styczynski, J; Wysocki, M. [Mechanisms of drug resistance in acute leukemias: therapeutic problem]. *Adv Clin Exp Med*, 2000, 9, 153-161.

[3] Den Boer, ML; Pieters, R; Veerman, AJ. Mechanisms of cellular anthracycline resistance in childhood acute leukemia. *Leukemia*, 1998, 12, 1657-1670.

[4] Marie, JP; Legrand, O. Drug resistance in acute leukemias.; In: Pui C (ed), *Treatment of acute leukemias. New directions for clinical research*. Totowa, Humana Press, 2003, 497-505.

[5] Deangelo, DJ. The treatment of adolescents and young adults with acute lymphoblastic leukemia. *Hematology* (Am Soc Hematol Educ Program), 2005, 123-130.

[6] Pui, CH; Evans, WE. Treatment of acute lymphoblastic leukemia. *N Engl J Med*, 2006, 354, 166-178.

[7] Styczynski, J; Wysocki, M. In vitro drug resistance profiles of adult acute lymphoblastic leukemia: possible explanation for difference in outcome to similar therapeutic regimens. *Leuk Lymphoma*, 2002, 43, 301-307.

[8] Plasschaert, SL; Kamps, WA; Vellenga, E; de Vries, EG; de Bont, ES. Prognosis in childhood and adult acute lymphoblastic leukaemia: a question of maturation? *Cancer Treat Rev.*, 2004, 30, 37-51.

[9] Styczynski, J; Gil, L. Acute lymphoblastic leukemia: differences between children and adults. *Acta Haematol Pol.*, 2006, 37, 185-201.

[10] Kuchinskaya, E; Heyman, M; Grander, D; Linderholm, M; Soderhall, S; Zaritskey, A; Nordgren, A; Porwit-Macdonald, A; Zueva, E; Pawitan, Y; Corcoran, M; Nordenskjold, M; Blennow, E. Children and adults with acute lymphoblastic leukaemia have similar gene expression profiles. *Eur J Haematol*, 2005, 74, 466-480.

[11] Cox, CV; Martin, HM; Kearns, PR; Virgo, P; Evely, RS; Blair, A. Characterization of a progenitor cell population in childhood T-cell acute lymphoblastic leukemia. *Blood*, 2007, 109, 674-682.

[12] Cox, CV; Evely, RS; Oakhill, A; Pamphilon, DH; Goulden, NJ; Blair, A. Characterization of acute lymphoblastic leukemia progenitor cells. *Blood*, 2004, 104, 2919-2925.

[13] Styczynski, J; Drewa, T. Leukemic stem cells: from metabolic pathways and signaling to a new concept of drug resistance targeting. *Acta Biochim Pol*, 2007, 54, 717-726.

[14] Kaspers, GJ; Zwaan, CM; Veerman, AJ; Rots, MG; Pieters, R; Bucsky, P; Domula, M; Gobel, U; Graf, N; Havers, W; Jorch, N; Kabisch, K; Spaar, HJ; Ritter, J; Creutzig, U. Cellular drug resistance in acute myeloid leukemia: literature review and preliminary analysis of an ongoing collaborative study. *Klin Padiatr*, 1999, 211, 239-244.

[15] Kaspers, GJ; Zwaan, CM; Pieters, R; Veerman, AJ. Cellular drug resistance in childhood acute myeloid leukemia. A mini-review with emphasis on cell culture assays. *Adv Exp Med Biol.*, 1999, 457, 415-421.

[16] Ravindranath, Y; Chang, M; Steuber, CP; Becton, D; Dahl, G; Civin, C; Camitta, B; Carroll, A; Raimondi, SC; Weinstein, HJ. Pediatric Oncology Group (POG) studies of acute myeloid leukemia (AML): a review of four consecutive childhood AML trials conducted between 1981 and 2000. *Leukemia*, 2005, 19, 2101-2116.

[17] Proctor, SJ; Taylor, PR. Age cohort subgroups in adult acute myeloid leukaemia studies--the population perspective. *Leukemia*, 2001, 15, 188-189.

[18] Tallman, MS. New agents for the treatment of acute myeloid leukemia. *Best Pract Res Clin Haematol*, 2006, 19, 311-320.

[19] Pieters, R; Huismans, DR; Loonen, AH; Hahlen, K; van der Does-van den Berg, A; van Wering, ER; Veerman, AJ. Relation of cellular drug resistance to long-term clinical outcome in childhood acute lymphoblastic leukaemia. *Lancet*, 1991, 338, 399-403.

[20] Frost, BM; Nygren, P; Gustafsson, G; Forestier, E; Jonsson, OG; Kanerva, J; Nygaard, R; Schmiegelow, K; Larsson, R; Lonnerholm, G. Increased in vitro cellular drug resistance is related to poor outcome in high-risk childhood acute lymphoblastic leukaemia. *Br J Haematol*, 2003, 122, 376-385.

[21] Den Boer, ML; Harms, DO; Pieters, R; Kazemier, KM; Gobel, U; Korholz, D; Graubner, U; Haas, RJ; Jorch, N; Spaar, HJ; Kaspers, GJ; Kamps, WA; Van der Does-

Van den Berg, A; Van Wering, ER; Veerman, AJ; Janka-Schaub, GE. Patient stratification based on prednisolone-vincristine-asparaginase resistance profiles in children with acute lymphoblastic leukemia. *J Clin Oncol*, 2003, 21, 3262-3268.

[22] Holleman, A; Cheok, MH; den Boer, ML; Yang, W; Veerman, AJ; Kazemier, KM; Pei, D; Cheng, C; Pui, CH; Relling, MV; Janka-Schaub, GE; Pieters, R; Evans, WE. Gene-expression patterns in drug-resistant acute lymphoblastic leukemia cells and response to treatment. *N Engl J Med*, 2004, 351, 533-542.

[23] Styczynski, J; Toporski, J; Wysocki, M; Debski, R; Chybicka, A; Boruczkowski, D; Wachowiak, J; Wojcik, B; Kowalczyk, J; Gil, L; Balwierz, W; Matysiak, M; Krawczuk-Rybak, M; Balcerska, A; Sonta-Jakimczyk, D. Fludarabine, treosulfan and etoposide sensitivity and the outcome of hematopoietic stem cell transplantation in childhood acute myeloid leukemia. *Anticancer Res.*, 2007, 27, 1547-1551.

[24] Styczynski, J; Wysocki, M; Dluzniewska, A; Juraszewska, E; Balwierz, W; Czyzewski, K; Wieczorek, M; Olejnik, I; Krawczuk-Rybak, M; Kuzmicz, M; Kowalczyk, J; Stefaniak, J; Badowska, W; Sonta-Jakimczyk, D; Szczepanski, T; Matysiak, M; Stanczak, E; Malinowska, I; Wachowiak, J; Konatkowska, B; Gil, L; Balcerska, A; Kapuscinska, L; Szczepanek, J; Kolodziej, B; Rafinska, B; Kubicka, M. Prognostic impact of combined fludarabine, treosulfan and mitoxantrone resistance profile in childhood acute myeloid leukemia. *Anticancer Res.*, 2008, 28, 1927-1931.

[25] Ramakers-van Woerden, NL; Pieters, R; Kaspers, GJL; Loonen, AH; Van Zantwijk, CH; Ludwig, WD; Veerman, AJP. The Philadelphia chromosome t(9;22) is associated with in vitro prednisolone and daunorubicin resistance in adult acute lymphoblastic leukaemia [abstract]. *Ann Hematol*, 1997, 74, A38.

[26] Ramakers-van, Woerden, NL; Pieters, R; Hoelzer, D; Slater, RM; den Boer, ML; Loonen, AH; Harbott, J; Janka-Schaub, GE; Ludwig, WD; Ossenkoppele, GJ; van Wering, ER; Veerman, AJ. In vitro drug resistance profile of Philadelphia positive acute lymphoblastic leukemia is heterogeneous and related to age: a report of the Dutch and German Leukemia Study Groups. *Med Pediatr Oncol*, 2002, 38, 379-386.

[27] Ramakers-Van Woerden, NL; Beverloo, HB; Veerman, AJ; Camitta, BM; Loonen, AH; Van Wering, ER; Slater, RM; Harbott, J; Den Boer, ML; Ludwig, WD; Haas, OA; Janka-Schaub, GE; Pieters, R. In vitro drug-resistance profile in infant acute lymphoblastic leukemia in relation to age, MLL rearrangements and immunophenotype. *Leukemia*, 2004, 18, 521-529.

[28] Ramakers-van Woerden, NL; Pieters, R; Loonen, AH; Hubeek, I; van Drunen, E; Beverloo, HB; Slater, RM; Harbott, J; Seyfarth, J; van Wering, ER; Hahlen, K; Schmiegelow, K; Janka-Schaub, GE; Veerman, AJ. TEL/AML1 gene fusion is related to in vitro drug sensitivity for L-asparaginase in childhood acute lymphoblastic leukemia. *Blood*, 2000, 96, 1094-1099.

[29] Frost, BM; Forestier, E; Gustafsson, G; Nygren, P; Hellebostad, M; Jonsson, OG; Kanerva, J; Schmiegelow, K; Larsson, R; Lonnerholm, G. Translocation t(12,21) is related to in vitro cellular drug sensitivity to doxorubicin and etoposide in childhood acute lymphoblastic leukemia. *Blood*, 2004, 104, 2452-2457.

[30] Frost, BM; Forestier, E; Gustafsson, G; Nygren, P; Hellebostad, M; Jonmundsson, G; Kanerva, J; Schmiegelow, K; Larsson, R; Lonnerholm, G. Translocation t(1,19) is

related to low cellular drug resistance in childhood acute lymphoblastic leukaemia. *Leukemia*, 2005, 19, 165-169.

[31] Raimondi, SC; Pui, CH; Hancock, ML; Behm, FG; Filatov, L; Rivera, GK. Heterogeneity of hyperdiploid (51-67) childhood acute lymphoblastic leukemia. *Leukemia*, 1996, 10, 213-224.

[32] Kaspers, GJ; Smets, LA; Pieters, R; Van Zantwijk, CH; Van Wering, ER; Veerman, AJ. Favorable prognosis of hyperdiploid common acute lymphoblastic leukemia may be explained by sensitivity to antimetabolites and other drugs: results of an in vitro study. *Blood*, 1995, 85, 751-756.

[33] Whitehead, VM; Vuchich, MJ; Cooley, LD; Lauer, SJ; Mahoney, DH; Shuster, JJ; Payment, C; Koch, PA; Akabutu, JJ; Bowen, T; Kamen, BA; Ravindranath, Y; Emami, A; Look, AT; Beardsley, GP; Pullen, DJ; Camitta, B. Accumulation of methotrexate polyglutamates; ploidy and trisomies of both chromosomes 4 and 10 in lymphoblasts from children with B-progenitor cell acute lymphoblastic leukemia: a Pediatric Oncology Group Study. *Leuk Lymphoma*, 1998, 31, 507-519.

[34] Matherly, LH; Taub, JW, Methotrexate pharmacology and resistance in childhood acute lymphoblastic leukemia. *Leuk Lymphoma*, 1996, 21, 359-368.

[35] Synold, TW; Relling, MV; Boyett, JM; Rivera, GK; Sandlund, JT; Mahmoud, H; Crist, WM; Pui, CH; Evans, WE. Blast cell methotrexate-polyglutamate accumulation in vivo differs by lineage, ploidy, and methotrexate dose in acute lymphoblastic leukemia. *J Clin Invest*, 1994, 94, 1996-2001.

[36] Belkov, VM; Krynetski, EY; Schuetz, JD; Yanishevski, Y; Masson, E; Mathew, S; Raimondi, S; Pui, CH; Relling, MV; Evans, WE. Reduced folate carrier expression in acute lymphoblastic leukemia: a mechanism for ploidy but not lineage differences in methotrexate accumulation. *Blood*, 1999, 93, 1643-1650.

[37] Zwaan, CM; Kaspers, GJ; Pieters, R; Ramakers-Van Woerden, NL; den Boer, ML; Wunsche, R; Rottier, MM; Hahlen, K; van, Wering, ER; Janka-Schaub, GE; Creutzig, U; Veerman, AJ. Cellular drug resistance profiles in childhood acute myeloid leukemia: differences between FAB types and comparison with acute lymphoblastic leukemia. *Blood*, 2000, 96, 2879-2886.

[38] Zwaan, CM; Kaspers, GJ; Pieters, R; Hahlen, K; Huismans, DR; Zimmermann, M; Harbott, J; Slater, RM; Creutzig, U; Veerman, AJ. Cellular drug resistance in childhood acute myeloid leukemia is related to chromosomal abnormalities. *Blood*, 2002, 100,3352-3360.

[39] Styczynski, J; Pieters, R; Huismans, DR; Schuurhuis, GJ; Wysocki, M; Veerman, AJ. In vitro drug resistance profiles of adult versus childhood acute lymphoblastic leukaemia. *Br J Haematol*, 2000, 110, 813-818.

[40] Pui, CH; Evans, WE. Acute lymphoblastic leukemia. *N Engl J Med*, 1998, 339, 605-615.

[41] Styczynski, J; Wysocki, M. Ex vivo modulation of response to prednisolone in childhood acute lymphoblastic leukaemia. *Br J Haematol*, 2006, 133, 397-399.

[42] Styczynski, J; Koltan, A; Wysocki, M. Resistance to glucocorticoids in childhood acute lymphoblastic leukemia: impact of relationship between ex vivo sensitivity and in vivo concentration on risk factor analysis. *Neoplasma*, 2006, 53, 168-173.

[43] Grimwade, D; Walker, H; Oliver, F; Wheatley, K; Harrison, C; Harrison, G; Rees, J; Hann, I; Stevens, R; Burnett, A; Goldstone, A. The importance of diagnostic cytogenetics on outcome in AML: analysis of 1,612 patients entered into the MRC AML 10 trial. The Medical Research Council Adult and Children's Leukaemia Working Parties. *Blood*, 1998, 92, 2322-2333.

[44] Grimwade, D. The clinical significance of cytogenetic abnormalities in acute myeloid leukaemia. *Best Pract Res Clin Haematol*, 2001, 14, 497-529.

[45] Grimwade, D; Walker, H; Harrison, G; Oliver, F; Chatters, S; Harrison, CJ; Wheatley, K; Burnett, AK; Goldstone, AH. The predictive value of hierarchical cytogenetic classification in older adults with acute myeloid leukemia (AML): analysis of 1065 patients entered into the United Kingdom Medical Research Council AML11 trial. *Blood*, 2001, 98, 1312-1320.

[46] Mrozek, K; Heerema, NA; Bloomfield, CD. Cytogenetics in acute leukemia. *Blood Rev*, 2004, 18, 115-136.

[47] Sakhinia, E; Faranghpour, M; Liu, Yin, JA; Brady, G; Hoyland, JA; Byers, RJ. Routine expression profiling of microarray gene signatures in acute leukaemia by real-time PCR of human bone marrow. *Br J Haematol*, 2005, 130, 233-248.

[48] Willenbrock, H; Juncker, AS; Schmiegelow, K; Knudsen, S; Ryder, LP. Prediction of immunophenotype, treatment response, and relapse in childhood acute lymphoblastic leukemia using DNA microarrays. *Leukemia*, 2004, 18, 1270-1277.

[49] Mullighan, CG; Flotho, C; Downing, JR. Genomic assessment of pediatric acute leukemia. *Cancer J*, 2005, 11, 268-282.

[50] Haferlach, T; Kern, W; Schnittger, S; Schoch, C. Modern diagnostics in acute leukemias. *Crit Rev Oncol Hematol*, 2005, 56, 223-234.

[51] Gershon, D. Microarray technology: an array of opportunities. *Nature*, 2002, 416, 885-891.

[52] Fuscoe, JC; Tong, W; Shi, L. QA/QC issues to aid regulatory acceptance of microarray gene expression data. *Environ Mol Mutagen*, 2007, 48, 349-353.

[53] Chung, CH; Levy, S; Chaurand, P; Carbone, DP. Genomics and proteomics: emerging technologies in clinical cancer research. *Crit Rev Oncol Hematol*, 2007, 61, 1-25.

[54] Han, T; Melvin, CD; Shi, L; Branham, WS; Moland, CL; Pine, PS; Thompson, KL; Fuscoe, JC. Improvement in the Reproducibility and Accuracy of DNA Microarray Quantification by Optimizing Hybridization Conditions. *BMC Bioinformatics*, 2006, 7 Suppl, 2, S17.

[55] Churchill, GA. Fundamentals of experimental design for cDNA microarrays. *Nat Genet*, 2002, 32, Suppl, 490-495.

[56] Barrett, JC; Kawasaki, ES. Microarrays: the use of oligonucleotides and cDNA for the analysis of gene expression. *Drug Discov Today*, 2003, 8, 134-141.

[57] Cussenot, O. DNA microarrays in clinical practice: present or future? *Eur J Intern Med*, 2002, 13, 225-226.

[58] Robert, J; Vekris, A; Pourquier, P; Bonnet, J. Predicting drug response based on gene expression. *Crit Rev Oncol Hematol*, 2004, 51, 205-227.

[59] Bullinger, L; Dohner, K; Bair, E; Frohling, S; Schlenk, RF; Tibshirani, R; Dohner, H; Pollack, JR. Use of gene-expression profiling to identify prognostic subclasses in adult acute myeloid leukemia. *N Engl J Med*, 2004, 350, 1605-1616.

[60] Bullinger, L; Valk, PJ. Gene expression profiling in acute myeloid leukemia. *J Clin Oncol*, 2005, 23, 6296-6305.

[61] Ross, ME; Mahfouz, R; Onciu, M; Liu, HC; Zhou, X; Song, G; Shurtleff, SA; Pounds, S; Cheng, C; Ma, J; Ribeiro, RC; Rubnitz, JE; Girtman, K; Williams, WK; Raimondi, SC; Liang, DC; Shih, LY; Pui, CH; Downing, JR. Gene expression profiling of pediatric acute myelogenous leukemia. *Blood*, 2004, 104, 3679-3687.

[62] Ross, ME; Zhou, X; Song, G; Shurtleff, SA; Girtman, K; Williams, WK; Liu, HC; Mahfouz, R; Raimondi, SC; Lenny, N; Patel, A; Downing, JR. Classification of pediatric acute lymphoblastic leukemia by gene expression profiling. *Blood*, 2003, 102, 2951-2959.

[63] Yeoh, EJ; Ross, ME; Shurtleff, SA; Williams, WK; Patel, D; Mahfouz, R; Behm, FG; Raimondi, SC; Relling, MV; Patel, A; Cheng, C; Campana, D; Wilkins, D; Zhou, X; Li, J; Liu, H; Pui, CH; Evans, WE; Naeve, C; Wong, L; Downing, JR. Classification, subtype discovery, and prediction of outcome in pediatric acute lymphoblastic leukemia by gene expression profiling. *Cancer Cell*, 2002, 1, 133-143.

[64] Carroll, WL; Bhojwani, D; Min, DJ; Moskowitz, N; Raetz, EA. Childhood acute lymphoblastic leukemia in the age of genomics. *Pediatr Blood Cancer*, 2006, 46, 570-578.

[65] Cario, G; Stanulla, M; Fine, BM; Teuffel, O; Neuhoff, NV; Schrauder, A; Flohr, T; Schafer, BW; Bartram, CR; Welte, K; Schlegelberger, B; Schrappe, M. Distinct gene expression profiles determine molecular treatment response in childhood acute lymphoblastic leukemia. *Blood*, 2005, 105, 821-826.

[66] Teuffel, O; Dettling, M; Cario, G; Stanulla, M; Schrappe, M; Buhlmann, P; Niggli, FK; Schafer, BW. Gene expression profiles and risk stratification in childhood acute lymphoblastic leukemia. *Haematologica*, 2004, 89, 801-808.

[67] Yagi, T; Morimoto, A; Eguchi, M; Hibi, S; Sako, M; Ishii, E; Mizutani, S; Imashuku, S; Ohki, M; Ichikawa, H. Identification of a gene expression signature associated with pediatric AML prognosis. *Blood*, 2003, 102, 1849-1856.

[68] Alaoui-Jamali, MA; Dupre, I; Qiang, H. Prediction of drug sensitivity and drug resistance in cancer by transcriptional and proteomic profiling. *Drug Resist Updat*, 2004, 7, 245-255.

[69] Lugthart, S; Cheok, MH; den Boer, ML; Yang, W; Holleman, A; Cheng, C; Pui, CH; Relling, MV; Janka-Schaub, GE; Pieters, R; Evans, WE. Identification of genes associated with chemotherapy crossresistance and treatment response in childhood acute lymphoblastic leukemia. *Cancer Cell*, 2005, 7, 375-386.

[70] Holleman, A; den Boer, ML; de Menezes, RX; Cheok, MH; Cheng, C; Kazemier, KM; Janka-Schaub, GE; Gobel, U; Graubner, UB; Evans, WE; Pieters, R. The expression of 70 apoptosis genes in relation to lineage, genetic subtype, cellular drug resistance, and outcome in childhood acute lymphoblastic leukemia. *Blood*, 2006, 107, 769-776.

[71] Sorich, MJ; Pottier, N; Pei, D; Yang, W; Kager, L; Stocco, G; Cheng, C; Panetta, JC; Pui, CH; Relling, MV; Cheok, MH; Evans, WE. In vivo response to methotrexate

forecasts outcome of acute lymphoblastic leukemia and has a distinct gene expression profile. *PLoS Med*, 2008, 5, e83.

[72] Tissing, WJ; den Boer, ML; Meijerink, JP; Menezes, RX; Swagemakers, S; van der Spek, PJ; Sallan, SE; Armstrong, SA; Pieters, R. Genomewide identification of prednisolone-responsive genes in acute lymphoblastic leukemia cells. *Blood*, 2007, 109, 3929-3935.

[73] Stams, WA; den Boer, ML; Holleman, A; Appel, IM; Beverloo, HB; van Wering, ER; Janka-Schaub, GE; Evans, WE; Pieters, R. Asparagine synthetase expression is linked with L-asparaginase resistance in TEL-AML1-negative but not TEL-AML1-positive pediatric acute lymphoblastic leukemia. *Blood*, 2005, 105, 4223-4225.

[74] Beesley, AH; Cummings, AJ; Freitas, JR; Hoffmann, K; Firth, MJ; Ford, J; de Klerk, NH; Kees, UR. The gene expression signature of relapse in paediatric acute lymphoblastic leukaemia: implications for mechanisms of therapy failure. *Br J Haematol*, 2005, 131, 447-456.

[75] Chiaretti, S; Li, X; Gentleman, R; Vitale, A; Wang, KS; Mandelli, F; Foa, R; Ritz, J. Gene expression profiles of B-lineage adult acute lymphocytic leukemia reveal genetic patterns that identify lineage derivation and distinct mechanisms of transformation. *Clin Cancer Res.*, 2005, 11, 7209-7219.

[76] Bogni, A; Cheng, C; Liu, W; Yang, W; Pfeffer, J; Mukatira, S; French, D; Downing, JR; Pui, CH; Relling, MV. Genome-wide approach to identify risk factors for therapy-related myeloid leukemia. *Leukemia*, 2006, 20, 239-246.

[77] Mrozek, K; Bloomfield, CD. Chromosome aberrations, gene mutations and expression changes, and prognosis in adult acute myeloid leukemia. *Hematology Am Soc Hematol Educ Program*, 2006, 169-177.

[78] Chiaretti, S; Li, X; Gentleman, R; Vitale, A; Vignetti, M; Mandelli, F; Ritz, J; Foa, R. Gene expression profile of adult T-cell acute lymphocytic leukemia identifies distinct subsets of patients with different response to therapy and survival. *Blood*, 2004,103, 2771-2778.

[79] Virtaneva, K; Wright, FA; Tanner, SM; Yuan, B; Lemon, WJ; Caligiuri, MA; Bloomfield, CD; de La Chapelle, A; Krahe, R. Expression profiling reveals fundamental biological differences in acute myeloid leukemia with isolated trisomy 8 and normal cytogenetics. *Proc Natl Acad Sci U S A*, 2001, 98, 1124-1129.

[80] Valk, PJ; Verhaak, RG; Beijen, MA; Erpelinck, CA. Barjesteh van Waalwijk van Doorn-Khosrovani, S; Boer, JM; Beverloo, HB; Moorhouse, MJ; van der Spek, PJ; Lowenberg, B; Delwel, R. Prognostically useful gene-expression profiles in acute myeloid leukemia. *N Engl J Med*, 2004, 350, 1617-1628.

[81] Bhojwani, D; Kang, H; Moskowitz, NP; Min, DJ; Lee, H; Potter, JW; Davidson, G; Willman, CL; Borowitz, MJ; Belitskaya-Levy, I; Hunger, SP; Raetz, EA; Carroll, WL. Biologic pathways associated with relapse in childhood acute lymphoblastic leukemia: a Children's Oncology Group study. *Blood*, 2006, 108, 711-717.

[82] Andersson, A; Ritz, C; Lindgren, D; Eden, P; Lassen, C; Heldrup, J; Olofsson, T; Rade, J; Fontes, M; Porwit-Macdonald, A; Behrendtz, M; Hoglund, M; Johansson, B; Fioretos, T. Microarray-based classification of a consecutive series of 121 childhood

acute leukemias: prediction of leukemic and genetic subtype as well as of minimal residual disease status. *Leukemia*, 2007, 21, 1198-1203.

[83] Staal, FJ; van der Burg, M; Wessels, LF; Barendregt, BH; Baert, MR; van den Burg, CM; van Huffel, C; Langerak, AW; van der Velden, VH; Reinders, MJ; van Dongen, JJ. DNA microarrays for comparison of gene expression profiles between diagnosis and relapse in precursor-B acute lymphoblastic leukemia: choice of technique and purification influence the identification of potential diagnostic markers. *Leukemia*, 2003, 17, 1324-1332.

In: Multiple Drug Resistance
Editors: A. Meszaros, G. Balogh, pp. 31-63
ISBN: 978-1-60741-595-4

Chapter II

Multidrug- Resistant *Acinetobacter baumannii* Infections: Characteristics and Treatment Options

A. Rodríguez- Guardado[1], A. Blanco[2], F. Pérez[3], M. Lantero[3], M. Álvarez Vega[4], JM Torres[4], and JA Cartón[1]
Hospital Universitario Central de Asturias. Spain.
[1] Infectious Diseases Unit
[2] Intensive Care Unit
[3] Microbiology Unit
[4] Neurosurgery Unit

Introduction

Interest in *Acinetobacter spp.* has been growing for the past 30 years. One of the main reasons for the present increased interest in this genus is the emergence of multiresistant strains, some of which are pan-resistant to antibiotics that suddenly cause an outbreak of infection involving [1].

Multidrug-resistant *Acinetobacter baumannii* is a rapidly emerging pathogen in the health care setting, where it causes infections that include bacteraemia, pneumonia, meningitis, urinary tract infection, and wound infection. The mortality associated with these infections is high. The crude mortality rate associated with bacteremia is approximately 52% and that associated with pneumonia ranges from 23% to 73% [2,3].It is recognized to be among the most difficult antimicrobial-resistant gram negative bacilli to control and treat due to the organism' ability to survive under a wide range of environmental conditions and to persist for extended periods of time on surfaces make it a frequent cause of outbreaks of infection and an endemic, health care-associated pathogens. Recently an increased rate of infections caused by *A.baumanii* strains resistant to the antibiotics traditionally used in this therapy has been reported [3-5]. This is an especially severe event in some infections like post-surgical meningitis because the election of the antibiotic depends not only to the sensitivity of *A.baumanii* but also to the penetrability of the chosen antibiotic through the blood-brain barrier. This multidrug-resistant complicates the treatment of these infections makes imperative the search of new agents and the return of old drugs as we consider the optimal treatment of these multidrug-resistant organism.

The focus of this review is to summarize the current state of knowledge regarding *Acinetobacter baumannii* in relation to this role, including their taxonomy, identification, microbiology, epidemiology, infections, and resistance to antibiotics and the potential therapeutic approaches.

Microbiological Characteristics

The genus *Acinetobacter* consists of ubiquitous gram-negative bacilli that were originally identified in the 1930s [3, 6]. Subsequently, several changes were introduced into the taxonomic classification of *Acinetobacter* species. The genus *Acinetobacter* initially encompassed a heterogeneous collection of non-pigmented, oxidase-positive and oxidase-negative gram-negative rods [3, 6-8]. The genus *Acinetobacter* is now defined as including gramnegative (but sometimes difficult to distain) coccobacilli, with a DNA G1C content of 39 to 47 mol%, that are strictly aerobic, nonmotile, nonfermentative, catalase-positive, and oxidase-negative. The good growth occurs on 40° C without growth factor requirements, while nitrates are reduced only rarely [3].In the rapid growth phase it appears as bacilli and in the stationary phase as cocobacilli [9].

Over 20 species belonging to the genus *Acinetobacter* have been identified [10]. *Acinetobacter baumannii* (genomic species 2) is the species of greatest clinical importance, and is typically associated with outbreaks in the hospital setting [11]. Other species that have been associated with disease in humans belong to the *A. calcoaceticus-A. baumannii* complex that includes *Acinetobacter* genomic species 3, *A. johnsonii*, *A. lwoffii*, and *A. calcoaceticus subsp anitratus* [9].

Epidemiology

Increasing isolation of multidrug-resistant *Acinetobacter baumannii* (MDR-ab) has been reported worldwide, and it is now one of the most difficult nosocomially acquired gram-negative pathogens to control and treat [12]. *Acinetobacter baumannii* have the ability to use various sources of nutrition which accounts for its growth on routine laboratory media. This explains its survival as an environemental pathogen. Some strains of *Acinetobacter* can survive environmental desiccation for weeks, a characteristic that promotes transmission through fomite contamination in hospitals [13]. The capacity of *Acinetobacter* species to survive on most environmental surfaces for long periods of time suggests that all animate and inanimate entities should be considered reservoirs.

In health-care settings, colonized and infected patients are often the sources of *A. baumannii* infections; however, the ability of the organism to survive for prolonged periods on environmental surfaces also has contributed to protracted outbreaks in these settings [12].

Acinetobacter has been isolated from pasteurized milk, frozen foods, chilled poultry, foundry, and hospital air, vaporizer mist, tap water faucets, peritoneal dyalisate baths, bedside urinals, washcloths, door handles, keyboards, angiography catheters, ventilators, contaminated gloves, duodenoscopes, laryngoscope blades, plasma protein fraction, and hospital pillows [14-16]. This ability to grown on medical equipment and hospital environmental emphasizing the need for special attention to desinfection of this place as they were in a later chapter [17-20].

Certain strains (clones) have been shown to be distributed between hospitals in wide geographical areas [21]. However, the origin of a suddenly appearing epidemic A. *baumannii* strain in a hospital is often unknown, and it remains possible that A. *baumannii* has a reservoir in the nonhospitalised human population, from which strains can be introduced into a hospital. In humans, *Acinetobacter* can colonize skin, wounds, and the respiratory and gastrointestinal tracts. Up to 25% of healthy ambulatory adults exhibit cutaneous colonization and 7% of adults and infants have transient pharyngeal colonization. It is the most common gram-negative organism persistently carried on the skin of hospital personnel and it has been found to colonizate 45% of inpatient tracheostomy sites and 41% of fecal samples in intensive care unit [22-23].

Acinetobacter baumannii can cause community-acquired infections although less frequently than nosocomially infections. Multidrug-resistant *Acinetobacter* infection has been reported among patients residing in rehabilitation and long-term care facilities, as well as in acute care hospitals [24-26]. Several factors maintain the presence of multidrug-resistant *Acinetobacter* species in the health care setting including the presence of susceptible patients, the presence of patients already colonized or infected with the organism, selective pressure from antimicrobial use and incomplete compliance with infection control procedures [27].

In addition to transmission emergence of resistance occurs in the context of selective pressure from broad-spectrum antimicrobial therapy, such as therapy involving carbapenems or third-generation cephalosporins. The relative contributions of antimicrobial selective pressure and transmission between patients on the emergence of multidrug-resistance *Acinetobacter* species are not known [28-30].

Recently multidrug resistant *Acinetobacter* deep wound infections, osteomyelitis and bacteraemia have been reported among military personnel with traumatic injuries during the war in Irak and Afghanistan [31-34]. Theories that previously colonized soldiers are autoinoculated or that *Acinetobacter* species from local soil or water are introducing during traumatic injury have not been supported by cultures of specimens obtained from healthy soldiers, soil samples water samples, or samples from fresh wounds. Current literature suggest that these infections are associated with health care and are acquired by soldiers in medical facilities during the processes of stabilization, emergency treatment and evacuation through the military medical system [35-39]. There is a possibility of transmission of these strains to hospitals destination of these patients so the Public Health Agency of Canada, in conjunction with the Canadian Forces, have developed an alert to inform hospitals of the potential for importation of *Acinetobacter baumannii*, and the appropriate precautionary measures that should be taken to prevent secondary spread within hospitals [34,40-42].

Antimicrobial Resistance

Acinetobacter spp. display mechanisms of resistance to all existing antibiotic classes as well as a prodigious capacity to acquire new determinants of resistance [43]. The capacity of *Acinetobacter* species for extensive antimicrobial resistance may be due in part to the organism's relatively impermeable outer membrane and its environmental exposure to large reservoir genes.

Various terms have been used (sometimes interchangeably) to denote antimicrobial-resistant phenotypes of *Acinetobacter spp.* The most common definitions of multidrug resitance are carbapenem resistance or resistance to ≥ 3 classes of antimicrobials [44].

The frequently observed multiresistance of *Acinetobacter spp.* isolates complicates antibiotic therapy and varies greatly between geographical regions, institutions, and even hospital wards [45]. Some studies have reported an average rate of carbapenem resistance of 27% among *Acinetobacter spp.* in European countries [46].

Mechanisms of Resistance

Resistance mechanisms for *Acinetobacter* species generally fall into 3 categories: a) antimicrobial-inactiving enzymes; b) reduced access to bacterial targets or c) mutations that change targets or cellular functions. Because the *Acinetobacter spp* are gram-negative organism, they posses an additional outer membrane that acts as a permeation barrier [2].

Resistance mechanisms that are expressed frequently in nosocomial strains of *Acinetobacter* include β-lactamases, alterations in cell-wall channels (porins), and efflux pumps. *A. baumannii* can become resistant to quinolones through mutations in the genes *gyrA* and *parC* and can become resistant to aminoglycosides by expressing aminoglycoside-modifying enzymes [13,44].

Resistance to Beta-Lactams

The mechanism of resistance to ß-lactams involve a) their hydrolysis by beta-lactamases, b) changes in penicillin-binding proteins (PBPs) that prevent their action, c) alterations in the structure and number of porin proteins that result in decreased permeability to antibiotics through the outer membrane of the bacterial cell, and (iv) the activity of efflux pumps that further decrease the concentration of antibiotic within the bacterial cell [47].

AmpC β-lactamases are chromosomally encoded cephalosporinases intrinsic to all *A. baumannii*. Usually, such β-lactamases have a low level of expression that does not cause clinically appreciable resistance; however, the addition of a promoterinsertion sequence, IS*Aba*1, next to the *ampC* gene increases β-lactamase production, causing treatment- limiting resistance to cephalosporins [48] Although porin channels in *A. baumannii* are poorly characterized, it is known that reduced expression or mutations of bacterial porin proteins can hinder passage of β-lactam antibiotics into the periplasmic space, leading to antibiotic resistance.

In addition to the class C cephalosporinase discussed above, other β-lactamases have been reported in *A. baumannii* [44]. These include the TEM-1 type [49,50], SHV type [3,51], CTX-M type [52], PER-1 [53,54], and VEB-1 [55,56] b-lactamases. Although they are important, it is difficult to assess their impact on resistance in the presence of the AmpC cephalosporinase.

The most important problem in multidrug-resistant *Acinetobacter* is the resistance to carbapenems. This resistance is mediated for various mechanisms:

- Metallo-β-lactamase (VIM, IMP)
- OXA carbapenemases (class D).
- Cell permeability changes.
- Target (PBPs) change.

The metallo-β-lactamases and OXA carbapenemases are the most important mechanism of resistant in *Acinetobacter baumannii* because confer resistance to carbapenems. These enzymes belong to either Ambler Class B (metalo-beta-lactamases) or class D (oxacillinases). Metalo-β-Lactamases are efficient carbapenemases and three groups of this enzyme class have been found in *Acinetobacter spp* the IMP-like MBL, the VIM-like MBL or SIM-1. IMP and VIM confer high-level resistance to carbapenems and most other B-lactams with the exception of aztreonam. MBL are located in class-1 integrons and may be transferred and expressed along with resistance genes to other antimicrobials such as aminoglycosides [45,47,57-59].

The other group of enzymes (carbapenem-hydrolysing oxacillinases) consists of oxacillinases with intrinsic carbapenemase activity. The significant contribution of these enzymes to carbapenem resistance in *A. baumannii* has been emphasized, particularly when they are accompanied by IS*Aba1* and IS*Aba3* in the naturally occurring plasmid [60-62].

A third mechanism of carbapenem resistance involves porins, which are outer-membrane proteins that allow antimicrobials, such as β-lactams, to permeate into the bacterial cell. Loss or modification of porin proteins has been shown to confer carbapenem resistance and high-level resistance is observed in the presence of both loss of porin function and expression and production of carbapenemases [47,63].

Additionally mechanism that contribute to carbapenem resistance is the overexpression of bacterial efflux pumps that decrease the concentration of β-lactam antibiotics in the periplasmic space [64]. To cause clinical resistance in *Acinetobacter spp*, efflux pumps usually act in association with overexpression of AmpC β-lactamases or carbapenemases. With less β-lactam entering the periplasmic space, the weak enzymatic activity of the β-lactamase is amplified In addition to removing β-lactam antibiotics, efflux pumps can actively expel quinolones, tetracyclines, chloramphenicol, disinfectants, and tigecycline [65].

The resistance of *A. baumannii* to carbapenems is also explained by reduced expression of PBP-2 [62]. Establishing the relative contribution of the action of beta-lactamases, beta-lactam penetration through OMPs, and interaction with other mechanisms of resistance, and the control of their expression presents important questions to the future [47].

Resistance to Aminoglycosides

Resistance to aminoglycosides is mediated by 3 mechanisms: alteration of the ribosomal target, reduction of uptake, and enzymatic modification of the drug. Alteration of the ribosomal target only affects streptomycin. The second mechanism is fairly common in *Acinetobacter spp*, but resistance to aminoglycosides in *A. baumannii* is mediated principally by aminoglycoside- modifying enzymes. These include aminoglycoside o-phosphotransferases, aminoglycoside N-acetyltransferases, and aminoglycoside o-nucleotidyltransferases and are mediated primarily by plasmids or transposons that can play a role in the spread of resistance. These enzymes may also be chromosomally located [3, 66,67].

Resistance to Quinolones

Resistance of *A. baumannii* to quinolones is often caused by modifications in the structure of DNA gyrase secondary to mutations in the quinolone resistance-determining regions of the *gyrA* and *parC* genes [68,69]. These changes result in a lower affinity for the binding of the quinolone to the enzyme-DNA complex. As mentioned above, a second mechanism of resistance to the quinolones is mediated by efflux systems that decrease intracellular drug accumulation [47].

Resistance to Tetracyclines

Two different mechanisms of resistance to tetracyclines have been described in *A. baumannii*. TetA and TetB are specific transposon-mediated efflux pumps; TetB determines the efflux of both tetracycline and minocycline, whereas TetA drives only the efflux of tetracycline. The second mechanism is the ribosomal protection protein, which shields the ribosome from the action of tetracycline. The *tet*(M) gene encodes this protein, which serves to protect the ribosome from tetracycline, doxycycline, and minocycline [3,47].

Tygecycline is the first antibiotic of a new class called glycylcyclines that may be useful for multidrug-resistant *Acinetobacter* [70]. Tigecycline overcomes the two major mechanisms of resistance to tetracyclines (ribosomal protection and efflux), but tigecycline resistance emerging during therapy has been reported [71]. This resistance appears to be attributable to the overexpression of AdeABC multidrug efflux pump [72]. Probably this mechanism can be upregulated by the previous use of other antibiotics (eg, fluoroquinolones, aminoglycosides) that are administered frequently in patients with serious infections [73].

Resistance to Polymyxins

There are several suggested mechanisms of resistance to colistin/polymyxin B in Gram-negative bacteria, most of which involve changes in the outer membrane. The mechanism of resistance to colistin likely resides in modifications in the lipopolysaccharide of *A. baumannii* (acidification, acylation, or presence of antigens that interfere with binding of the antibiotic to the cell membrane) [3]. It had been reported a strong association between the use of colistin and the development of resistance in *A.baumannii* clinical isolates [74].

Virulence and Pathogenicity

A. baumannii is regarded as a low-grade pathogen, with limited virulence. However, this organism has certain features that allow it to increase the virulence of those strains implicated in infections. The invasiveness of the bacteria may be related to substances that protect the surface of phagocytosis, as is the polysaccharide capsule. The presence of fimbriae along with the dish allows the adhesion to human epithelial cells. It has studied the production of enzymes as butyrate esterase, caprylate esterase, leucine and aryl amidasa which may damage tissue lipids and the potentially toxic role of the lipopolysaccharide component of the cell wall and the presence of lipid A. Apart from owning factors *Acinetobacter spp* in common with other gram-negative bacteria produce a lipopolysaccharide that can take effect endotoxigénico through the lipid A and that would highlight the ability of these microorganisms to capture the iron through the secretion of siderophores, which allows them to survive in the body human. On the other hand, some strains of *Acinetobacter spp* can producing slime which was considered to be the main factor responsible for the enhancement of virulence in mixed infections [1,3, 75].

All this factors acts together in the pathogenicity of *Acinetobacter spp*. The capsular polysaccharides and lipopolysaccharides (LPSs) act in synergy by blocking the access of the human complement to the bacterial cell wall, thus preventing its lytic activity on bacterial membranes. Furthermore, the hydrophilicity conferred by the presence of capsular polysaccharides, together with other nonspecific adherence factors (i.e., fimbriae), prompts the colonization of human epithelial cells by pathogen strains [76]. Enzymes able to damage tissue lipids are also produced during infectious stages of the colonization. Interestingly, the action of LPSs in the pathogenicity of *Acinetobacter* is not limited to the protection of bacterial cells from host defenses; these molecules are in fact provided with a powerful endotoxic activity, and their production in vivo is thought to be related to *Acinetobacter* septicemia symptoms, given the ability of *Acinetobacter* LPSs to induce lethal toxicity in mice and pyrogenicity in rabbits [77].

LPSs are characteristic of the Gram-negative bacteria outer membrane. Their chemical nature affects the physical properties of the cell envelope, thus determining the interactions with the surrounding environment as well as the host-pathogen recognition mechanism. From a structural point of view can be divided in two categories: smooth-type LPSs, composed of the glycolipid portion of lipid A, the core oligosaccharide, and the *O*-polysaccharide or *O*-specific chain; and rough-type LPSs (R-LPSs), in which the *O*-polysaccharide is missing. The structural variability that characterizes the polysaccharide decreases in the core oligosaccharide and primarily in lipid A, whose architecture is usually conserved within the genus. All virulent strains of *Acinetobacter spp* have been found to possess smooth-type LPSs. Nevertheless, the most powerful immunostimulator center of the LPS is the lipid A glycolipid moiety, which is able to activate the innate immune system, triggering cytokine production that, when uncontrolled, can lead to septic shock [78].

Antibiotic Useful on Acinetobacter Infections

There is distint classes of antimicrobial agents that are considered as potentially effective for the treatment of *A baumannii* infections that include: Sulbactam, Anti-pseudomonal penicillins or cephalosporins, carbapenems, monobactams, aminoglycosides, fluoroquinolones, glycylcyclines and colistin [79]. However the apparition of strains with high resistance to carbapenems, aminoglycosides and fluoroquinolones [80,81] presents a challenge to the clinician so sulbactam, tigecycline and colistin represent the current therapeutic approaches, which are associated with satisfactory efficacy.

Carbapenems

Imipenem and meropenem, have been regarded as the treatment of choice for severe *A. baumannii* infections [3], although the increase of resistance rated of *A baumannii* isolates to carbapenems, especially in Europe and North America have diminished its usefulness. In a recent surveillance study [82] about 2,902 strains of *A. baumannii* the susceptibility of imipenem varied across the regions, from fairly good in North America and Europe (74%) to poor or moderate in Latin America (60.6%) and Asia/Pacific Rim (69.2% and 59.6%, respectively). On the other hand carbapenem-resistant *A baumannii* strains might only rarely be susceptible to other antipseudomonal [79] and the treatment became very difficult.

As described in previous chapters Carbapenem resistance in *A baumannii* is mediated by several mechanism including plasmid or chromosomally encoded carbapenemases (mainly OXA-23-like, OXA-24-like, or OXA-58-like class D β-lactamases), as well as metallo-β lactamases (class B β lactamases), efflux pump mechanisms, penicillin binding protein alterations, and modifications or loss of outer membrane proteins (porins) [48,79]. More than one of these resistance determinants could be present in the same strain conferring high-level resistance.

Recently a new carbapenem has been development. Doripenem is a novel forthcoming carbapenem that possesses a broad spectrum of activity against Gram-negative bacteria, similar to that of meropenem, while retaining the spectrum of imipenem against Gram-positive pathogens [83]. It has approved for the treatment of complicated urinary tract and complicated intra-abdominal infections. An indication for hospital-acquired pneumonia including ventilator-associated pneumonia is pending. Its principal features are: a) bactericidal action against most species; b) β-lactamase stability to commonly occurring enzymes, including the emerging extended spectrum β-lactamases (ESBLs); (c) pharmacokinetic and pharmacodynamic qualities similar to those of meropenem (half-life of 1 h) with minimal risk of convulsive adverse reactions; d) postantibiotic effects of nearly 2 h in vitro for *P.aeruginosa*; and e) low serum protein binding (8.9%). Doripenem is stable enough in the presence of renal dehydropeptidase I that it need not be coadministered with a dehydropeptidase I inhibitor such as cilastatin. Pharmacokinetic studies have supported a 3-times-daily dosing schedule [84].

The most frequents adverse reactions are: nausea, diarrhea, headache, phlebitis, hypersensitivity reaction and *C. difficile*-associated colitis. In contrast to imipenem, doripenem did not cause EEG changes and seizures in animal studies [85].

Doripenem may be have a important role in the treatment of *Acinetobacter* infection because have a lower MIC than ertapenem or imipenem when tested against *Acinetobacter spp*.[86,87] and some isolates that are intermediate or resistant to other carbapenems may be susceptible to doripenem and will require additional susceptibility testing [88,89]. In a recent study [87] realized about 12,581 isolates collected between 2005 and 2006 and tested by doripenem, imipenem and meropenem, the MIC(90) of doripenem (0.12) was comparable to that of meropenem (0.12) and superior to that of imipenem (2), though susceptibility of isolates exceeded 99% for all evaluated carbapenems. Against imipenem-susceptible *Acinetobacter spp*., doripenem (MIC(90) = 2, 89.1%S) was twice as active by MIC(90) as were imipenem and meropenem. However none of the carbapenems was active against *A. baumannii* strains expressing plasmid-mediated carbapenemases [88].

Colistin

Colistin belongs to Polymyxins group and is available in two forms, colistin sulfate and colistimethate sodium. Colistimethate sodium is a non-active prodrug that is used for parenteral administration because of its lower toxicity [90]. Polymyxins show bactericidal activity against A *baumannii* that acts by interacting with anionic lipopolysaccharide moieties on the bacterial cell membrane, thereby leading to increase membrane permeability [91,92] and resistance rates against these agents have remained low despite of its more frequent use and the presence of carbapenem-resistant strains [93,94,95].

The dose of colistin is 2.5-5 mg/Kg/day of colistin base in two to four divided doses. In persons with > 60 Kg bodyweight the doses more frequent used is 80-160 mg/8 hours. The bactericidal activity of colistin is concentration dependent; therefore administering large doses in less frequent intervals may be a favourable approach [96-99]. Isolated case report described the cure of *Acinetobacter baumannii* bacteraemia with continuous intravenous colistin (2,000,000 units per 24 h) in patients with allergic reactions to other treatment. In this context colistin may be a useful salvage regimen [100].

Dose adjustment is required in presence of renal failure.

Colistin had demonstrated alone or in combination with other antimicrobials like rifampicin, its usefulness in several infections due to *A. baumannii* as ventilator- associated pneumonia, meningitis, bacteraemia, etc. [100-104]

The most common toxic effects of colistin are nephrotoxicity and the emergence of polyneuropathy. For this reason, the systemic administration of polymyxins had been abandoned for about 20 years in most areas of the world. However, the problem of infections due to multidrug-resistant (MDR) Gram-negative bacteria such us *Pseudomonas aeruginosa* and *Acinetobacter baumanniii* has led to the re-use of polymyxins. Recent studies showed that the rate of development of nephrotoxicity in patients treated with colistin for Gramnegative bacterial infections is similar to that related to other antimicrobial agents [105-109]. Most non-comparative studies have reported a rate of renal toxicity associated with polymyxin therapy of between 8% and 21%. Patients with pre-existing renal dysfunction seem to be more susceptible to the renal adverse effects of polymyxins [108-109]. Other side effects are the apparition of neurotoxicity, bronchoconstriction, chest tightness or cough following administration via the respiratory tract, and chemical meningitis with intraventricular or intrathecal use but has been infrequently reported [110-111].

Resistance to colistin is very lower but it has already report. In recent report risk factors significantly associated with the isolation of colistin-resistant isolates were age, duration of intensive care unit stay, surgical procedures, use of colistin, use of monobactams, duration of use of colistin although in the multivariable model, the use of colistin was identified as the only independent risk factor [112]. To prevent this phenomenon, colistin should be used judiciously, given that treatment options for colistin-resistant gram-negative bacteria are limited.

Sulbactam

Sulbactam was introduced in the eighties as a beta-lactamase inhibitor in combination with beta-lactamic antibiotics [4,5]. Sulbactam have bacteriostatic activity against *Acinetobacter spp* through binding to PBP2. The most frequent used combination is ampicillin/sulbactam (ratio 2:1) although the two agents are not synergetic [103-105]. The combination of ampicillin-sulbactam has been used by some authors in doses of 2 gr to 6-8 hours [45,113].

The use of ampicillim/sulbactam had been described in the literature in retrospective series. The combination therapy has shown similar effectiveness to imipenem therapy in *A baumannii* ventilator-associated pneumonia or bacteraemia caused by multidrug-resistant [113-118]. Favourable clinical outcomes have also been reported with sulbactam or combination ampicillin/sulbactam therapy in patients with other types of nosocomial infections like meningitis [119]. Recent studies compared the efficacy of ampicillin/sulbactam to polymyxins therapy and appears to be more efficacious than polymyxins, which was an independent factor associated with mortality during treatment [120].

Therefore, ampicillin-sulbactam is a sensible option for the treatment of life-threatening *Acinetobacter* infections. However the role of sulbactam in the treatment of *Acinetobacter* infections is limited due to the apparition of multidrug-resistant strains.

Glycylcyclines

Glycylcyclines are a novel class of antimicrobial agents related to the tetracyclines. Tigecycline, a semisynthetic derivative of minocycline, is the first commercially available agent of this class. It has a similar mechanism of action to that of the tetracyclines, and shows bacteriostatic activity against *A baumannii* because interfere with bacterial protein synthesis through ribosomal binding and thus exhibits time dependent bactetericidal activity [121-122].

Tigecycline is extensively distributed into many tissues, resulting in a prolonged half-life that justifies twice-daily dosing. Fifty-nine percent of a tigecycline dose is excreted through the liver, and 33% is excreted through the kidney. In patients with severe hepatic impairment (Child's class C), the normal dose of tigecycline (100-mg initial dose, then 50 mg twice daily) should be reduced to 25 mg twice daily after the normal loading dose. No adjustments are required for any level of renal impairment [123].

Tigecycline is able to evade the most common mechanisms of resistance to tetracyclines in *A baumannii*, including efflux pumps encoded by the *tet*(A) and *tet*(B) determinants, and ribosomal protection mechanisms. Nevertheless several unique multidrug efflux pumps have been shown to reduce organism susceptibility to tygecycline and the rate of resistance is nearly 6% in strains of Europe and America [124]. In-vitro studies have shown that resistance to tigecycline is mediated by the expression of resistance-nodulation division-type multidrug efflux pumps in *A. baumannii* suggests that resistance may emerge during therapy [125].

Clinical experience regarding the use of tigecycline for the treatment of patients with multidrug-resistant *A baumannii* infections is accumulating. In the available relevant reports, tigecycline has been used in a small number of critically ill patients—mainly as part of combination antibiotic regimens—for the treatment of various types of infections, including ventilator-associated pneumonia and primary or secondary bacteraemia [126-128]. In first case series, most patients had a good clinical outcome. However, failure of tigecycline to clear *A baumannii* bacteraemia was reported in a few cases [129-130]. On the other hand pharmacokinetic and pharmacodynamic data indicate that tigecycline blood concentrations seem to be suboptimal for maximal antibacterial activity to be exerted at this compartment. The emergence of resistance in *A baumannii* during tigecycline therapy is an additional point for consideration. There is a crescent number of reports which indicate that resistance to tigecycline developed during the treatment. In recent review reporting retrospective data regarding 42 severely ill patients, among whom 31 had respiratory tract infection (in 4 cases with secondary bacteraemia) and 4 had bacteraemia , tigecycline therapy (in combination with other antibiotics in 28 patients) was effective in 32/42 cases but in three cases the resistance development during the treatment [129].

Clinicians should be aware that tigecycline MICs for A. *baumannii* isolates may increase during therapy with tigecycline after only brief exposure to the drug. Patients receiving tigecycline for *Acinetobacter* should be monitored for the development of clinical resistance, and isolates should be monitored for evidence of microbiologic resistance.

Aminoglycosides

Aminoglycosides have shown moderate rates of antimicrobial activity against *A baumannii.* In worldwide collections of *Acinetobacter spp* isolates, susceptibility rates to amikacin were approximately 60% [92] and the activity of aminoglycosides is lower for multidrug-resistant isolates of *A baumannii* compared with non-multidrugresistant ones [131].

Reports about the clinical use of aminoglycosides in human beings are scarce, and refer to cases of bacteraemia [132] or meningitis [104] in which aminoglycosides have been used in combination with other classes of antimicrobial agents.

Fluoroquinolones

Fluoroquinolones have moderate antimicrobial activity against *A baumannii.* Althought levofloxacin has been shown to yield a lower MIC compared with ciprofloxacin and ofloxacin against *Acinetobacter spp o*verall resistance rates to ciprofloxacin and levofloxacin in clinical isolates are around 50%. [133]. On the other hand the activity of fluoroquinolones against recent multidrug-resistant or imipenem-resistant isolates has been reported to be low [92,132].

The clinical dates are based on in vitro studies. In this studies levofloxacin has shown similar effectiveness to imipenem in a mouse pneumonia model against a strain susceptible to both agents [134]. However, no comprehensive evidence exists regarding the effectiveness of fluoroquinolones for the treatment of human infections caused by *A baumannii.*

Combination Therapy

Against infections multidrug- resistant *Acinetobacter baumannii* isolates several novel antibiotic combinations demonstrate increased activity in vitro compared with that of any single agent. Whether these combinations yield outcomes that are improved over those seen with a polymyxin or other agent alone remains to be determined. However, against infections with species resistant to all antibiotics, including polymyxins, novel combinations are the only remaining therapeutic option.Several drugs combinations havee been tested mostly involving colisitin, carbapenems, rifampicin, fluorquinolones and sulbactam [135].

Although most of the studies were done *in vitro* and in animal models of pneumonia, they show that the combined therapy, especially the combination with rifampin, obtained better results than monotherapy with carbapenems or colistin [136,137]. The colistin and rifampicin combination (colistin sulphomethate sodium 2 million IU three times a day and intravenous rifampicin 10 mg/kg every 12 h) has been probed in the treatment of ventilator-associated pneumonia or bacteremia caused by carbapenem-resistant *Acinetobacter baumannii* with clinical response of 76% and mortality of 21% [138,139]. Some studies [140] has compared the efficacy of intravenous and aerosolized colistin combined with rifampicin in the treatment of critically patients with nosocomial infections caused by multiresistant *A. baumannii* with good results.

The imipenem and ripampicin combination had been studied in some clinical papers.The combination of imipenem with rifampicin, although synergistic in vitro,was not associated with clinical benefits in a small study.[141] In a small retrospective cohort study of patients with infections caused by multidrug-resistant, including carbapenem-resistant, Gram-negative bacteria, the combination of colistin with meropenem was found to be inferior in terms of patient survival compared with colistin monotherapy, although infection-related outcomes did not differ. The combination of imipenem and tigecycline has not been shown to be synergistic [45]. The combination of imipenem with sulbactam has showed synergistic activity in vitro although the clinical usefulness of this combination in patients infected with carbapenem resistant *A baumannii* is not well established [142].

The assessment of in-vitro synergy of the combination of imipenem with a polymyxin against carbapenem-resistant *A baumannii* strains has provided mixed findings. Among other polymyxin-based combination regimens for multidrug-resistant *A baumannii*, the combination of colistin with a carbapenem has shown in vitro either synergistic or indiff rent activity [143,144] but clinical effectiveness has not been substantiated [145]. By contrast, the combination of polymyxin B and tigecycline has resulted in indifferent activity [146].

Clinical data are currently insufficient to favour the use of specific combination regimens for the treatment of multidrug-resistant *A baumannii* infections.

Specific Infections due to A. Baummanii

1. Nosocomial Infections

Acinetobacter baumannii is an important cause of nosocomial infections. Risk factors specific for nosocomial infection include length of hospital stay, surgery, wounds, underlying severity of illness, previous infection, fecal colonization with *Acinetobacter*, treatment with broad-spectrum antibiotics, parenteral nutrition, indwelling central intravenous or urinary catheters or other invasive procedures, admission to a burn unit or intensive care unit, parenteral nutrition, and mechanical ventilation [28,147].

Nosocomial meningitis

A. baumannii meningitis is an infrequent infection mostly associated with intraventricular catheters, CSF fistula or head trauma [148,149].

A. baummanii meningitis is more frequent in patients with intraventricular hemorrhages, head trauma, longer hospital stays and admitted to the intensive care unit [104,150,151]. Others risk factors are the presence of intraventricular catheters longer than 7 days like in all post-surgical meningitis ,[152], and the previous use of antimicrobials.

The clinical manifestations of *A. baumannii* post-surgical meningitis are unremarkable, mostly fever and progressive loss of consciousness. Therefore these manifestations are attributed to the underlying disease, delaying this way the final diagnosis of meningeal infection , and representing a prognostic factor of mortality [104,153].

Acinetobacter spp is a genus with tendence to quickly develop resistances to multiple antimicrobials. This complicates the treatment of these infections makes imperative the search of new agents and the return of old drugs. Until the apparition of resistances carbapenems alone or combined with amikacin was the gold standard in the treatment of this infection. However the resistance to the new antibiotics in the last years has determined the use of alternative agents such as ampicillin-sulbactam or colistin [154]. Sulbactam was introduced in the eighties as a beta-lactamase inhibitor in combination with beta-lactamic antibiotics [5] with "in vitro" activity against *Acinetobacter spp*, enhanced by its affinity for penicillin-binding proteins. Intravenous sulbactam penetrates only 1% the blood-brain barrier but increased up to 32% with meningeal inflammation [119]. The combination of ampicillin-sulbactam has been used by some authors in doses of 2 gr to 6-8 hours with mortalities of 20-25% [104,119].

The presence of multiresistance and the poor penetration of many drugs through the blood-brain barrier has forced the use of intrathecal therapies initially with aminoglycosides and most recently with colistin. The use of intrathecal and intravenous amikacin has been reported in the treatment of meningitis refractary to standard therapy in a small number of cases con rates of cure by 50-60%, [155,156]. The exact dose of intrathecal amikacin has not been established. In recent study a 20mg/day dose was used with cure rates of 83.4% and without side-effects [104,116].

Table 1. Main clinical studies on *A. baumannii meningitis* treatment.

Reference	Design	Patients	Treatment	Dosing	Cure
Levin et al (1999)[162]	Prospective nonrandomized	5 CNS infections	colistin	2.5-5 mg/kg/day iv divided into 3 doses	80%
Jiménez-Mejias et al (2000)[158]	Case report	1 meningits	colistin	5 mg/Kg/day iv in 3 dosis	Cure
Jiménez-Mejias et al (2002)[157]	Case report	1 meningitis	colistin	5 mg/Kg/day iv in 4 dosis	Cure
Levin et al (2003) [117]	Prospective nonrandomized	2 CNS infections	Ampicillin-sulbactam	6 gr/ day in 3 dosis	None
Jimenez-Mejias et al (1997)[119]	Retrospective	8 pos-tsurgical meningitis	Ampicillin-sulbactam	2 gr/iv every 6-8 hours	75% cure
Cawley et al (2002)[166]	Case reprort	Meningitis	Ampicillin-sulbactam	2 gr/iv every 3 hours	Cure
Siegman-Igra et al(1993) [148]	Retrospective	25 nosocomial meningitis	Various	Not reported	3 death
Nguyen et al (1994) [155]	Retrospective	7 post-surrgical meningitis	2 imipenem+ amikacin 3 imipenem+ amikacin + intrathecal aminoglicosides 2 others treatments	-Not reported	86%
Benifla M et al (2004) [166]	Case report	1 Surgical meningitis	intrathecal colistin	40.000 U/day	Cure
Gleeson T et al (2005) [167]	Case report	Surgical meningitis	Rifampin Meropenem	600 mg/24 hours Dose not reported	cure
Vasen W et al (2000) [168]	Case report	Post-surgical meningitis	Intrathecal Colistin	10 mg/24 hours 21 days	Cure
Karakitsos et al (2006) [169]	Retrospective	Postsurgical meningitis	Ripampin Colistin	10 mg/Kg/12h 10-20 mg day	Cure
Rodriguez-Guardado et al (2008) [104]	Retrospective	51 Postsurgical meningitis	Intravenous and Intrathecal colistin Carbapenems Ampicillin-Sulbactam Various	160 mg/8h+10 mg/12 Various 3 gr/8 hours	17 death

The role of colistin in the treatment of meningitis was initially limited due to its poor CSF penetration (25% of serum levels) without modification in the presence of meningeal inflammation [157]. However it has been used in isolated clinical cases by intrathecal and IV routes with good results [104,158]. The dose of intrathecal colistin is variable, most of the authors use 5mg/12 hours. In recent study the doses were 10 mg/12 hours without increasing side-effects [104].In this paper all the patients treated with intravenous and intrathecal colistin survived. Although the small number of cases limit the statistical meaning of this findings the data show that colistin can be an effective and safe alternative for this infection [104].

New antibiotics have recently appeared such as tigecycline, member of a new class of antibiotics, the glycines. In animal studies of meningitis, tigecycline in a unique dose of 20 mg/kg/ day has shown CSF concentrations higher than 1μg/ml 3 hours after the infusion. However enough data regarding its ability to pass the blood-brain barrier and its future use in the treatment of meningitis are lacking [159-160]. Polymyxins have also been used for the treatment of nosocomial meningitis caused by multidrug-resistant *A baumannii.* [161]. Clinical effectiveness has been reported for treatment via the intravenous route alone, although studies have only included a small number of patients [157,158,162]. Because of suboptimal penetration through the blood–brain barrier [157] colistin has been used via the intraventricular or the intrathecal route in addition to systemically administered colistin [104,110,163,164] or other antibacterial agents, such as amino glycosides [104,110,163,164].

In the series the lack of removal of the intraventricular catheters is associated with higher mortality. Therefore the early removal of the intraventricular devices is imperative to obtain the cure of the infection. Other of the factors conditioning a higher mortality was the absence of an adequate treatment and the delay in starting therapy emphasizing the value of an adequate empirical treatment [104].

Hospital acquired/ventilator associated pneumonia (VAP)

Acinetobacter spp are a major cause of VAP and are associated with mortality rates up to 50-70% [170] in some cases associated to inappropriate initial antibiotic therapy [171]. The incidence of this microorganism varies from site to site, but it is the second commonest aetiological agent among the gram-negative bacteria. Longer periods of hospitalization, longer time on mechanical ventilation and prior use of antibiotics are the recognized factors increasing the risk of VAP due to *Acinetobacter spp* [172]. The presentation of VAP due to *Acinetobacter baumannii* only sensitive to colistin is associated with previous treatment with carbapenems [173], previous episode of VAP, prior antimicrobial therapy for >10 days [174,175]. Treatment needs to clearly differentiate infection from colonization, and the agents with the most antimicrobial activity are imipenem/cilastatin, amikacin, colistin, ampicillin/sulbactam and tigecycline.

The treatment with imipenen is considerated the treatment of choice in carbapenems-susceptible strains. However a experimental study about the useful of combination treatment with amikacina showed that the combination of imipenem plus amikacin was inferior to imipenem alone with the imipenem-susceptible strain, despite their in-vitro synergy, and was inferior to amikacin alone with the imipenem-resistant strain. Combined use of imipenem with amikacin was less efficacious than monotherapy, probably because of a drug-drug interaction that resulted in decreased pharmacokinetic and pharmacodynamic parameters for both antimicrobial agents[176].Further studies assessed prospectively or retrospectively treatment with colistin for patients with ventilator-associated pneumonia caused by *A baumannii* [101,106,107]. Specifically, no difference in clinical response was reported between patients treated with intravenous colistin for infections caused by organisms susceptible only to polymyxins and those treated with other agents, mainly carbapenems, for infections caused by carbapenem-susceptible organisms.

Colistin may also be administered by inhalation. The dose of aerosolized colistin may range between 500,000 UI every 12 hours and 2,000,000 IU every 8 hours. Several studies have reported favourable clinical outcomes with the use of aerosolised colistin along with intravenous colistin or other parenteral antimicrobial agents for nosocomial pneumonia caused by multidrug-resistant *A baumannii* [102,177]. In recent study about sixty critically ill patients that received aerosolized colistin (2,000,000 million international units) during 16 days in concomitant intravenous treatment with colistin or other antimicrobial agents the bacteriological and clinical response of VAP was observed in 83.3% patients. No adverse effects related to inhaled colistin were recorded. Aerosolized colistin may be considered as adjunctive to intravenous treatment in patients with VAP due to MDR Gram-negative bacteria susceptible to colistin in critically ill patients [178].

Reports of patients with polymyxin-only susceptible gram-negative nosocomial pneumonia treated with inhaled, but without concurrent intravenous treatment are rare. Notably, in some of the few relevant cases reported in the literature, administration of nebulised colistin as the sole microbiologically active treatment against *A baumannii* nosocomial pneumonia has shown clinical effectiveness nearly to 60% [179-180].

The efficacy and safety of ampicillin-sulbactam for MDR *Acinetobacter baumannii* VAP has been evaluated in a few reports with clinical improvement of 67%. [181] and high-dose ampicillin/sulbactam were comparably safe and effective treatments respect to colistin for critically ill patients with MDR *A. baumannii* VAP [182].

The role of tigecycline alone or in combination with other antimicrobials for treatment of ventilator-associated pneumonia (VAP) had showed best clinical response (84%) in a little retrospective case series. However four patients had clinical failure: three with VAP and one with VAP plus bacteremia that developed resistance to tigecycline during therapy and three patients with VAP had a recurrence of infection Tigecycline may be effective when used alone or in combination with other antimicrobials for VAP caused by multidrug-resistant A. *baumannii*. However the emergence of a resistant strain while one patient was receiving therapy is concerning [126].

A very important item on hospital associated pneumonia is the prevention. There is convincing evidence to suggest that specific interventions can be employed to prevent HAP/VAP. The evidence-based interventions focus on the prevention of aerodigestive tract colonization (avoidance of unnecessary antibiotics and stress ulcer prophylaxis, use of sucralfate for stress ulcer prophylaxis, chlorhexidine oral rinse, selective digestive decontamination, short-course parenteral prophylactic antibiotics in high-risk patients) and the prevention of aspiration of contaminated secretions (preferred oral intubation, appropriate intensive care unit staffing, avoidance of tracheal intubation with the use of mask ventilation, application of weaning protocols and optimal use of sedation to shorten the duration of mechanical ventilation, semirecumbent positioning, minimization of gastric distension, subglottic suctioning, avoidance of ventilator circuit changes/manipulation, routine drainage of ventilator circuit condensate) [183].

Bloodstream infections

Bacteremia, followed by respiratory tract and surgical wound infections, is the most significant infection caused by *A. baumannii* [184]. The known risk factors for A. *baumannii* bacteremia are previous colonization with *A. baumannii*, invasive procedures and the use of broad-spectrum antimicrobials [185,186]. In other series found risk factors are immunosupression and mechanical ventilation [187-188]. Consequently, episodes of bacteremia due to *A. baumannii* occur most frequently in critically-ill patients admitted to an intensive care unit [189]. The clinical manifestations of bacteremia by *A. baumannii* are not specific. The most common sources of bacteremia are intravascular catheters and the respiratory tract [189-191]. *A. baumannii* bacteremia is associated with a high crude mortality rate, but it is difficult to distinguish morbidity and mortality attributable to *A. baumannii* from that attributable to the common and severe co-morbidity in these patients. The risk factors associated with higher mortality are: presence of inappropriate antimicrobial treatment, age > 65 years, development of septic shock and the severity of the underlying disease [192-196].

Generally, imipenem is the most active agent against *A. baumannii.* However, the description of imipenem-resistant *A. baumannii* strains is becoming increasingly common. Among the different antimicrobial regimens prescribed, the combination of a carbapenem and ampicillin-sulbactam was associated with a better outcome than the combination of a carbapenem and amikacin, or a carbapenem alone [190,192,197,198].The imipenem resistance has a significant impact on the mortality rate among patients with *Acinetobacter* bacteraemia [199].

2. Community-Acquired Infections

Although *Acinetobacter* infections have been attracting increasing attention during recent years because they cause nosocomial infections, the available literature suggests that the pathogen can cause community-acquired infections [200]. The most frequent community-acquired *Acinetobacter baumannii* infections are pneumonia and bacteremia [201,202] and occasionally have been described meningitis, empyema or endocarditis [203,204]. These infections have high mortality (56%). Most community-acquired *Acinetobacter* infections have been reported from countries with tropical or subtropical climate [201]. Comorbidity was commonly present in all patients mainly chronic obstructive pulmonary disease, renal disease, liver cirrhosis, diabetes mellitus, heavy smoking and excess alcohol consumption [205]. The most important infection is pneumonia because have a high mortality. This is a distinct syndrome with a high incidence of bacteremia nearly 100%. It is most frequent during the wet season. Nineteen-two percent of patients had a fulminant course presenting with septic shock and respiratory failure. *A. baumannii* should be considered as a possible etiologic agent in community-acquired lobar pneumonia when (1) patients with a fulminant course present during the warmer and more humid months of the year, and (2) patients are younger alcoholics. Early antibiotherapy is required because of the fulminant clinical course, with approximatively 50% fatality rate [206].

Infection control and prevention

Several studies have indicated that colonization with multidrug-resistant gram-negative bacilli is a frequent precursor of true infection. Specific sites of colonization may be amenable to eradication strategies. Hand colonization contributes significantly to *Acinetobacter* transmission and can be controlled by proper hand washing, glove use, and use of antiseptic- or alcohol-based soaps [207].

The digestive tract has only rarely been implicated as a major site for *Acinetobacter* colonization [208,209]. If this is documented during an outbreak, selective decolonization with polymyxin B, or aminoglycosides could be attempted.

The strategies for infection control and prevention of outbreaks caused by multiresistant *A.baumanii.* need to be simultaneous and multiples to be useful. Identification of colonized and infected patients, combined with implementation of infection-control measures such as hand-hygiene and contact-isolation precautions, might help prevent transmission of this organism within medical facilities These strategies have included [210-215]:

- Institution of active surveillance of groin, axillary, and/or wound cultures for *A. baumannii* for all patients.
- Use of contact precautions for colonized or infected patients
- Increased availability and use of alcohol-based hand rubs,daily review of antibiotic susceptibility of all clinical isolates
- Select cefepime or carbapenem-resistant isolates
- Review patient records prospectively to determine geographic location, nosocomial acquisition, and presence of clinical infection
- Emphasize contact precautions to prevent transmission of isolates
- Assign a dedicated infection-control nurse to affected area or areas
- Use polymyxin B to selectively decontaminate colonized wounds
- Consider inhaled polymyxin B for pulmonary colonization or infection (to supplement parenteral therapy)
- Use surveillance techniques to monitor personnel, equipment, and environmental contamination
- Instruct housekeeping to decontaminate the inanimate environment on a regular schedule
- Close contaminated unit if necessary
- Use molecular epidemiologic techniques to determine clonality of isolates

Bibliography

[1] Joly-Guillou, ML. Clinical impact and pathogenicity of *Acinetobacter. Clin Microbiol Infect.* 2005; 11:868-73.

[2] Jain, R; Danziger, LH. Multidrug-resistant *Acinetobacter* infections: an emerging challenge to clinicians. *Ann Pharmacother* 2004; 38: 1449-59.

[3] Bergogne-Berezin, E; Towner, KJ. *Acinetobacter spp.* As nosocomial pathogens: microbiological, clinical, and epidemiological features. *Clin Microbiol Rev* 1996; 9:148-165.

[4] Levin, AS. Multiresistant *Acinetobacter* infections. A role for sulbactam combinations in overcoming an emerging worldwide problem. *Clinical and Microbiological Infection* 2002; 8: 144-153

[5] Fernandez-Viladrich, P; Corbella, X; Corral, L; Tubau, F; Mateu, A. Successful treatment of ventriculitis due to carbapenem-resistant *Acinetobacter baumannii* with intraventricular colistin sulfomethate sodium. *Clin Infect Dis* 1999; 28: 916-917.

[6] Cowan, ST. Unusual infections following cerebral operations: with a description of Diplococcus mucosus (von Lingelsheim). *Lancet* 1938; 2:1052.

[7] Brisou, J; Prevot, AR. *Studies on bacterial taxonomy.* X. The revision of species under Acromobacter group. Ann Inst Pasteur (Paris) 1954; 86:722.

[8] Ingran, M; Shewan, JW. Introductory reflections on the *Pseudomonas-Acinetobacter* group. *J Appl Bacteriol* 1960; 23: 373-378.

[9] Juni, E. Genetics and physiology of *Acinetobacter. Annu Rev Microbiol* 1978; 32:349

[10] Dijkshoorn, L; van der, Toorn J. *Acinetobacter* species: which do we mean?. *Clin Infect Dis* 1992; 15:748.

[11] Seifert, H; Baginski, R; Schulze, A; Pulverer, G. The distribution of *Acinetobacter* species in clinical culture materials. *Zentralbl Bakteriol* 1993; 279:544.

[12] Urban, C; Segal-Maurer, S; Rahal, JJ. Considerations in control and treatment of nosocomial infections due to multidrug-resistant *Acinetobacter baumannii. Clin Infect Dis* 2003; 36:1268-74.

[13] Muñoz-Price, SL; Weinstein, RA. *Acinetobacter* Infection. *N Engl J Med* 2008; 358:1271-81.

[14] Allen, DM; Hartman, BJ. *Acinetobacter* species. In Mandell, Douglas and Bennett's.Principles and Practice of Infectious Diseases.5th Edition.

[15] Cordes, LG; Brink, EW; Checo, PJ; et al. A cluster of *Acinetobacter* pneumonia in foundry workers. *Ann Intern Med* 1981;95:688-693

[16] Allen, KD; Green, HT. Hospital outbreak of multi-resistant *Acinetobacter anitratus:* An airborne mode of spread? *J Hosp Infect* 1987; 9:110-119.

[17] Bernards, AT; Harinck, HI; Dijkshoorn, L; van der Reijden, TJ; van den Broek, PJ. Persistent *Acinetobacter baumannii*? Look inside your medical equipment. *Infect Control Hosp Epidemiol*. 2004; 25:1002-4.

[18] Maragakis, LL; Cosgrove, SE; Song, X; Kim, D; Rosenbaum, P; Ciesla, N; Srinivasan, A; Ross, T; Carroll, K; Perl, TM. An outbreak of multidrug-resistant *Acinetobacter baumannii* associated with pulsatile lavage wound treatment. *JAMA*. 2004; 292:3006-11.

[19] Das, I; Lambert, P; Hill, D; Noy, M; Bion, J; Elliott, T. Carbapenem-resistant *Acinetobacter* and role of curtains in an outbreak in intensive care units. *J Hosp Infect.* 2002; 50:110-4.

[20] Wilks, M; Wilson, A; Warwick, S; et al. Control of an outbreak of multidrug-resistant *Acinetobacter baumannii-calcoaceticus* colonization and infection in an intensive care unit (ICU) without closing the ICU or placing patients in isolation. *Infect Control Hosp Epidemiol* 2006; 27:654-658.

[21] Dijkshoorn, L; van Aken, E; Shunburne, L; van der Reijden, TJ; Bernards, AT; Nemec, A; Towner, KJ. Prevalence of *Acinetobacter baumannii* and other *Acinetobacter* spp. in faecal samples from non-hospitalised individuals. *Clin Microbiol Infect.* 2005; 11:329-32.

[22] Larson, EL. Persistent carriage of gram-negative bacteria on hands. *Am J Infect Control* 1981; 9:112-119.

[23] Corbella, X; Pujol, M; Ayats, J; et al. Relevance of digestive tract colonization in the epidemiology of nosocomial infections due to multiresistant *Acinetobacter baumannii. Clin Infect Dis* 1996; 23: 329–334.

[24] Furuno, JP; Hebden, JN; Standiford, HC; Perencevich, EN; Miller, RR; Moore, AC; Strauss, SM; Harris, AD. Prevalence of methicillin-resistant *Staphylococcus aureus* and *Acinetobacter baumannii* in a long-term acute care facility. *Am J Infect Control.* 2008; 36:468-71.

[25] Apisarnthanarak, A; Pinitchai, U; Thongphubeth, K; Yuekyen, C; Warren, DK; Fraser, VJ; Thammasat University Pandrug-Resistant *Acinetobacter baumannii* Control Group. A multifaceted intervention to reduce pandrug-resistant *Acinetobacter baumannii* colonization and infection in 3 intensive care units in a Thai tertiary care center: a 3-year study. *Clin Infect Dis.* 2008; 47:760-7.

[26] Stephens, C; Francis, SJ; Abell, V; DiPersio, JR; Wells, P. Emergence of resistant *Acinetobacter baumannii* in critically ill patients within an acute care teaching hospital and a long-term acute care hospital. *Am J Infect Control.* 2007; 35:212-5.

[27] Siegel, JD; Rhinehart, E; Jackson, M; Chiarello, L; Health Care Infection Control Practices Advisory Committee. 2007 Guideline for Isolation Precautions: Preventing Transmission of Infectious Agents in Health Care Settings. *Am J Infect Control.* 2007; 35 (10 Suppl 2):S65-164.

[28] Maragakis, LL; Perl, TM. *Acinetobacter baumannii*: Epidemiology, antimicrobial resistance, and treatment options. *Clin Infect Dis* 2008; 46:1254-63.

[29] Lee, SO; Kim, NJ; Choi, SH; Hyong Kim, T; Chung, JW; Woo, JH; Ryu, J; Kim, YS. Risk factors for acquisition of imipenem-resistant *Acinetobacter baumannii*: a case-control study. *Antimicrob Agents Chemother.* 2004; 48:224-8.

[30] Kim, YA; Choi, JY; Kim, CK; Kim, CO; Kim, MS; Choi, SH; Chin, BS; Han, SH; Lee, HS; Choi, HK; Jeoung, SJ; Song, YG; Yum, JH; Yong, D; Lee, K; Kim, JM. Risk factors and outcomes of bloodstream infections with metallo-beta-lactamase-producing *Acinetobacter. Scand J Infect Dis.* 2008; 40:234-40.

[31] Sebeny, PJ; Riddle, MS; Petersen, K. *Acinetobacter baumannii* skin and soft-tissue infection associated with war trauma. *Clin Infect Dis.* 2008; 47:444-9.

[32] Yun, HC; Branstetter, JG; Murray, CK. Osteomyelitis in military personnel wounded in Iraq and Afghanistan. *J Trauma.* 2008;64(2 Suppl):S163-8

[33] Calhoun, JH; Murray, CK; Manring, MM. Multidrug-resistant organisms in military wounds from Iraq and Afghanistan. *Clin Orthop Relat Res.* 2008; 466:1356-62.

[34] Stuart, TL; Mulvey, M; Simor, AE; Tien, HC; Battad, A; Taylor, G; Vayalumkal, JV; Weir, C; Ofner, M; Gravel, D; Paton, S. *Acinetobacter baumannii* in casualties returning from Afghanistan. *Can J Infect Control* 2007; 22:152-4.

[35] Griffith, ME; Lazarus, DR; Mann, PB; Boger, JA; Hospenthal, DR; Murray, CK. *Acinetobacter* skin carriage among US army soldiers deployed in Iraq. *Infect Control Hosp Epidemiol.* 2007; 28:720-2.

[36] Turton, JF; Kaufmann, ME; Gill, MJ; Pike, R; Scott, PT; Fishbain, J; Craft, D; Deye, G; Riddell, S; Lindler, LE; Pitt, TL. Comparison of *Acinetobacter baumannii* isolates from the United Kingdom and the United States that were associated with repatriated casualties of the Iraq conflict. *J Clin Microbiol.* 2006; 44:2630-4.

[37] Griffith, ME; Ceremuga, JM; Ellis, MW; Guymon, CH; Hospenthal, DR; Murray, CK. *Acinetobacter skin colonization of US Army Soldiers.Infect Control Hosp Epidemiol.* 2006; 27:659-61.

[38] Centers for Disease Control and Prevention (CDC). *Acinetobacter baumannii* infections among patients at military medical facilities treating injured U.S. service members, 2002-2004. *MMWR Morb Mortal Wkly Rep.* 2004; 53:1063-6.

[39] Griffith, ME; Gonzalez, RS; Holcomb, JB; Hospenthal, DR; Wortmann, GW; Murray, CK. Factors associated with recovery of *Acinetobacter baumannii* in a combat support hospital. *Infect Control Hosp Epidemiol.* 2008; 29:664-6.

[40] Whitman, TJ; Qasba, SS; Timpone, JG; Babel, BS; Kasper, MR; English, JF; Sanders, JW; Hujer, KM; Hujer, AM; Endimiani, A; Eshoo, MW; Bonomo, RA. Occupational transmission of *Acinetobacter baumannii* from a United States serviceman wounded in Iraq to a health care worker. *Clin Infect Dis.* 2008; 47:439-43.

[41] Wortmann, G; Weintrob, A; Barber, M; Scott, P; Zoll, ST; Eshoo, MW; Sampath, R; Ecker, DJ; Massire, C. Genotypic evolution of *Acinetobacter baumannii* strains in an outbreak associated with war trauma. *Infect Control Hosp Epidemiol* 2008; 29:553-5.

[42] Whitman, TJ. Infection control challenges related to war wound infections in the ICU setting. *J Trauma.* 2007; 62 (6 Suppl):S53.

[43] Falagas, ME; Koletsi, PK; Bliziotis, IA. The diversity of definitions of multidrug-resistant (MDR) and pandrug-resistant (PDR) *Acinetobacter baumannii* and *Pseudomonas aeruginosa. J Med Microbiol* 2006; 55:1619-29

[44] Bonomo, RA; Szabo, D. Mechanisms of multidrug resistance in *Acinetobacter* species and Pseudomonas aeruginosa. *Clin Infect Dis* 2006; 43: Suppl 2:S49-S56.

[45] Gilad, J; Carmeli, Y. Treatment Options for Multidrug-Resistant *Acinetobacter* species. *Drugs* 2008; 68: 165-189

[46] Van Looveren, M; Goossens, H; ARPAC Steering Group. Antimicrobial resistance of *Acinetobacter spp.* in Europe. *Clin Microbiol Infect.* 2004; 10:684-704.

[47] Perez, F; Hujer, AM; Hujer, KM; Decker, BK; Rather, PN; Bonomo, RA. Global challenge of multidrug-resistant *Acinetobacter baumannii. Antimicrob Agents Chemother.* 2007; 51:3471-84.

[48] Poirel, L; Nordmann, P.Carbapenem resistance in *Acinetobacter baumannii*; mechanisms and epidemiology. *Clin Microbiol Infect* 2006; 12:826-836

[49] Vila, J; Marcos, A; Marco, F; et al. In vitro antimicrobial production of ß-lactamases, aminoglycoside-modifying enzymes, and chloramphenicol acetyltransferase by and

susceptibility of clinical isolates of *Acinetobacter baumannii. Antimicrob Agents Chemother* 1993; 37: 138–41.

[50] Bou, G; Cervero, G; Dominguez, MA; Quereda, C; Martinez-Beltran, J. Characterization of a nosocomial outbreak caused by a multiresistant *Acinetobacter baumannii* strain with a carbapenem-hydrolyzing enzyme: high-level carbapenem resistance in *A. baumannii* is not due solely to the presence of b-lactamases. *J Clin Microbiol* 2000; 38:3299–305.

[51] Huang, ZM; Mao, PH; Chen, Y; Wu, L; Wu, J. Study on the molecular epidemiology of SHV type ß-lactamase-encoding genes of multiple drug-resistant *Acinetobacter baumannii*. Zhonghua Liu Xing Bing Xue Za Zhi 2004; 25:425–7.

[52] Vahaboglu, H; Ozturk, R; Aygun, G; et al. Widespread detection of PER-1-type extended-spectrum ß-lactamases among nosocomial *Acinetobacter* and *Pseudomonas aeruginosa* isolates in Turkey: a nationwide multicenter study. *Antimicrob Agents Chemother* 1997; 41:2265–9.

[53] Yong, D; Shin, JH; Kim, S; et al. High prevalence of PER-1 extended spectrum ß-lactamase-producing *Acinetobacter spp.* in Korea. *Antimicrob Agents Chemother* 2003; 47:1749–51.

[54] Poirel, L; Karim, A; Mercat, A; et al. Extended-spectrum ß-lactamase producing strain of *Acinetobacter baumannii* isolated from a patient in France. *J Antimicrob Chemother* 1999; 43:157–8.

[55] Poirel, L; Menuteau, O; Agoli, N; Cattoen, C; Nordmann, P. Outbreak of extended-spectrum ß-lactamase VEB-1-producing isolates of *Acinetobacter baumannii* in a French hospital. *J Clin Microbiol* 2003; 41:3542–7.

[56] Carbonne, A; Naas, T; Blanckaert, K; et al. Investigation of a nosocomial outbreak of extended-spectrum ß-lactamase VEB-1-producing isolates of *Acinetobacter baumannii* in a hospital setting. *J Hosp Infect* 2005; 60:14–8.

[57] Poirel, L; Nordmann, P. Carbapenem resistance in *Acinetobacter baumannii*: mechanisms and epidemiology. *Clin Microbiol Infect* 2006; 12:826-36.

[58] Walsh, TR. The emergence and implications of metallo-beta-lactamases in Gram-negative bacteria. *Clin. Microbiol. Infect* 2005; 11(Suppl. 6):2–9.

[59] Walsh, TR; MA. Toleman, L. Poirel, and P. Nordmann. Metallo-ß- lactamases: the quiet before the storm? *Clin. Microbiol. Rev.* 2005; 18:306–325.

[60] Walther-Rasmussen, JN. Hoiby. OXA-type carbapenemases. *J. Antimicrob Chemother.* 2006; 57:373–383.

[61] Coelho, J; Woodford, N; Afzal-Shah, M; et al. Occurrence of OXA-58-like carbapenemases in *Acinetobacter* spp. Collected over 10 years in three continents. *Antimicrob Agents Chemother* 2006; 50: 756-8

[62] Heritier, C; Poirel, L; Lambert, T; et al. Contribution of acquired -hydrolyzing oxacillinases to carbapenem resistance in *Acinetobacter baumannii. Antimicrob Agents Chemother* 2005 Aug; 49 (8): 3198-202

[63] Bou, G; Cervero, G; Dominguez, MA; et al. Characterization of a nosocomial outbreak caused by a multiresistant *Acinetobacter baumannii* strain with a carbapenem-hydrolyzing enzyme: high-level carbapenem resistance in *A. baumannii* is not due solely to the presence of beta-lactamases. *J Clin Microbiol* 2000; 38: 3299-305

[64] Fernandez-Cuenca, F; Martinez-Martinez, L; Conejo, MC; et al. Relationship between beta-lactamase production, outer membrane protein and penicillin-binding protein profiles on the activity of carbapenems against clinical isolates of *Acinetobacter baumannii*. *J Antimicrob Chemother* 2003; 51: 565-74

[65] Peleg, AY; Adams, J; Paterson, DL. Tigecycline efflux as a mechanism for nonsusceptibility in *Acinetobacter baumannii*. *Antimicrob Agents Chemother* 2007; 51: 2065-9.

[66] Seward, RJ; Lambert, T; Towner, KJ. Molecular epidemiology of aminoglycoside resistance in *Acinetobacter spp*. *J Med Microbiol* 1998; 47:455–62.

[67] Nemec, A; Dolzani, L; Brisse, S; van den Broek, P; Dijkshoorn, L. Diversity of aminoglycoside-resistance genes and their association with class 1 integrons among strains of pan-European *Acinetobacter baumannii* clones. *J Med Microbiol* 2004; 53:1233–40.

[68] Vila, J; Ruiz, J; Goni, P; Marcos, A; Jimenez de Anta, T. Mutation in the *gyrA* gene of quinolone-resistant clinical isolates of *Acinetobacter baumannii*. *Antimicrob Agents Chemother* 1995; 39:1201–3.

[69] Vila, J; Ruiz, J; Goni, P; Jimenez de Anta, T. Quinolone-resistance mutations in the topoisomerase IV *parC* gene of *Acinetobacter baumannii*. *J Antimicrob Chemother* 1997; 39:757–62.

[70] Karageorgopoulos, DE; Kelesidis, T; Kelesidis, I; Falagas, ME. Tigecycline for the treatment of multidrug-resistant (including carbapenem-resistant) *Acinetobacter* infections: a review of the scientific evidence. *J Antimicrob Chemother*. 2008; 62:45-55.

[71] Reid, GE; Grim, SA; Aldeza, CA; Janda, WN; Clark, NM. Rapid development of *Acinetobacter baumannii* resistance to tigecycline. *Pharmacotherapy* 2007; 27:1198-1201.

[72] Bosó-Ribelles, V; Romá-Sánchez, E; Carmena, J; Cáceres, C; Bautista, D. Tigecycline: a new treatment choice against *Acinetobacter baumannii.Recent Patents Anti-Infect Drug Disc*. 2008; 3:117-22.

[73] Gallagher, JC; Rouse, HM. Tigecycline for the treatment of *Acinetobacter* infections: a case series. *Ann Pharmacother* 2008; 42:1188-94.

[74] Gilad, J; Eskira, S; Riesenberg, K; Schlaeff er, F; Hyam, E; Borer, A. Emergence of nosocomial colistin-resistant *Acinetobacter baumannii*. *45th Interscience Conference on Antimicrobial Agents and Chemotherapy;* Washington, DC, USA; Dec 16–19, 2005.

[75] Goel, VK; Kapil, A. Monoclonal antibodies against the iron regulated outer membrane proteins of *Acinetobacter baumannii* are bactericidal. *BMC Microbiol* 2001; 1: 16–24.

[76] Bergogne-Bérézin, E; Joly-Guillou, ML; Towner, KJ. *Acinetobacter*: Microbiology, Epidemiology, *Infections, Management*. Editors CRC Press, 1996.

[77] Obana, Y. Pathogenic significance of *Acinetobacter calcoaceticus*: analysis of experimental infection in mice. *Microbiol. Immunol* 1986; 30:645–657.

[78] Leone, S; Sturiale, L; Pessione, E; Mazzoli, R; Giunta, C; Lanzetta, R; Garozzo, D; Molinaro, A; Parrilli, M. Detailed characterization of the lipid A fraction from the nonpathogen *Acinetobacter radioresistens* strain S13. *Journal of Lipid Research* 2007; 48: 1045-1051.

[79] Karageorgopoulos, DE; Falagas, ME. Current control and treatment of multidrug-resistant *Acinetobacter baumannii* infections. *Lancet Infect Dis* 2008; 8:751–762.

[80] Dijkshoorn, L; Nemec, A; Seifert, H. An increasing threat in hospitals: multidrug-resistant *Acinetobacter baumannii.Nat Rev Microbiol* 2007; 5: 939–51.

[81] Van Looveren, M; Goossens, H. Antimicrobial resistance of *Acinetobacter spp* in *Europe. Clin Microbiol Infect* 2004; 10: 684–704.

[82] Reinert, RR; Low, DE; Rossi, F; Zhang, X; Wattal, C; Dowzicky, MJ. Antimicrobial susceptibility among organisms from the Asia/ Pacific Rim, Europe and Latin and North America collected as part of TEST and the in vitro activity of tigecycline. *J Antimicrob Chemother* 2007; 60: 1018–29.

[83] Poulakou, G; Giamarellou, H. Doripenem: an expected arrival in the treatment of infections caused by multidrug-resistant Gram-negative pathogens. *Expert Opin Investig Drugs.* 2008; 17:749-71.

[84] Rice, LB. Challenges in identifying new antimicrobial agents effective for treating infections with *Acinetobacter baumannii* and *Pseudomonas aeruginosa. Clin Infect Dis* 2006; 43 Suppl 2:S100-5.

[85] Horiuchi, M; Kimura, M; Tokumura, M; Hasebe, N; Arai, T; Abe, K. Absence of convulsive liability of doripenem, a new carbapenem antibiotic, in comparison with beta-lactam antibiotics. *Toxicology* 2006;222:114-24

[86] Jones, RN; Sader, HS; Fritsche, TR. Comparative activity of doripenem and three other carbapenems tested against Gram-negative bacilli with various beta-lactamase resistance mechanisms. *Diagn Microbiol Infect Dis.* 2005;52:71-*4*

[87] Pillar, CM; Torres, MK; Brown, NP; Shah, D; Sahm, DF.In vitro activity of doripenem, a carbapenem for the treatment of challenging infections caused by gram-negative bacteria, against recent clinical isolates from the United States. *Antimicrob Agents Chemother.* 2008; 52:4388-99.

[88] Jones, RN; Huynh, HK; Biedenbach, DJ. Activities of doripenem (S-4661) against drug-resistant clinical pathogens. *Antimicrob Agents Chemother*. 2004; 48:3136-40.

[89] Zhanel, GG; Wiebe, R; Dilay, L; Thomson, K; Rubinstein, E; Hoban, DJ; Noreddin, AM; Karlowsky, JA. Comparative review of the carbapenems. *Drugs* 2007; 67:1027-52.

[90] Falagas, ME; Kasiakou, SK. Colistin: the revival of polymyxins for the management of multidrug-resistant Gram-negative bacterial infections. *Clin Infect Dis* 2005; 40: 1333–41.

[91] Giamarellou, H. Treatment options for multidrug-resistant bacteria. *Expert rev Anti Infect Ther* 2006;4: 601-18

[92] Gales, AC; Jones, RN; Sader, HS. Global assessment of the antimicrobial activity of polymyxin B against 54,731 clinical isolates of Gram-negative bacilli: report from the SENTRY antimicrobial surveillance programme (2001–2004). *Clin Microbiol Infect* 2006; 12: 315–21.

[93] Henwood, CJ; Gatward, T; Warner, M; et al. Antibiotic resistance among clinical isolates of *Acinetobacter* in the UK, and in vitro evaluation of tigecycline (GAR-936). *J Antimicrob Chemother* 2002; 49: 479–87.

[94] Song, JY; Kee, SY; Hwang, IS; et al. In vitro activities of carbapenem/sulbactam combination, colistin, colistin/rifampicin combination and tigecycline against carbapenem-resistant *Acinetobacter baumannii. J Antimicrob Chemother* 2007; 60: 317–22.

[95] Scheetz, MH; Qi, C; Warren, JR; et al. In vitro activities of various antimicrobials alone and in combination with tigecycline against carbapenem-intermediate or -resistant *Acinetobacter baumannii. Antimicrob Agents Chemother* 2007; 51: 1621–26.

[96] Falagas, ME; Kasiakou, SK. Colistin: the revival of polymyxins for the management of multidrug-resistant gram-negative bacterial infections. *Clin Infect Dis* 2005; 40: 1333–41.

[97] Li, J; Nation, RL; Turnidge, JD; et al. Colistin: the re-emerging antibiotic for multidrug-resistant Gram-negative bacterial infections. *Lancet Infect Dis* 2006; 6: 589–601.

[98] Falagas, ME; Kasiakou, SK; Tsiodras, S; et al. The use of intravenous and aerosolized polymyxins for the treatment of infections in critically ill patients: a review of the recent literature. *Clin Med Res 2*006; 4: 138–46.

[99] Li, J; Nation, RL; Milne, RW; et al. Evaluation of colistin as an agent against multi-resistant Gram-negative bacteria. *Int J Antimicrob Agents* 2005; 25: 11–25.

[100] Michalopoulos, A; Kasiakou, SK; Rosmarakis, ES; Falagas, ME. Cure of multidrug-resistant *Acinetobacter baumannii* bacteraemia with continuous intravenous infusion of colistin. *Scand J Infect Dis*. 2005; 37:142-5.

[101] Kallel, H; Hergafi, L; Bahloul, M; et al. Safety and efficacy of colistin compared with imipenem in the treatment of ventilator-associated pneumonia: a matched case-control study. *Intensive Care Med* 2007; 33:1162–67.

[102] Falagas, ME; Kasiakou, SK; Kofteridis, DP; Roditakis, G; Samonis, G. Effectiveness and nephrotoxicity of intravenous colistin for treatment of patients with infections due to polymyxin-onlysusceptible (POS) Gram-negative bacteria. *Eur J Clin Microbiol Infect Dis* 2006; 25: 596–99.

[103] Michalopoulos, A; Kasiakou, SK; Mastora, Z; Rellos, K; Kapaskelis, AM; Falagas, ME. Aerosolized colistin for the treatment of nosocomial pneumonia due to multidrug-resistant Gram-negative bacteria in patients without cystic fibrosis. *Crit Care* 2005; 9: R53–59.

[104] Rodríguez Guardado, A; Blanco, A; Asensi, V; et al. Multidrugresistant *Acinetobacter* meningitis in neurosurgical patients with intraventricular catheters: assessment of different treatments. *J Antimicrob Chemother* 2008; 61: 908–13.

[105] Falagas, ME; Rizos, M; Bliziotis, IA; Rellos, K; Kasiakou, SK; Michalopoulos, A. Toxicity after prolonged (more than four weeks) administration of intravenous colistin. *BMC Infect Dis*.2005; 5:1.

[106] Garnacho-Montero, J; Ortiz-Leyba, C; Jimenez-Jimenez, FJ; et al. Treatment of multidrug-resistant *Acinetobacter baumannii* ventilator associated pneumonia (VAP) with intravenous colistin: a comparison with imipenem-susceptible VAP. *Clin Infect Dis* 2003; 36: 1111–18.

[107] Reina, R; Estenssoro, E; Saenz, G; et al. Safety and efficacy of colistin in *Acinetobacter* and Pseudomonas infections: a prospective cohort study. *Intensive Care Med* 2005; 31: 1058–65.

[108] Falagas, ME; Kasiakou, SK. Toxicity of polymyxins: a systematic review of the evidence from old and recent studies. *Crit Care* 2006; 10: R27.

[109] Falagas, ME; Fragoulis, KN; Kasiakou, SK; Sermaidis, GJ; Michalopoulos, A. Nephrotoxicity of intravenous colistin: a prospective evaluation. *Int J Antimicrob Agents* 2005; 26: 504–07.

[110] Ng, J; Gosbell, IB; Kelly, JA; Boyle, MJ; Ferguson, JK. Cure of multiresistant *Acinetobacter baumannii* central nervous system infections with intraventricular or intrathecal colistin: case series and literature review. *J Antimicrob Chemother* 2006; 58: 1078–81.

[111] Evagelopoulou, P; Katsaros, A; Myrianthefs, P; et al. Colistin and rhabdomyolysis: a causative agent or an innocent bystander? *Intensive Care Med* 2007; 33: 556–7.

[112] Matthaiou, DK; Michalopoulos, A; Rafailidis, PI; Karageorgopoulos, DE; Papaioannou, V; Ntani, G; Samonis, G, Falagas, ME. Risk factors associated with the isolation of colistin-resistant gram-negative bacteria: a matched case-control study. *Crit Care Med.* 2008; 36:807-11.

[113] Rafailidis, PI; Ioannidou, EN; Falagas, ME. Ampicillin/sulbactam: current status in severe bacterial infections. *Drugs* 2007; 67: 1829–49.

[114] Ko, WC; Lee, HC; Chiang, SR; et al. In vitro and in vivo activity of meropenem and sulbactam against a multidrug-resistant *Acinetobacter baumannii* strain. *J Antimicrob Chemother* 2004; 53: 393–95.

[115] Corbella, X; Ariza, J; Ardanuy, C; et al. Efficacy of sulbactam alone and in combination with ampicillin in nosocomial infections caused by multiresistant *Acinetobacter baumannii. J Antimicrob Chemother* 1998; 42: 793–802.

[116] Wood, GC; Hanes, SD; Croce, MA; Fabian, TC; Boucher, BA. Comparison of ampicillin-sulbactam and imipenem-cilastatin for the treatment of *Acinetobacter* ventilator-associated pneumonia. *Clin Infect Dis* 2002; 34: 1425–30.

[117] Levin, AS; Levy, CE; Manrique, AE; Medeiros, EA; Costa, SF. Severe nosocomial infections with imipenem-resistant *Acinetobacter baumannii* treated with ampicillin/sulbactam. *Int J Antimicrob Agents* 2003; 21: 58–62.

[118] Betrosian, AP; Frantzeskaki, F; Xanthaki, A; Georgiadis, G. High-dose ampicillin-sulbactam as an alternative treatment of late-onset VAP from multidrug-resistant *Acinetobacter baumannii. Scand J Infect Dis* 2007; 39: 38–43.

[119] Jimenez-Mejias, ME; Pachon, J; Becerril, B; Palomino-Nicas, J; Rodriguez-Corbacho, A; Revuelta, M. Treatment of multidrug-resistant *Acinetobacter baumannii* meningitis with ampicillin/sulbactam. *Clin Infect Dis* 1997; 24: 932–35.

[120] Oliveira, MS; Prado, GV; Costa, SF; Grinbaum, RS; Levin, AS. Ampicillin/sulbactam compared with polymyxins for the treatment of infections caused by carbapenem-resistant *Acinetobacter spp. J Antimicrob Chemother.* 2008; 61:1369-75.

[121] Fraise, AP. Tigecycline: the answer to beta-lactam and fluorquinolone resistance? *J Infect* 2006; 53: 293-300;

[122] Nathwani, D. Tigecycline: clinical evidence and formulary positioning. *Int J Antimicrobial Agents* 2005; 25: 185-92.

[123] Rice, LB. Challenges in identifying new antimicrobial agents effective for treating infections with *Acinetobacter baumannii* and *Pseudomonas aeruginosa. Clin Infect Dis.*2006; 43 Suppl 2:S100-5.

[124] Seifert, H; Stefanik, D; Wisplinghoff, H. Comparative in vitro activities of tygecycline and 11 other antimicrobial agents against 215 epidemiologically defined multidrug – resistant *Acinetobacter baumannii* isolates. *J Antimicrob Chemother* 2006; 58: 1099-100.

[125] Peleg, AY; Adams, J; Paterson, DL. Tigecycline efflux as a mechanism for nonsusceptibility in *Acinetobacter baumannii. Antimicrob Agents Chemother* 2007; 51: 2065–69.

[126] Schafer, JJ; Goff, DA; Stevenson, KB; Mangino, JE. Early experience with tigecycline for ventilator-associated pneumonia and bacteremia caused by multidrug-resistant *Acinetobacter baumannii. Pharmacotherapy* 2007; 27: 980–87.

[127] Karageorgopoulos, DE; Kelesidis, T; Kelesidis, I; Falagas, ME. Tigecycline for the treatment of multidrug-resistant (including carbapenem-resistant) *Acinetobacter* infections: a review of the scientific evidence. *J Antimicrob Chemother* 2008; 62: 45–55.

[128] Anthony, KB; Fishman, NO; Linkin, DR; Gasink, LB; Edelstein, PH; Lautenbach, E. Clinical and microbiological outcomes of serious infections with multidrug-resistant Gram-negative organisms treated with tigecycline. *Clin Infect Dis* 2008; 46: 567–70.

[129] Gallagher, JC; Rouse, HM. Tigecycline for the treatment of *Acinetobacter* infections: a case series. *Ann Pharmacother.*2008; 42:1188-94.

[130] Reid, GE; Grim, SA; Aldeza, CA; Janda, WM; Clark, NM.. Rapid development of *Acinetobacter baumannii* resistance to tigecycline. *Pharmacotherapy.*2007; 27:1198-201.

[131] Halstead, DC; Abid, J; Dowzicky, MJ. Antimicrobial susceptibility among *Acinetobacter calcoaceticus-baumannii* complex and Enterobacteriaceae collected as part of the Tigecycline Evaluation and Surveillance Trial. *J Infect* 2007; 55: 49–57

[132] Kuo, LC; Lai, CC; Liao, CH; et al. Multidrug-resistant *Acinetobacter baumannii* bacteraemia: clinical features, antimicrobial therapy and outcome. *Clin Microbiol Infect* 2007; 13: 196–98

[133] Sahm, DF; Critchley, IA; Kelly, LJ; et al. Evaluation of current activities of fluorquinolones against gram-negative bacilli using centralized in vitro testing and electronic surveillance. *Antimicrob Agents Chemother* 2001; 45:267-74.

[134] Joly-Guillou, ML; Wolff, M; Farinotti, R; Bryskier, A; Carbon, C. In vivo activity of levofl oxacin alone or in combination with imipenem or amikacin in a mouse model of *Acinetobacter baumannii* pneumonia. *J Antimicrob Chemother* 2000; 46: 827–30.

[135] Rahal, JJ. Novel antibiotic combinations against infections with almost completely resistant *Pseudomonas aeruginosa* and *Acinetobacter species. Clin Infect Dis.* 2006; 43 Suppl 2:S95-9.

[136] Song, JY; Cheong, HJ; Lee, J; Sung, AK; Kim, WJ. Efficacy of monotherapy and combined antibiotic therapy for carbapenem-resistant *Acinetobacter baumannii*

pneumonia in an immunosuppressed mouse model. *Int J Antimicrob Agents*. 2009; 33:33-9.

[137] Montero, A; Ariza, J; Corbella, X; Doménech, A; Cabellos, C; Ayats, J; Tubau, F; Borraz, C; Gudiol, F. Antibiotic combinations for serious infections caused by carbapenem-resistant *Acinetobacter baumannii* in a mouse pneumonia model. *J Antimicrob Chemother*. 2004; 54:1085-91.

[138] Song, JY; Lee, J; Heo, JY; Noh, JY; Kim, WJ; Cheong, HJ; Hwang, IS. Colistin and rifampicin combination in the treatment of ventilator-associated pneumonia caused by carbapenem-resistant *Acinetobacter baumannii*. *Int J Antimicrob Agents*. 2008; 32:281-4.

[139] Bassetti, M; Repetto, E; Righi, E; Boni, S; Diverio, M; Molinari, MP; Mussap, M; Artioli, S; Ansaldi, F; Durando, P; Orengo, G; Bobbio Pallavicini, F; Viscoli, C. Colistin and rifampicin in the treatment of multidrug-resistant *Acinetobacter baumannii* infections. *J Antimicrob Chemother*. 2008; 61:417-20.

[140] Motaouakkil, S; Charra, B; Hachimi, A; Nejmi, H; Benslama, A; Elmdaghri, N; Belabbes, H; Benbachir, M. Colistin and rifampicin in the treatment of nosocomial infections from multiresistant *Acinetobacter baumannii*. *J Infect*.2006; 53:274-8.

[141] Saballs, M; Pujol, M; Tubau, F; Peña, C; Montero, A; Domínguez, MA; Gudiol, F; Ariza, J. Rifampicin/imipenem combination in the treatment of carbapenem-resistant *Acinetobacter baumannii* infections. *J Antimicrob Chemother*.2006; 58:697-700.

[142] Lee, NY; Wang, CL; Chuang, YC; et al. Combination carbapenem-sulbactam therapy for critically ill patients with multidrug-resistant *Acinetobacter baumannii* bacteremia: four case reports and an in vitro combination synergy study. *Pharmacotherapy* 2007; 27: 1506–11.

[143] Timurkaynak, F; Can, F; Azap, OK; Demirbilek, M; Arslan, H; Karaman, SO. In vitro activities of non-traditional antimicrobials alone or in combination against multidrug-resistant strains of *Pseudomonas aeruginosa* and *Acinetobacter baumannii* isolated from intensive care units. *Int J Antimicrob Agents* 2006; 27: 224–28.

[144] Yoon, J; Urban, C; Terzian, C; Mariano, N; Rahal, JJ. In vitro double and triple synergistic activities of polymyxin B, imipenem, and rifampin against multidrug-resistant *Acinetobacter baumannii*. *Antimicrob Agents Chemother* 2004; 48: 753–57.

[145] Falagas, ME; Rafailidis, PI; Kasiakou, SK; Hatzopoulou, P; Michalopoulos, A. Eff ectiveness and nephrotoxicity of colistin monotherapy *vs* colistin-meropenem combination therapy for multidrug-resistant Gram-negative bacterial infections. *Clin Microbiol Infect* 2006; 12: 1227–30.

[146] Scheetz, MH; Qi, C; Warren, JR; et al. In vitro activities of various antimicrobials alone and in combination with tigecycline against carbapenem-intermediate or -resistant *Acinetobacter baumannii*. *Antimicrob Agents Chemother* 2007; 51: 1621–26.

[147] Lortholary, O; Fagon, J-Y; Hoi, AB; et al. Nosocomial acquisition of multi-resistant *Acinetobacter baumannii*: Risk factors and prognosis.*Clin Infect Dis* 1995; 20:790-796.

[148] Siegman-Igra, Y; Bar Yosef, S; Gorea, A; Avram, J. Nosocomial A*cinetobacter* meningitis secondary to invasive procedures: report of 25 cases and review. *Clin Infect Dis* 1993; 17:843-849.

[149] Seifert, H; Ritcher, W; Pulverer, G. Clinical and bacteriological features of relapsing shunt-associated meningitis due to *Acinetobacter baumannii. Eur J Clin Microbiol Infect Dis* 1995; 14: 130-134.

[150] Chen, HP; Lai, Ch; Chan, Y; Chen, T; Liu Ch; Fung Ch; Liu Ch. Clinical significance of *Acinetobacter* species isolated from cerebrospinal fluid. Scand *J Infect Dis* 2005; 37: 669-675.

[151] Rodríguez-Guardado, A; Maradona, JA; Asensi, V; Cartón, JA; Pérez, F; Blanco, A; Arribas, JM. Meningitis postquirúrgica por *Acinetobacter baumannii*: estudio de 22 casos y revisión de la literatura. *Rev Clin Esp* 2001; 201: 497-500.

[152] Mayhall, CG; Archer, NH; Archer Lamb, V; Spadora, AC; Baggett, JW; Ward, JD; Narayan, RK. Ventriculostomy-related infections. A prospective epidemiologic study. *N Engl J Med* 1984; 310: 553-559.

[153] Wang, KW; Chang, WN- Huang CR; Tsai, NW; Tsui, HW; wang, HC; Su, TM; Rau, CS; Cheng, BC; et al. Post-neurosurgical nosocomial bacterial meningitis in adults: microbiology, clinical features, and outcomes. *J Clin NeuroSci* 2005; 12: 647-650.

[154] Mahgoub, S; Ahmed, J; Glatt, AE. Completely resistant *Acinetobacter baumannii* strains. *Infect control Hosp Epidemiol* 2002; 23:477-79.

[155] Nguyen, MH; Harris, SP; Muder, RR; Pasculle, AW. Antibiotic- resistant *Acinetobacter* meningitis in neurosurgical patients. *Neurosurgery* 1994; 35: 851-855.

[156] Gilbert, VE; Velas, Jr JD; Natelson, SE; Tyler, WA. Treatment of cerebrospinal fluid leaks and gram-negative bacillary meningitis with large doses of intratecal amikacin and systemic antibiotics. *Neurosurgery* 1986; 18: 402-406.

[157] Jiménez-Mejías, ME; Pichardo-Guerrero, C; Marquez-Rivas, FJ; Martin-Lozano, D; Prados, T; Pachón, J. Cerebrospinal fluid penetration and pharmacokinetic /pharmacodynamic parameters of intravenously administered colistin in a case of multidrug-resistant *Acinetobacter baumannii* meningitis. *Eur J Clin Microbiol Infect Dis* 2002; 21: 212-214.

[158] Jiménez-Mejías, ME; Becerril, B; Marquez-Rivas, FJ; Pichardo, C; Cuberos, L; Pachón, J. Sucessfull treatment of multidrug- resistant *Acinetobacter baumannii* meningitis with intravenous colisitn sulfomethate sodium. *Eur J Clin Microbiol Infect Dis* 2000; 19: 970-1.

[159] Pankey, GA. Tigecycline. *J Antimicrob Chemother 2*005;56: 470-480.

[160] Noskin, GA. Tigecycline: A new glycylcycline for treatment of serious infections. *Clin Infect Dis* 2005; 41: S303-14.

[161] Falagas, ME; Bliziotis, IA; Tam, VH. Intraventricular or intrathecal use of polymyxins in patients with Gram-negative meningitis: a systematic review of the available evidence. *Int J Antimicrob Agents* 2007; 29: 9–25.

[162] Levin, AS; Barone, AA; Penco, J; et al. Intravenous colistin as therapy for nosocomial infections caused by multidrug-resistant *Pseudomonas aeruginosa* and *Acinetobacter baumannii. Clin Infect Dis* 1999; 28: 1008–11.

[163] Katragkou, A; Roilides, E. Successful treatment of multidrugresistant *Acinetobacter baumannii* central nervous system infections with colistin. *J Clin Microbiol* 2005; 43: 4916–17.

[164] Paramythiotou, E; Karakitsos, D; Aggelopoulou, H; Sioutos, P; Samonis, G; Karabinis, A. Post-surgical meningitis due to multiresistant *Acinetobacter baumannii*. Effective treatment with intravenous and/or intraventricular colistin and therapeutic dilemmas. *Med Mal Infect* 2007; 37: 124–25.
[165] Cawley, MJ; Suh, C; Lee, S; Ackerman, BH. Nontraditional dosing of ampicillin-sulbactam for multidrug-resistant *Acinetobacter baumannii* meningitis. *Pharmacotherapy* 2002; 22:527-532.
[166] Benifla, M; Zucker, G; Cohen, A; Alkan, M. Successful treatment of *Acinetobacter* meningitis with intrathecal polymixyn E. J Antimicrob Chemother 2004; 54: 290-292.
[167] Gleeson, T; Petersen, K; Mascola, J. Successful treatment of *Acinetobacter* meningitis with meropenm and rifampicin. *J Antimicrob chemother* 2005: 56: 602-603.
[168] Vasen, W; Desmery, P; Ilutovich, S; Di Martino, A. Intrathecal use of colistin. *Journal of Clinical Microbiology* 2000; 38: 3523.
[169] Karakitsos, D; Paramythiotou, E; Samonis, G; et al. Is intraventricular colistin an effective and safe treatment for post-surgical ventriculitis in the intensive care unit? *Acta Anaesthesiol Scand* 2006; 50:1309-1310.
[170] Montero, A; Corbella, X; Ariza, J. Clinical relevance of *Acinetobacter baumanni*i ventilator-associated pneumonia. *Crit Care Med* 2003; 31:2557-9.
[171] Kollef, KE; Schramm, GE; Wills, AR; Reichley, RM; Micek, ST; Kollef, MH. Predictors of 30-day mortality and hospital costs in patients with ventilator-associated pneumonia attributed to potentially antibiotic-resistant gram-negative bacteria. *Chest.* 2008; 134:281-7.
[172] Luna, CM; Aruj, PK. Nosocomial *Acinetobacter* pneumonia. *Respirology.* 2007;12:787-91.
[173] Garnacho-Montero, J; Ortiz-Leyba, C; Fernández-Hinojosa, E; Aldabó-Pallás, T, Cayuela A, Marquez-Vácaro JA, Garcia-Curiel A, Jiménez-Jiménez FJ. *Acinetobacter baumannii* ventilator-associated pneumonia: epidemiological and clinical findings. *Intensive Care Med.* 2005; 31:649-55.
[174] Medina, J; Formento, C; Pontet, J; Curbelo, A; Bazet, C; Gerez, J; Larrañaga, E. Prospective study of risk factors for ventilator-associated pneumonia caused by *Acinetobacter species*. *J Crit Care.* 2007; 22:18-26.
[175] Rios, FG; Luna, CM; Maskin, B; Saenz Valiente, A; Lloria, M; Gando, S; Sosa, C; Baquero, S; Llerena, C; Petrati, C; Apezteguia, C. Ventilator-associated pneumonia due to colistin susceptible-only microorganisms. *Eur Respir J.* 2007; 30:307-13.
[176] Bernabeu-Wittel, M; Pichardo, C; García-Curiel, A; Pachón-Ibáñez, ME; Ibáñez-Martínez, J; Jiménez-Mejías, ME; Pachón, J. Pharmacokinetic/pharmacodynamic assessment of the in-vivo efficacy of imipenem alone or in combination with amikacin for the treatment of experimental multiresistant *Acinetobacter baumannii* pneumonia. *Clin Microbiol Infect.* 2005; 11:319-25.
[177] Berlana, D; Llop, JM; Fort, E; Badia, MB; Jodar, R. Use of colistin in the treatment of multiple-drug-resistant Gram-negative infections. *Am J Health Syst Pharm* 2005; 62: 39–47.

[178] Michalopoulos, A; Fotakis, D; Virtzili, S; et al. Aerosolized colistin as adjunctive treatment of ventilator-associated pneumonia due to multidrug-resistant Gram-negative bacteria: a prospective study. *Respir Med* 2008; 102: 407–12.

[179] Kwa, AL; Loh, C; Low, JG; Kurup, A; Tam, VH. Nebulized colistin in the treatment of pneumonia due to multidrug-resistant *Acinetobacter baumannii* and *Pseudomonas aeruginosa*. *Clin Infect Dis* 2005; 41: 754–57.

[180] Michalopoulos, A; Kasiakou, SK; Mastora, Z; et al. Aerosolized colistin for the treatment of nosocomial pneumoniae due to multidrug-resistant Gram-negative bacteria in patients without cystic fibrosis. *Crit Care* 2005; 9: R53-59.

[181] Betrosian, AP; Frantzeskaki, F; Xanthaki, A; Georgiadis, G. High-dose ampicillin-sulbactam as an alternative treatment of late-onset VAP from multidrug-resistant *Acinetobacter baumannii*. *Scand J Infect Dis.*2007;39:38-43.

[182] Betrosian, AP; Frantzeskaki, F; Xanthaki, A; Douzinas, EE. Efficacy and safety of high-dose ampicillin/sulbactam vs. colistin as monotherapy for the treatment of multidrug resistant *Acinetobacter baumannii* ventilator-associated pneumonia. *J Infect.* 2008; 56:432-6.

[183] Kollef, MH. Prevention of hospital-associated pneumonia and ventilator-associated pneumonia. *Crit Care Med.* 2004; 32:1396-405.

[184] Cisneros, JM; Rodríguez-Baño, J. Nosocomial bacteremia due to *Acinetobacter baumannii*: epidemiology, clinical features and treatment. *Clin Microbiol Infect.* 2002; 8:687-93.

[185] Shih, MJ; Lee, NY; Lee, HC; Chang, CM; Wu, CJ; Chen, PL; Ko, NY; Ko, WC. Risk factors of multidrug resistance in nosocomial bacteremia due to *Acinetobacter baumannii*: a case-control study. *J Microbiol Immunol Infect.*2008; 41:118-23.

[186] Wareham, DW; Bean, DC; Khanna, P; Hennessy, EM; Krahe, D; Ely, A; Millar, M. Bloodstream infection due to *Acinetobacter spp*: epidemiology, risk factors and impact of multi-drug resistance. *Eur J Clin Microbiol Infect Dis.* 2008; 27:607-12.

[187] Wisplinghoff, H; Edmond, MB; Pfaller, MA; Jones, RN; Wenzel, RP; Seifert, H. Nosocomial bloodstream infections caused by *Acinetobacter* species in United States hospitals: clinical features, molecular epidemiology, and antimicrobial susceptibility. *Clin Infect Dis.*2000; 31:690-7.

[188] García-Garmendia, JL; Ortiz-Leyba, C; Garnacho-Montero, J; Jiménez-Jiménez, FJ; Pérez-Paredes, C; Barrero-Almodóvar, AE; Gili-Miner, M. Risk factors for *Acinetobacter baumannii* nosocomial bacteremia in critically ill patients: a cohort study. *Clin Infect Dis.*2001;33:939-46.

[189] Kuo, LC; Lai, CC; Liao, CH; Hsu, CK; Chang, YL; Chang, CY; Hsueh, PR. Multidrug-resistant *Acinetobacter baumannii* bacteraemia: clinical features, antimicrobial therapy and outcome. *Clin Microbiol Infect.*2007; 13:196-8.

[190] Wisplinghoff, H; Edmond, MB; Pfaller, MA; Jones, RN; Wenzel, RP; Seifert, H. Nosocomial bloodstream infections caused by *Acinetobacter species* in United States hospitals: clinical features, molecular epidemiology, and antimicrobial susceptibility. *Clin Infect Dis.*2000; 31:690-7.

[191] Tseng, YC; Wang, JT; Wu, FL; Chen, YC; Chie, WC; Chang, SC. Prognosis of adult patients with bacteremia caused by extensively resistant *Acinetobacter baumannii. Diagn Microbiol Infect Dis.* 2007; 59:181-90.

[192] Cisneros, JM; Reyes, MJ; Pachón, J; Becerril, B; Caballero, FJ; García-Garmendía, JL; Ortiz, C; Cobacho, AR. Bacteremia due to *Acinetobacter baumannii:* epidemiology, clinical findings, and prognostic features. *Clin Infect Dis.*1996; 22:1026-32.

[193] Poutanen, SM; Louie, M; Simor, AE. Risk factors, clinical features and outcome of *Acinetobacter* bacteremia in adults. *Eur J Clin Microbiol Infect Dis.*1997;16:737-40.

[194] Valero, C; García Palomo, JD; Matorras, P; Fernández-Mazarrasa, C; González Fernández, C; Fariñas, MC. *Acinetobacter* bacteraemia in a teaching hospital, 1989-1998. *Eur J Intern Med.*2001;12:425-429.

[195] Choi, JY; Park, YS; Kim, CO; Park, YS; Yoon, HJ; Shin, SY; Kim, YA; Song, YG; Yong, D; Lee, K; Kim, JM. Mortality risk factors of *Acinetobacter baumannii* bacteraemia. *Intern Med J.*2005;35:599-603.

[196] Grupper, M; Sprecher, H; Mashiach, T; Finkelstein, R. Attributable mortality of nosocomial *Acinetobacter* bacteremia. *Infect Control Hosp Epidemiol.*2007;28:293-8.

[197] Kuo, LC; Lai, CC; Liao, CH; Hsu, CK; Chang, YL; Chang, CY; Hsueh, PR. Multidrug-resistant *Acinetobacter baumannii* bacteraemia: clinical features, antimicrobial therapy and outcome. *Clin Microbiol Infect.* 2007;13:196-8.

[198] Jellison, TK; Mckinnon, PS; Rybak, MJ. Epidemiology, resistance, and outcomes of *Acinetobacter baumannii* bacteremia treated with imipenem-cilastatin or ampicillin-sulbactam. *Pharmacotherapy.*2001;21:142-8.

[199] Kwon, KT; Oh, WS; Song, JH; Chang, HH; Jung, SI; Kim, SW; Ryu, SY; Heo, ST; Jung, DS; Rhee, JY; Shin, SY; Ko, KS; Peck, KR; Lee, NY. Impact of imipenem resistance on mortality in patients with *Acinetobacter* bacteraemia. *J Antimicrob Chemother.* 2007; 59:525-30.

[200] Falagas, ME; Karveli, EA; Kelesidis, I; Kelesidis, T. Community-acquired *Acinetobacter* infections. *Eur J Clin Microbiol Infect Dis.*2007;26:857-68.

[201] Wang, JT; McDonald, LC; Chang, SC; Ho, M. Community-acquired *Acinetobacter baumannii* bacteremia in adult patients in Taiwan. *J Clin Microbiol.*2002;40:1526-9.

[202] Chen, MZ; Hsueh, PR; Lee, LN; Yu, CJ; Yang, PC; Luh, KT. Severe community-acquired pneumonia due to *Acinetobacter baumannii. Chest.*2001; 120:1072-7.

[203] Chang, WN; Lu, CH; Huang, CR; Chuang, YC. Community-acquired *Acinetobacter* meningitis in adults. *Infection.*2000; 28:395-7.

[204] Alonso Fernández, A; Alvarez-Sala Walter, R; Prados Sánchez, C; Mayoralas Alises, S; Villamor León, J. Community-acquired empyema caused by *Acinetobacter baumannii. An Med Interna.*2001; 18:529-30.

[205] Leung, WS; Chu, CM; Tsang, KY; Lo, FH; Lo, KF; Ho, PL. Fulminant community-acquired *Acinetobacter baumannii* pneumonia as a distinct clinical syndrome. *Chest.* 2006; 129:102-9.

[206] Drault, JN; Herbland, A; Kaidomar, S; Mehdaoui, H; Olive, C; Jouanelle, J. Community-acquired *Acinetobacter baumannii* pneumonia. *Ann Fr Anesth Reanim.*2001;20:795-8.

[207] Kollef, MH; Fraser, VJ. Antibiotic resistance in the intensive care unit. *Ann Intern Med* 2001; 134:298–314.

[208] Timsit, JF; Garrait, V; Misset, B; et al. The digestive tract is a major site for *Acinetobacter baumannii* colonization in intensive care unit patients. *J Infect Dis* 1993; 168:1336–7.

[209] Agusti, C; Pujol, M; Argerich, MJ; et al. Short-term effect of the application of selective decontamination of the digestive tract on different body site reservoir ICU patients colonized by multi-resistant *Acinetobacter baumannii. J Antimicrob Chemother* 2002; 49:205–8.

[210] Podnos, YD; Cinat, ME; Wilson, SE; Cooke, J; Gornick, W; Thrupp, LD. Eradication of multi-drug resistant *Acinetobacter* from an intensive care unit. *Surg Infect* (Larchmt) 2001; 2:297-301.

[211] Aygun, G; Demirkiran, O; Utku, T; et al. Environmental contamination during a carbapenem-resistant *Acinetobacter baumannii* outbreak in an intensive care unit. *J Hosp Infect* 2002; 52:259-62.

[212] Zanetti, G; Blanc, DS; Federli, I; et al. Importation of *Acinetobacter baumannii* into a burn unit: a recurrent outbreak of infection associated with widespread environmental contamination. *Infect Control Hosp Epidemiol* 2007; 28:723-725.

[213] Wang, SH; Sheng, WH; Chang, YY; et al. Healthcare-associated outbreak due to pan-drug resistant *Acinetobacter baumannii* in a surgical intensive care unit.*J Hosp Infect* 2003; 53:97-102

[214] Urban, C; Segal-Maurer, S; Rahal, JJ. Considerations in control and treatment of nosocomial infections due to multidrug-resistant *Acinetobacter baumannii. Clin Infect Dis* 2003; 36:1268-74

[215] Siegel, JD; Rhinehart, E; Jackson, M; Chiarello, L. Healthcare Infection Control Practices Advisory Committee. Management of multidrug-resistant organisms in healthcare settings. Atlanta: Centers for Disease Control and Prevention, 2006. Available at: *http://www.cdc.gov/ncidod/dhqp/pdf/ar/mdroguideline2006.pdf* Accessed 9 March 2007.

In: Multiple Drug Resistance
Editors: A. Meszaros, G. Balogh, pp. 65-98 ISBN: 978-1-60741-595-4

Chapter III

Multiple Drug Resistance

Paul D. Brown*
University of the West Indies, Kingston, Jamaica

Abstract

The problem of multiple drug resistance is a significant public health problem as health officials try to contain drug resistance in bacteria, fungi, viruses, including HIV and influenza, and particularly complicates the therapeutics for control and limits what is available for emerging infections. While most multiple drug resistant (MDR) pathogens were traditionally associated with nosocomial infections, including methicillin-resistant *Staphylococcus* species (MRSA and CoNS) and several MDR organisms, including penicillin-resistant *Streptococcus pneumoniae* and MRSA, have recently been isolated from community sources, and some of these have begun to cause problems in the hospital setting. Nosocomial infections affect a significant proportion of patients in intensive care units (ICUs) and are associated with substantial morbidity and mortality, and increased costs. Furthermore, the prevalence of antibiotic-resistant pathogens isolated in the ICU is usually significantly higher than in other hospital wards. This has precipitated a plethora of strategies to contain these organisms, while the scientific community struggle to keep pace with the need to devise new combinations of drugs.

In Jamaica, the traditional approach has been to assess the prevalence of multiple drug resistance among important nosocomial pathogens, primarily in the intensive care units. However, in more recent times, attention has been given to investigation of molecular resistance determinants, such as the presence of plasmids, such as *qnr* plasmids in *E. coli* and genetic elements, such as the staphylococcal cassette chromosome *mec* (SCCmec) elements in community- and hospital-acquired MRSA. This paper will assess the molecular and cellular mechanisms of bacterial resistance, some of the overlooked aspects concerning development and spread of antimicrobial resistance, the local situation in Jamaica, and implications for clinical practice.

---

* Department of Basic Medical Sciences, University of the West Indies, Mona, Kingston 7, Jamaica, paul.brown@uwimona.edu.jm

1. Introduction

Antibiotics are naturally occurring, semi-synthetic compounds that have antimicrobial activity such as bactericidal or bacteriostatic effects and are used for the prevention and treatment of clinical infections in both human and veterinary medicine (Phillips *et al.,* 2004; Yang *et al.,* 2004). While antimicrobial resistance is an inevitable evolutionary response to antimicrobial use, it has become a major threat to public health. For many years, we have been faced with the emergence and spread of microorganisms resistant to one or more antimicrobial agents commonly used in the treatment of infections, caused by both Gram-positive and negative bacteria, fungi, and viruses. In some cases, pathogens have become resistant to all anti-infectious drugs, e.g., multiple drug resistant *Mycobacterium tuberculosis*, leading to therapeutic failure. Initially limited to hospital environments and nosocomial infections, the resistance phenomenon is now a major concern in community infections. Multiple drug-resistant (MDR) organisms that cause serious hospital or community infections and are now difficult to treat include methicillin- and multiple-resistant *Staphylococcus aureus* (MRSA) and coagulase-negative *Staphylococcus* species, vancomycin-resistant enterococci (VRE), penicillin-resistant pneumococci, and multi-resistant Gram-negative bacilli such as *Escherichia coli*, *Klebsiella* and *Enterobacter* spp., and *Pseudomonas aeruginosa*. (CDC, 2003)

In Jamaica, health services are delivered through four semiautonomous regional health authorities (RHA) that have direct management responsibility within a geographically defined region. The Northeast RHA comprises the parishes of St. Ann, St. Mary and Portland; the Southeast RHA includes Kingston and St. Andrew, St. Catherine and St. Thomas; the Southern RHA comprises St. Elizabeth, Manchester and Clarendon; and the Western RHA manages the parishes of Westmoreland, Hanover, St. James and Trelawney (See Figure 1).

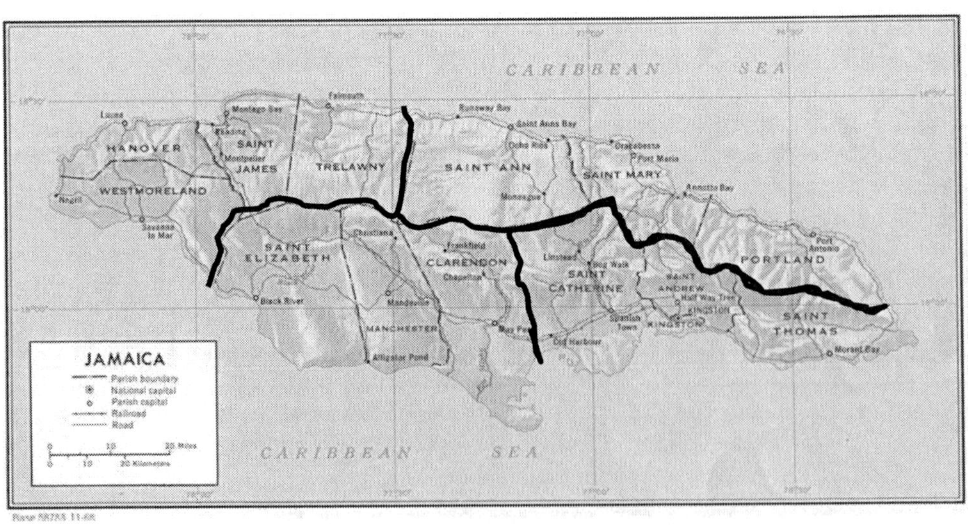

Figure 1. A shaded relief physical map that pictures Jamaica, and including parish boundaries, parish capitals, and the divisions of the four Regional Health Authorities and the parishes served.

2. Molecular and Cellular Mechanisms of Bacterial Resistance

Molecular mechanisms of the actions of antimicrobial agents must be recalled for better understanding of bacterial resistance mechanisms. There are four main mechanisms of antimicrobial action (Figure 2)

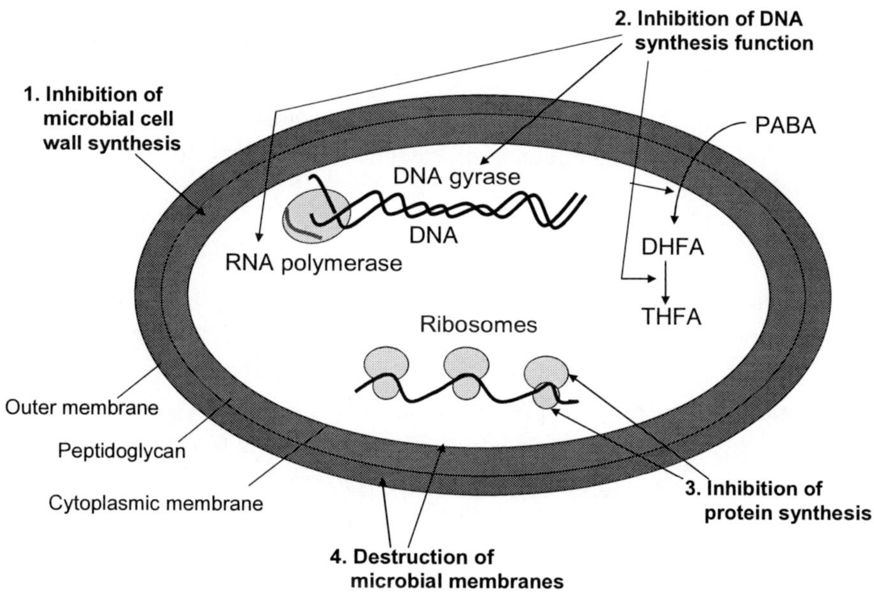

Figure 2. The four main mechanisms of antimicrobial action

2.1. Inhibition of Synthesis of Microbial Cell Wall

Examples of antimicrobial agents that inhibit the synthesis of microbial cell wall include beta-lactam and glycopeptides antibiotics as well as fosfomycin and bacitracin. Beta-lactams inhibit interpeptide bond formation, which is the last step of peptidoglycan synthesis, through the binding of enzymes (transpeptidases and DD-peptidases). The resulting acyl-enzyme complex has no physiological activity, leading to a bactericidal effect. Beta lactams do not need to make their way through the cytoplasmic membrane to reach their targets, penicillin-binding proteins (PBPs), since these are located on the external face of the cytoplasmic membrane. Glycopeptide antibiotics, such as vancomycin and teicoplanin, also act at the last step of peptidoglycan synthesis, through inhibition of peptidoglycan polymerization. Fosfomycin acts at the first step polymerization by inhibiting pyruvyl transferase, an intra-cytoplasmic enzyme which is involved in the synthesis of UDP-N-acetylmuramyl pentapeptide (NAMP) precursor. Fosfomycin crosses the cytoplasmic membrane through two systems of active transport. Bacitracin also acts early in the peptidoglycan synthesis process, through the inhibition of the phospholipid dephosphorylation which is required for the synthesis of the peptidoglycan longitudinal chain.

2.1.1. Inhibition of DNA synthesis or function

Quinolone drugs induce rapid inhibition of DNA synthesis and then bacterial death through binding to DNA gyrase, a topoisomerase, thus forming a DNA-enzyme-quinolone complex which inhibits the enzyme function. DNA gyrase is not only required for DNA compaction, but also for the replication and transcription process. Recently, quinolone drugs have been shown to inhibit DNA topoisomerase IV, a second bacterial topoisomerase. Rifampicin belongs to the ansamycin family, and is a hydrophobic antibiotic that blocks RNA polymerase, which transcribes DNA into mRNA, leading to a bacteriostatic effect. Its selective toxicity for bacteria relies on its absence of activity on eukaryotic cells. Nitroimidazole and nitrofuran drugs induce direct DNA damage. Sulfonamides and trimethoprim inhibit the synthesis of folates, which are required for the synthesis of purines and pyrimidines, the major constituents of nucleic acids, thus leading to reduction or cessation of bacterial growth.

2.1.2. Inhibition of synthesis of bacterial proteins

Aminoglycoside antibiotics inhibit DNA replication initiation by binding to the 16S ribosomal RNA, one of the components of the ribosomal 30S subunit. All the steps of translation are altered, leading to translation inhibition. Moreover, abnormal proteins are synthesized because of numerous reading mistakes. Tetracyclines have bacteriostatic activity by inhibiting the elongation step of translation. They bind to the ribosomal 30S subunit, thus preventing fixation of new aminoacyl-tRNA on ribosomal site A. They have a broad spectrum of activity. Macrolide, streptogramin and lincosamide antibiotics bind to the ribosomal 50S subunit, thus resulting in inhibition of peptide elongation through blockage of either peptide transfer or translocation steps. Chloramphenicol binds to the 50S subunit and prevents the aminoacid of the aminoacyl-tRNA complex from binding normally to the ribosome. It thus inhibits peptide transfer from the P site to the A site, and therefore incorporation of the aminoacid present in the A site. It displays a broad spectrum of activity. Fusidic acid appears to block the translocation step.

2.1.3. Lesion or destruction of microbial membranes

Polymixin antibiotics bind to lipid membranes, which induces structural alterations and leads to rapid bacterial death.

2.2. Mechanisms of Antimicrobial Resistance

The mechanisms responsible for resistance developed towards antimicrobial agents have been elucidated in most cases. In each class of antimicrobial agents, there is at least one mechanism that allows the bacteria to protect themselves against antimicrobial activity. The most frequent mechanisms are antimicrobial inactivation; altered antimicrobial target or overproduction of target; reduced antimicrobial accumulation (facilitated by impaired uptake or enhanced efflux); and bypass antimicrobial-sensitive step (table 1).

Table 1. Chart showing mechanisms of microbial resistance to antimicrobial agents

Inactivation	Altered target	Reduced accumulation	Bypass
Aminoglycosides β-lactams Chloramphenicol Macrolides	Aminoglycosides Ansamycins β-lactams Glycopeptides Macrolides Quinolones Trimethoprim Sulphonamides	Ansamycins Chloramphenicol Macrolides Quinolones Tetracyclines Trimethoprim Sulphonamides	Trimethoprim Sulphonamides

2.3. Genetic Determinants for Resistance

Genes encoding resistance mechanisms may be housed on chromosomes which are inherited by successive generations of the bacterial species (vertical transmission). In this case, microbial resistance is stable, but is generally poorly transmitted from one bacterium to another (horizontal transmission). Resistance may be due to the presence of certain chromosomal genes (e.g., β-lactamase genes of Gram negative bacteria); mutations in chromosomal genes (e.g., point mutations at N-terminus of the GyrA protein reduce nalidixic acid binding in *E. coli*); or due to foreign genes integrated in the microbial chromosome (e.g., the genes encoding PBPs in Gram-positive cocci).

On the other hand, genes encoding resistance may belong to mobile elements such as plasmids, transposons and gene cassettes integrated into integrons (Chang *et al.,* 2000; Reyes *et al.,* 2003; Saenz *et al.,* 2004; Zhang *et al.,* 2004). In this case, transmission of resistance to descendants is possible but tends to be unstable in the absence of the selective antibiotics involved. Bacteria that have acquired such a mobile element may be cured and become susceptible again to antibiotics. By means of these mobile genetic elements, antibiotic resistance genes can be horizontally transferred among different bacterial strains (Chang *et al.,* 2000; Bywater *et al.,* 2004). Nowadays, the global dissemination of antibiotic resistance genes has created the problem of rapid emergence of antibiotic resistance among bacterial species and has complicated the treatment of infections (Chang *et al.,* 2000).

2.3.1. Integrons

Integrons act as a major expression vector in the dissemination of antibiotic resistance genes. They possess an effective site-specific recombination system that is able to capture and express the gene cassettes. Such gene cassettes are always associated with antimicrobial resistance genes (Liebert *et al.,* 1999; Reyes *et al.,* 2003; Solberg *et al.,* 2006). Chromosomal and broad-host-range plasmid-borne integrons are commonly found among the family of *Enterobacteriaceae* and thus enhance the interspecies dissemination (Bass *et al.,* 1999; Liebert *et al.,* 1999).

According to the types of respective integrase (*intl*), integrons can be broadly divided into four different classes, including class 1, 2, 3, and 4 integrons, and they can carry integrase *intl1*, *intl2*, *intl3*, and *intl4* genes, respectively (Bass *et al.*, 1999; Goldstein *et al.*, 2001; White *et al.*, 2001). Among these classes of integrons, class 1 integrons are the most widely spread among gram-negative organisms and are also the most extensively characterized (White *et al.*, 2001; Reyes *et al.*, 2003; Yang *et al.* 2004; Zhang *et al.*, 2004).

Class 1 integrons were first described by 1993 (Hall and Stokes, 1993; Zhang *et al.*, 2004). It has been identified from bacterial chromosomes and transposable elements such as Tn*21*, a mercury resistance transposon and its relatives (Bennett *et al.*, 1999; Goldstein *et al.*, 2001). Class 2 integrons are found on the transposon Tn*7* and its integrase (*intl2*) seems to be confined in their distribution between *E. coli* and *Salmonella* species (Goldstein *et al.*, 2001). Class 3 integrons have been described from the *Serratia marcescens* isolated from Japan that are associated with the metallo-beta-lactamase gene bla_{IMP}. (Arakawa *et al.*, 1995; Goldstein *et al.*, 2001). Class 4 integron is a distinctive class of integrons and is only found on *Vibrio cholerae* (Mazel *et al.*, 1998). On the other hand, class 4 integrase is not identified from any veterinary isolates (Goldstein *et al.*, 2001). Finally, a super-integron was identified from *V. cholerae* and it harbors hundreds of gene cassettes (Rowe-Magnus *et al.*, 1999; Mazel *et al.*, 2004).

By means of Southern hybridization with *intl* gene specific oligonucleotide probe, the location of an integron can be found whether it is present on the plasmids or chromosome (Chang *et al.*, 2000). Genetic mobilization can occur through the process of transformation, transduction, and conjugation (Salyers, 1995).

2.3.2. Plasmids

Antibiotic resistance plasmid was first described in 1960 (Watanabe and Fukasawa 1960). It is ubiquitous among the diverse bacterial communities. It can exist as circular, extra-chromosomal, and double-stranded DNA fragments, and the acquisition of new genes can be achieved through the lateral transfer between bacterial cells by means of conjugation or genetic transformation (Carattoli 2003; Caratolli *et al.*, 2005). Small non-conjugative plasmids also carry antibiotic-resistance genes and can be mobilized by a large conjugative plasmid

Plasmids can be classified through an incompatibility (Inc) replicon typing (Carattoli, 2003; Carattoli *et al.*, 2005). It consists of IncF, FIA, FIB, FIC, HI1, HI2, I1-Iγ, L/M, N, P, W, T, A/C, K, B/O, X, Y, and FIIA (Carattoli *et al.*, 2005). Plasmids that cannot coexist in the same cell are said to be incompatible. In particular, plasmids that replicate by the same mechanism are incompatible, whereas plasmids that replicate by other mechanisms belong to the same incompatibility group as they are compatible (Carattoli *et al.*, 2005).

2.3.3. Transposons

Transposons are mobile genetic elements that can migrate from one genetic location to another (Horak *et al.*, 1998). Similar to integrons, antibiotic resistance genes can be integrated into the transposons and thus enhance the dissemination of antibiotic resistance (Guerra *et al.*, 2002). In addition, class 1 integrons are often found within the transposons and are either chromosomal or plasmid located (Guerra *et al.*, 2002). They are frequently carried by conjugative or board-host-range plasmids and hence enhance their dissemination among bacterial communities (Dahlberg and Hermansson, 1995).

Among the different classes of transposons, class II is the one that is extensively characterized (Dahlberg and Hermansson, 1995). These are also called Tn*3* family transposons that include Tn*3*, Tn*21*, Tn*917*, and Tn*501* (Ward *et al.*, 1987; Dahlberg and Hermansson, 1995). Moreover, Tn*3* can carry resistant gene bla_{TEM} that encoded for ampicillin resistance and associated with other extended-spectrum beta-lactamases (ESBLs), while Tn*21* is associated with multi-antibiotic determinants such as antibiotic resistance genes like *sul* and *aadA* (Zuhlsdorf and Wiedemann, 1992; Dahlberg and Hermansson, 1995; Liebert *et al.*, 1999).

2.4. Multi-Drug Resistance and Cross-Resistance

Multi-drug resistance (MDR) to different antimicrobial agents generally results from a combination of different independent mechanisms of resistance. Regarding the resistance mechanisms, multi-drug resistance may occur naturally or is acquired.

Two examples are particularly representative of natural multi-drug resistance. The first, *Pseudomonas aeruginosa*, is resistant to β-lactams, including 3rd generation cephalosporins; quinolones; chloramphenicol, and tetracyclines. The major cause is the vey low cell wall permeability; at least 100 times lower than *E. coli*. In addition, this organism is characterized by the production of inducible cephalosporinase, active efflux and poor target affinity for the target (DNA gyrase), three mechanisms which act synergistically with the poor permeability of the cell wall (Li et al., 1994). The second example is mycobacteria, which express resistance to β-lactams and tetracyclines as a result of low cell wall permeability, production of antimicrobial-inactivating enzymes (β-lactamases, enzymes inactivating aminoglycosides), and poor target affinity (PBP, DNA gyrase) (Jarlier et al., 1994).

Acquired multi-drug resistance corresponds to the epidemiologic situation of strains which have acquired resistance to one antimicrobial agent, and then tend to acquire resistance to other agents which may belong to different families. In other words, several mechanisms of acquired resistance (or natural and acquired resistance) may coexist simultaneously in the same organism. In most cases, several genes, which determine different mechanisms of resistance, may be borne by the same plasmid, such as genes encoding β-lactamases; enzymes inactivating aminoglycosides; or resistance to sulphonamides or chloramphenicol. In addition, mechanisms of acquired resistance that are independent and involve different genetic carriers may be present in the same strain. The best example is given by hospital strains of MRSA, with prevalence rates of 43% in the USA (Keuhnert et al., 2005), up to 48% in European countries (Tiermersma et al., 2004), up to 54% in Japan (Lotsu et al., 1995) and 23% in Jamaica (Brown and Ngeno, 2007).

Fortunately, vancomycin, a glycopeptides antibiotic, together with teicoplanin, remains active against *S. aureus*. The first resistant strain to vancomycin was described in Japan in 1996 in the sputum of a patient with *S. aureus*-mediated pneumonia, and clinical failure (CDC 1997a). The two strains were isolated in the USA in 1997 (CDC 1997b), and one strain in Europe in 1997 in an immunocompromised child with Job syndrome (Krémëry et al., 1997). Although no resistance to vancomycin was found in common strains, up to 20% of the strains are heterogeneously resistant with reduced susceptibility to vancomycin (MIC = 3 mg/L). Fortunately, all MRSA isolated in Jamaica to date have been susceptible to vancomycin (Brown and Ngeno, 2007; Nicholson, pers. comm.).

Cross-resistance generally occurs in antimicrobials of the same family, for example between penicillins, and more widely between all β-lactams including the cephalosporins.

The range of resistance exchange is illustrated in Figure 3, which highlight the fact that conjugative Gram-negative and Gram-positive bacteria are the main drivers of the process of genetic exchange in nature.

Table 2. Frequency of Resistance in MRSA

Antimicrobial	% of resistant strains[1]	% of resistant strains[2]
Aminoglycosides	35-40	10
Macrolides	40	18
Fluoroquinolones	40	13
Tetracyclines	40	21
Chloramphenicol	10	13
Trimethoprim-sulfamethoxazole	40	26
Rifampicin	>30	N/A
Fosfomycin	20	N/A

[1] Swartz,1994;
[2] Brown & Ngeno, 2007
N/A not assessed

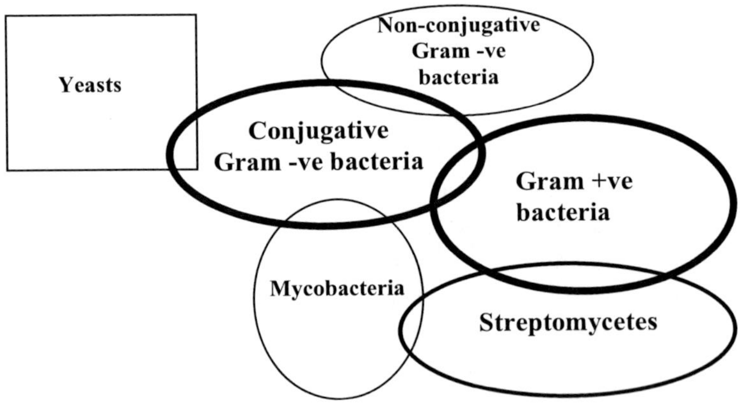

Figure 3.

2.5. Expression of Resistance to Specific Agents

2.5.1. Resistance to sulphonamides

Antifolate resistance is relatively widespread throughout the world. These antifolate antibiotics in particular, trimethoprim and its combination with the sulphonamide sulphamethoxazole (co-trimoxazole, SXT) are widely accessible and provide treatment for many types of Gram negative infections.

Resistance to trimethoprim and sulphonamides is in some cases caused by chromosomal alterations. In the case of trimethoprim, the chromosomal resistance can be of three types: first, by loss of thymidylate synthase activity making the dihydrofolate reductases redundant for the bacteria since it will depend on external supply of thymine. Second, changes in the structure or expression of porins have been shown to affect the susceptibility of some Gram negative strains of *Klebsiella*, *Enterobacter* and *Serratia* to trimethoprim. Third, mutations in the *fol*A gene encoding the bacterial dihydrofolate reductase DHFR, leads to a lower affinity of the drug to the enzyme and thus a lower level of enzyme inhibition (Sköld, 2000, 2001).

The clinically most important trimethoprim resistance in Gram negative bacteria is conferred by alternative resistant dihydrofolate reductases which are encoded by a number of different *dfr* genes. The majority of these 29 known genes are carried as gene cassettes in integrons. However, another group of *dfr* genes have recently been defined as located in a region connected to a putative recombinase in which genes conferring resistance to several antibiotics seem to have accumulated (Hall and Stokes, 1990; Stokes et al., 1993; Toleman et al., 2006). Some of the *dfr* genes are also disseminated by more or less defined independent mechanisms. The *dfr* genes are divided into two phylogenetic families, with the majority belonging to *dfrA*. These genes are very diverse and share homology among themselves and with several housekeeping genes (20 to 95%), resulting in the recognition of subfamilies. Such subfamilies include the *dfrA1* group, which consists of *drfA1, 5, 6, 7, 14, 15, 16, 17* and *25* and the *dfrA12* family, including *dfrA12, 12, 21* and *22*. The second group is designated *dfrB* or *dfr2* genes, and include *dfrB1, 2, 3, 4*, and *5* (or *dfr2a* to *e*), and encodes peptides that are 65% identical and have no relationship with any other known dihydrofolate reductases. While *dfrA* genes encode proteins consisting of dimers of 152 to 189 aminoacids conferring different levels of resistance to TMP, the *dfrB* genes encode tetrameric proteins of 78 peptides which always confer a very high level of TMP resistance upon their hosts.

The horizontally transferred sulphonamide resistance genes are very few in contrast to *dfr* genes. Only three *sul* genes are known, however, these genes seem to be efficiently spread and have been implicated in the resistance of most sulphonamide resistance in Gram negative bacteria. The first two genes, *sul1* and *sul2* have been known to be plasmid borne since the 1960s and have been described as equally distributed among resistant isolates (Sköld, 2000; Swedberg and Sköld, 1980, 1983). The more recently described *sul3* was first identified in *E. coli* from pigs in 2003 (Perreten and Boerlin, 2003). The sulphonamide-resistant dihydropterotate synthases encoded by these genes are identical to 34%, are fairly different from housekeeping DHPS enzymes and are 263-279 aminoacids long. While the *sul1* gene is located in the 3' end of class 1 integrons, with a defective *attC* element, the s*ul2* gene is often seen associated with a streptomycin-resistance gene in small conjugative plasmids, or on several other plasmids, which indicate proper recombination are associated with this gene (Rådström et al., 1991). Neither *sul2* nor *sul3* have been reported to be parts of or genetically linked to integrons.

2.5.2. Resistance to Quinolones

Quinolone resistance has become a serious problem in the clinical treatment of human infections since the introduction of nalidixic acid in the 1960s (Tran and Jacoby, 2002). In the past, quinolone resistance was noted as a result of several mechanisms: (i) chromosomal mutations in the target type II topoisomerase enzymes, including DNA gyrase (both subunits of GyrA and GyrB) in gram-negative organisms and topoisomerase IV (subunits ParC and ParE) in gram-positive organisms. The most common site for amino acid substitution was located around the region of Quinolone Resistance Determining Region (QRDR) (Tran and Jacoby, 2002; Nordmann and Poirel, 2005); (ii) chromosomal mutations in active efflux system that reduced the drug accumulation (Martinez-Martinez *et al.*, 1998; Tran and Poirel, 2002; Wang *et al.*, 2003); (iii) deficiencies in outer membrane porin channels (Martinez-Martinez *et al.*, 2003; Poirel *et al.*, 2005a). More recently, plasmid-mediated resistance to quinolone was also described after the identification of a *qnr* gene (later termed *qnr*A) from a 1994 isolate of *Klebsiella pneumoniae* in Birmingham, AL, USA (Martinez-Martinez *et al.*, 1998).

Plasmid-quinolone resistance gene (*qnr*A) was identified from a multi-resistance plasmid (pMG252) that encodes a protein (namely Qnr, lately termed QnrA) and consisted of 218 amino acids that belong to the pentapeptide repeat family (Martinez-Martinez *et al.*, 1998; Tran and Jacoby, 2002; Poirel *et al.*, 2005a; Nordmann and Poirel, 2005). This protein conferred a low level resistance to quinolone with 4 to 32-fold increase in MICs (Martinez-Martinez *et al.*, 1998; Rodriguez-Martinez *et al.*, 2003; Wang *et al.*, 2004a). In addition to the *qnr*, the protein was found on the broad-host-range plasmids with sizes ranging from 50 to 200 kb (Wang *et al.*, 2004b; Poirel *et al.*, 2005a; Nazic *et al.*, 2005). Moreover, *qnr* was also found worldwide in many different clinical isolates including *K. pneumoniae*, *E. coli*, *Providencia stuartii*, *Salmonella enterica*, *Enterobacter cloacae*, *Citrobacter freundii*, and *Shigella flexneri* (Wang *et al.*, 2003, 2004b; Cheung *et al.*, 2005; Hata *et al.*, 2005; Jeong *et al.*, 2005; Jonas *et al.*, 2005; Nazic *et al.*, 2005; Poirel *et al.*, 2005a; Robicsek *et al.*, 2005). However, *qnr* was not found in non-enterobacterial gram-negative strains such as *Pseudomonas aeruginosa* and *Acinebacter baumanni* (Nordmann and Poirel, 2005). Other *qnr*-like genes were also identified such as *qnr*B and *qnr*S (Hata *et al.*, 2005; Nordmann and Poirel, 2005).

2.5.3. Resistance to Aminoglycosides

Aminoglycosides comprise a large family of antibiotics, which includes gentamicin, netilmicin, amikacin, tobramycin, dibekacin, isepamicin, arbekacin, and older compounds such as kanamycin and streptomycin (Vakulenko and Mobashery, 2003). It has a synergistic effect when working with beta-lactam antibiotics and vancomycin. Moreover, it is still the preferred therapeutic option for the treatment of life-threatening infections in hospitalized patients (Vanhoof *et al*., 1992; Magnet *et al*., 2003; Vakulenko and Mobashery, 2003). Nowadays, bacterial resistance to aminoglycoside is quite common. There are several mechanisms leading to the cause of antimicrobial resistance for this class of antibiotics: (1) Decrease uptake of antibiotic through the modification in drug permeability, leading to an insufficient intracellular concentration of antibiotics. Thus, the bactericidal activity of aminoglycoside will be reduced as it is concentration dependent; (2) Point mutation in the primary ribosomal target site; (3) Efflux system and pump out the aminoglycoside from the bacterial cells; (4) Enzymatic modification of aminoglycoside by means of aminoglycoside-modifying enzymes (AME); and (5) It has been speculated that aminoglycoside resistance genes can potentially come from originated aminoglycoside producing organism like actinomycetes (Chaslus-Dancla *et al.*, 1987; Gaynes *et al.*, 1987; Vilegenthart *et al.*, 1991; Shaw *et al.*, 1993; Vakulenko and Mobashery, 2003; Magnet *et al.*, 2003). Resistance genes that encoded AME can be interspecies transferred through transposable genetic elements such as plasmids, transposons (i.e., Tn*21*), and integrons (Chaslus-Dancla *et al.*, 1987; Ho *et al.*, 1993; Shaw *et al.*, 1993; Choi *et al.*, 2003; Nemec *et al.*, 2004).

2.5.4. Resistance to Tetracycline

Tetracyclines were discovered in the 1940s and have been used clinically to treat a variety of infections since the 1950s and are still widely used today (Bartlett, 2004; Roberts, 2003). Since the original reports of TetA-mediated efflux of and resistance to tetracycline in *E. coli*, numerous other Tet proteins have been described, in Gram-negative and Gram positive organisms, with at least 20 different types presently known (reviewed in Butaye et al., 2003 and Roberts, 2005). These MF family exporters are almost invariably encoded by genes present on mobile genetic elements (Butaye et al., 2003 and Roberts, 2003), often together with additional resistance genes, e.g., in multidrug-resistant *S. enterica* (Guerra et al., 2001; Doublet et al., 2004; Gebreyes and Thakur, 2005; Randall et al., 2004), *E. coli* (Maynard et al., 2004) and *V. cholerae* (Iwanaga et al., 2004).

Recently, a chromosomal *tet* efflux determinant, tet38, was reported in *Staphylococcus aureus*, its overexpression in a mutant strain providing for markedly enhanced tetracycline resistance (Truong et al., 2005). The vast majority of the different Tet proteins have been reported in Gram-negative bacteria and includes the Tet proteins A–E, G, H, I, J, Z and Tet(30), which are found exclusively in Gram-negative bacteria (Butaye et al., 2003; Roberts, 2005) with two, TetK and TetL, found predominantly in Gram-positive bacteria (Roberts, 2005).

Novel Tet efflux proteins, Tet(V) and Tet(39) have also been reported in *Mycobacterium smegmatis* and *Mycobacterium fortuitum* (Viveiros et al., 2003) and *Acinetobacter* spp. (Agersø and Guardabassi, 2005), respectively. Still, efflux is a very uncommon mechanism of tetracycline resistance in Gram-positive pathogens, e.g., *Streptococcus* (Poyart et al., 2003; Lancaster et al., 2003; Matsumoto et al., 2005; Rodriguez-Avial et al., 2003) and *Enterococcus* spp. (Peterson and Dalsgaard, 2003; Huys et al., 2004) though it is reported in pathogenic staphylococci (Strommenger et al., 2003; Sekiguchi et al., 2004). In Gram negative pathogens, efflux is the predominant mechanism of tetracycline resistance in several organisms, e.g., *Salmonella* spp. (Gebreyes and Thakur, 2005, Aarestrup et al., 2003; Poppe et al., 2002) *Shigella* spp. (Hartman et al., 2001; Toro et al., 2005) *E. coli* (Hartman et al., 2003; Guerra et al., 2003; Miles et al., 2006) *Acinetobacter* spp. (Guardabassi et al., 2000) and *Chlamydia* spp. (Dugan et al., 2004).

The Tet efflux proteins typically export and provide resistance to tetracycline, oxytetracycline and chlortetracycline, with TetB and TetL the only known Tet family exporters of minocycline (Butaye et al., 2003; Roberts, 2003). Unfortunately, however, TetB has the widest host range among Gram-negative pathogens (Roberts, 2003). Expression of the various *tet* genes is inducible by tetracyclines, although the induction mechanisms differ for Gram-negative versus Gram-positive tetracycline efflux genes; Gram-negative *tet* genes are controlled by the tetracycline responsive TetR repressor whereas Gram-positive *tet* genes are controlled by a 'translational attenuation' mechanism (Butaye et al., 2003).

2.5.5. Resistance to Beta-Lactam Antibiotics

Antibiotic resistance to beta-lactam antibiotics is mainly mediated by β-lactamases that are capable of hydrolyzing the beta-lactam ring and cause the antibiotic to malfunction (Brinas *et al.*, 2002). Beta-lactam antibiotics include penicillin, first, second, and third generation cephalosporins, and aztreonam (Paterson and Bonomo 2005). Beta-lactam antibiotics are commonly used among humans as well as veterinary medicine (Brinas *et al.*, 2002). Table 3 shows the identification scheme of Bush-Jacoby-Medeiros for the different classes of β-lactamases.

Plasmid-mediated β-lactamase TEM-1 can be encoded by resistance genes $bla_{\text{TEM-1a}}$, $bla_{\text{TEM-1b}}$, $bla_{\text{TEM-1c}}$, $bla_{\text{TEM-1d}}$, $bla_{\text{TEM-1e}}$, and $bla_{\text{TEM-1f}}$ (Brinas *et al.*, 2002; Baraniak *et al.*, 2005). There are four different types of promoter described in the bla_{TEM} gene that are responsible for the initiation of transcription, including weak promoter (P3) for $bla_{\text{TEM-1a}}$ in transposon Tn*3,* strong promoter (P4 and overlapping promoter Pa/Pb), and P5 (Goussard and Courvalin 1999; Leflon-Guibout *et al.*, 2000; Brinas *et al.*, 2002; Lartigue *et al.*, 2002). According to the study by Brinas *et al.*, promoter P3 is most commonly found in PCR bla_{TEM} amplicons and $bla_{\text{TEM-1b}}$ is most frequently found among ampicillin-resistant *E. coli* isolates (Brinas *et al.*, 2002; Hasman *et al.*, 2005).

The worldwide problem of expression of ESBL in gram-negative bacteria has drawn the global attention as it complicated the treatment of human infections (Bou *et al.*, 2002). The enzymes of CTX-M-type β-lactamase are non-TEM, non-SHV-derived ESBL that are identified globally with increasing frequency since the mid 1990s (Brigante *et al.*, 2005; Pitout *et al.*, 2005; Duan *et al.*, 2006). This family comprises more than 40 types of enzymes and mainly classified into five groups according to their amino acid identities, it includes CTX-M-1, CTX-M-2, CTX-M-8, CTX-M-9, and CTX-M-25 groups. (Brigante *et al.*, 2005; Duan *et al.*, 2006).

Table 3. Identification scheme of Bush-Jacoby-Medeiros for different classes of β-lactamases

Different groups of β-lactamase enzymes	Description	Representative enzymes
Group 1 cephalosporinases	Not completely inhibited by β-lactamase inhibitor, clavulanic acid	AmpC type β-lactamase
Group 2 cephalosporinases, penicillinases & broad spectrum β-lactamase	Inhibited by β-lactamase inhibitor that target the active site directly	TEM-1, TEM-2, SHV-1, OXA-1 & CTX-M
Group 3 metallo-β-lactamase	Inhibited by β-lactamase inhibitor poorly	CcrA (*Bacteroides fragilis*) & L1 (*Stenotrophomonas maltophilia*)
Group 4 penicillinases	Resistant to the hydrolysis by β-lactamase inhibitor	Penicillinase (*Burkholderia cepacia*)

3. Some Overlooked Aspects Concerning Development and Spread of Antimicrobial Resistance

Part of the challenge of antimicrobial resistance in general and multiple drug resistance in particular is the fact that there are several overlooked aspects, which are at least as important as surveillance of the multiple drug resistant organisms themselves. These include antimicrobial misuse associated with patients' non-compliance, the spread of antimicrobial resistance by disposal of industrial antimicrobial waste and/or hospital effluent, the role of pets as reservoirs, and the role of the environment as reservoirs of antibiotic resistance genes.

3.1. Patients' Contribution to Antimicrobial Misuse

While there is general admission that antibiotic resistance is a consequence of antibiotic use, there is hesitancy in some quarters of the significance of the role of antibiotic misuse. However, what is now clear is that patients' non-compliance in antibiotic therapy can significantly enhance the emergence of antibiotic resistant organisms during treatment because of the low antimicrobial concentration or short antimicrobial exposure attained in body tissues. Patient's non-compliance is a worldwide phenomenon, but has been only properly studied in some countries, for example, Branthwaite and Pechere (1996) in a study of 3610 individuals from six countries in Europe, reported that 25% of patients miss at least one dose, 31% of patients stop before the end of the course, and 44% of patients saved part of course for future. These figures might be higher in developing countries where cost and availability of effective antibiotics might be important issues in compliance. Further Pechere et al (2002) noted that good communication between patient and physician seemed to contribute to a more appropriate use of antimicrobials, although a lot depends on the patient's attitude in relating to their doctor. However, the problem of non-compliance is further compounded by the fact that there is a significant portion of drugs that are excreted unchanged, and 20-30% of drugs not consumed by patients are disposed of in household drains (Kummerer, 2001).

If the drugs are not degraded or eliminated during sewage treatment, in soil or in other environmental compartments, they will reach surface water and ground water, and, potentially, drinking water. Unmetabolized antibiotic substances are often passed into the aquatic environment in wastewater. Antibiotics used for veterinary purposes or as growth promoters are excreted by the animals and end up in manure. Manure is used as an agricultural fertilizer; thus, the antibiotics seep through the soil and enter ground water. However, very little is known about the occurrence, fate and risks associated with antibiotics entering the environment after being used in human and veterinary medicine and as growth promoters; 95% community use is reported for the UK, while 75% is reported for the USA. In Germany, 75% of antimicrobials are used in the community and 25% in hospitals (Kummerer, 2003).

3.2. Impact of Industrial Antimicrobial Production and Hospital Effluent on the Spread of Resistance

Industrial antimicrobial production generates large volumes of waste containing antimicrobial residues. Because the recovery yield in the antimicrobial production can be as low as 20%, 1-4 kg of antimicrobials can be discharged into sewage system for each kg of antimicrobial produced. This considerable amount of antimicrobials is likely to select for resistant bacteria in the bacterial flora of sewage (Guardabassi et al., 1998), and/or the sewage may act as an enrichment medium for the resistant bacteria as well as a vehicle for their dispersal. This medium has been associated with the spread of vancomycin-resistant Enterococci (VRE), which is an important nosocomial pathogen (Guardabassi et al., 2002).

Hospital effluent contributes significantly to the pool of environmental sources of multidrug resistant microorganisms. Chitnis et al. (2000) found that the multidrug resistant bacteria population in hospital effluents ranged from 0.6% to 40% for 10 hospitals studied, compared to <0.00002 to 0.025% for 11 sewage samples from residential areas. The authors felt that a high percentage of the MDR in some of the hospital effluents could be due to excessive use of antibiotics resulting in increased selective pressure and in turn increase in the prevalence of MDR bacteria. Further, there was a pattern of simultaneous resistance to ampicillin, amoxicillin-clavulanate, piperacilllin, second and third generation cephalosporins, co-trimoxazole, gentamicin, netilmycin and quinolones like ciprofloxacin. This pattern was noted for *E. coli*, *Klebsiella, Enterobacter, Citrobacter* and *Pseudomonas*, and strongly suggested involvement of plasmids.

3.3. Role of Pets as Reservoirs of Resistant Bacteria

The close proximity of pets (treated with antibiotics, often for chronic skin infections and otitis externa) and owners provides opportunity for exchange of bacteria and resistance determinants among these populations. In fact, there is evidence of pets acting as reservoirs of MRSA within family households. For example, recurrent MRSA infection has been reported in a human patient with diabetes and his wife's wound; the source was the family dog that carried the same strain in its nares (Manian, 2003).

3.4. Environmental Reservoirs of Antimicrobial Resistance Genes

There is strong evidence that the use of antimicrobial agents can lead to the emergence and dissemination of resistant *E. coli* (Linton *et al.*, 1997; Levy *et al.*, 1976; van den Bogaard *et al.*, 2001; Galland *et al.*, 2001; Meng *et al.*, 1998; Schroeder *et al.*, 2002), which can then be passed onto people via food or through direct contact with animals. However, there are increasing numbers of reports detailing circulation and amplification of antimicrobial resistance genes, including tetracycline resistance in the environment (Adhikari et al., 2000; Cohen, 2000; Furushita *et al.*, 2003; Rysz and Alvarez, 2004; Sayah *et al.*, 2005), which could facilitate the emergence and spread of antibiotic resistance in bacteria. The finding of multiple drug resistant commensal *E. coli* isolates from broiler chickens from farms that did not report antibiotic use concurs with these latter reports. Rysz and Alvarez (2004) demonstrated that bacteria in the soil could acquire resistance to tetracycline from environmental exposure, possibly creating a reservoir of resistance factors generated outside host animals. Their finding suggests that collection of environmental samples from a farm is important for accessing exposure to resistance factors from farm runoff in watersheds, except in cases where soil is augmented with organic fertilizer. Sayah *et al.* (2005) reported that farm environmental isolates showed reduced susceptibility (as measured by disc diffusion zone sizes) compared to faecal sample isolates to most agents studied. They suggested that non-sampled sources, e.g., farm workers and wildlife with access to the farm environment, could be sources of resistance factors.

In a recent study in Jamaica, Miles *et al.*, (2006) investigated the prevalence and genetic basis of tetracycline resistance in faecal *Escherichia coli* isolates from healthy broiler chickens. In their finding of an 82.4% resistance frequency to tetracycline mediated by *tet*B and/or *tet*D genes and significant multiple drug resistance in the absence of selection pressure from antibiotics in feed or water supplies, they concluded that genes responsible are disseminated in the environment.

4. Multidrug Resistance in Specific Organisms in Jamaica

4.1 *Staphylococcus aureus*

S. aureus is naturally susceptible to many classes of antimicrobials but has great ability to develop multiple resistance (Shanson *et al.*, 1981). Penicillin resistance due to the production of plasmid-mediated penicillinase appeared in *S. aureus* soon after the introduction of penicillin and had affected 85% of both hospital and community isolates by the late 1970s. In the 1950s and early 1960s, hospital outbreaks with strains resistant to penicillin, tetracycline, erythromycin and chloramphenicol became common but disappeared after the introduction of methicillin and other penicillins resistant to breakdown by staphylococcal penicillinase.

Gentamicin resistance became common in the 1970s, and in the 1980s methicillin- and multiple-resistance emerged throughout the world (Brumfit and Hamilton-Miller, 1989). In both the US and Europe around 30–50% of hospital isolates of *S. aureus* are now methicillin- and multiple-resistant *S. aureus* (MRSA) (NNIS, 2002); although in the Netherlands and Scandinavia, MRSA rates are less than 1% (EARSS, 2001).

Many strains of MRSA remain reliably susceptible only to the glycopeptides vancomycin and teicoplanin, and vancomycin is the drug of choice for serious infection (French *et al.*, 1990; Michel and Gutman, 1997). Unfortunately, several types of glycopeptide resistance have emerged in MRSA in recent years. Some isolates show glycopeptide tolerance, that is, they are inhibited by normal concentrations of glycopeptides but are not killed (May *et al.*, 1998). Tolerance has been associated with treatment failures, but its exact clinical significance is unclear. Occasional strains of *S. aureus* with chromosomally encoded low-level or 'intermediate' resistance to vancomycin have appeared in Japan, North America and Europe (Liu and Chambers, 2004), associated with treatment failures and designated 'vancomycin-intermediate' or 'glycopeptide-intermediate' *S. aureus* (VISA or GISA). Up to the end of 2004, three isolates of MRSA have been reported (from the US) with high-level glycopeptide resistance of the VanA type, probably derived from vancomycin-resistant enterococci (CDC, 2004). Although still exceptionally rare, these dangerously resistant organisms may become more frequent in the future.

In Jamaica, MRSA was first recognized in 1991 at the University Hospital of the West Indies (Bodonaik and Nicholson, 2002; Figure). Previous work (Bodonaik *et al.*, 1984) reported that 82% of isolates from outpatients and 84% of those from inpatients at the University Hospital of the West Indies (UHWI) were resistant to penicillin. The UHWI is a 500-bed multi-disciplinary teaching hospital, which serves the metropolitan area of Kingston and St. Andrew. In that study, no methicillin-resistance was found. However, by 1991, the incidence was 5.1% and by 1997 this had increased to 9.3%. A more recent study in 2003 in Mandeville, situated about 124 km from Kingston and St. Andrew metropolis, noted that 87% of the *S. aureus* isolates were resistant to penicillin, and 24% were methicillin-resistant (Brown and Ngeno, 2007). Interestingly, all MRSA isolates were from community sources. Historically, methicilin-resistant isolates are also resistant to all beta-lactam agents, including the cephalosporins and carbapenems. Continuing active surveillance noted a fall in the incidence of MRSA in 2004, however, the frequency is on the increase again, reaching 8% during 2008.

There has been much debate over whether MRSA infections have a worse outcome than those caused by methicillin-sensitive strains (MSSA). However, this issue has been resolved by a recent meta-analysis by Cosgrove and colleagues (2003) who reviewed studies comparing MRSA and MSSA bacteraemia published between 1980 and 2000. Nearly 78% of these studies failed to show an effect of MRSA on mortality, probably because individual studies lacked statistical power. However, the pooled results showed a significant excess mortality associated with MRSA bacteraemia (OR, 1.93; 95% CI, 1.54–2.42). The authors thought that since the mean mortality rate for MSSA bacteraemia was 23%, the odds ratios might have overestimated the effect. They therefore calculated a pooled relative risk of 1.42, which they thought better reflected the magnitude of the effect. The increased mortality remained after adjusting for nosocomial infection, the presence of an outbreak, central venous catheterization and endocarditis. The effect of MRSA on mortality was lower in patients with central venous line infections, perhaps because these patients can be readily treated by removal of the focus of infection.

Similar results were found when surgical site infection with MRSA and MSSA were compared (Engemann *et al.*, 2003). Those with MRSA infection had a significantly greater 90-day mortality rate, a greater length of hospitalization and significantly increased hospital charges compared with patients with MSSA surgical site infection. In Jamaica, one-third of patients colonized by MRSA develop infection, and there is an increased risk of death from MRSA (OR=1.93). In addition, there is significant morbidity, particularly due to increased incidence of MRSA-associated bacteraemia and shock. Costs associated with MRSA hospitalization are significant, with cost of drugs between US$325 to US$574, and patients needing 14 to 36 bed-days. In addition, because these patients become a source of infection, there might be other persons to treat. For the patient, hospitalization fee/day can range from JM$3024 to JM$12,835, and while most of these costs can be recouped because of insurance, the emotional toll on the patient is often priceless.

Possible reasons why MRSA is associated with poor outcome include enhanced virulence, decreased effectiveness of vancomycin which is widely used to treat MRSA, and delay in institution of appropriate therapy. There is no evidence so far that MRSA are any more or less virulent than MSSA, although strains in each group appear to vary. The glycopeptides are relatively poor anti-staphylococcal antibiotics compared with β-lactams because of slow killing, development of low-level resistance as discussed previously, and poor tissue penetration. There is accumulating evidence that the new oxazolidone linezolid may have better clinical effectiveness against MRSA than the glycopeptides (Wilcox *et al.*, 2004; Wunderink *et al.*, 2003) despite being a bacteriostatic agent, perhaps because of its excellent tissue distribution.

MRSA infections are a very clear example of the adverse clinical effects of multiple antibiotic resistance. Compared with MSSA infections, they have a significantly increased mortality when adjusted for other co-morbidities, and alternative therapies are less effective (glycopeptides), more toxic (vancomycin), or more expensive (linezolid).

4.2. Enterobacteria

E. coli is the leading cause of urinary tract infection and Gram-negative bacteraemia, both in the community and in hospitals. It is naturally susceptible to ampicillin, but now about 50–60% of isolates are resistant worldwide, usually by the production of plasmid-encoded TEM-1 β-lactamase (Stapleton *et al.*, 1995; Wu *et al.*, 1992). Some strains produce TEM-2, a similar enzyme that differs from TEM-1 only by a single amino acid. Organisms producing TEM-1 or TEM-2 are resistant to ampicillin but susceptible to newer cephalosporins.

Mutations in TEM-1 and TEM-2 have resulted in new 'extended-spectrum' β-lactamases (ESBLs) that can break down newer cephalosporins and thus render *E. coli* resistant to them. These ESBLs are named TEM-3, TEM-4, etc., and more than 100 of them have been reported (Jacoby *et al.*, 1991; Phillipon *et al.*, 1989). They are often plasmid-borne and associated with other resistances such as aminoglycoside resistance. ESBL-producers may also mutate to chromosomal quinolone resistance. Multiple drug resistance in *E. coli* is now increasingly common in both community and hospital isolates (Leung *et al.*, 1997), although this is less common in *E. coli* compared with other enterobacteria and *E. coli* does not usually cause outbreaks of cross infection.

Several publications have reported case controlled studies comparing clinical outcomes of patients infected with ESBL-producing *E. coli* or *K. pneumoniae* with those infected with non-ESBL-producing strains. A limitation of many of these studies is the relatively small number of cases and a failure to analyse the contribution of susceptibility to other drugs than the cephalosporins. Various measures of outcome have been used, including mortality, other measures of response to therapy, delay of starting appropriate therapy, length of hospital stay, and costs of treatment. The results are not consistent, but most studies have shown some level of worse outcome in the ESBL groups.

Lautenbach and colleagues (2001) studied various infections with *E. coli* or *K. pneumoniae*. They found a significant delay in starting effective therapy in the ESBL group (a median delay of 72 h compared with 11.5 h), a significantly longer median duration of hospital stay (11 days vs. 2 days) and greater hospital charges (US$67,000 vs. US$22,000). However, there was no significant difference in mortality between the two groups. In a study of *E. coli* and *K. pneumoniae* bacteraemia (Du *et al.*, 2002) antibiotic treatment failure was the only independent risk factor for hospital mortality. ESBL production was associated with inappropriate antibiotic therapy but not with treatment failure. However, patients treated with the carbapenem imipenem were more likely to survive than those treated with cephalosporins. In a study of bacteraemia in paediatric patients (Kim *et al.*, 2002), the mortality rate in the ESBL group was significantly higher than in the non-ESBL group (27% vs. 6%). In patients treated with third-generation cephalosporins with or without an aminoglycoside, the outcome was significantly better in the non-ESBL group. In contrast, Pena *et al.* (2001) studied hospital-acquired *K. pneumoniae* bacteraemia and did not find ESBL-production or inadequate or delayed antibiotic therapy to be associated with a significantly worse outcome when adjusted for other risk factors.

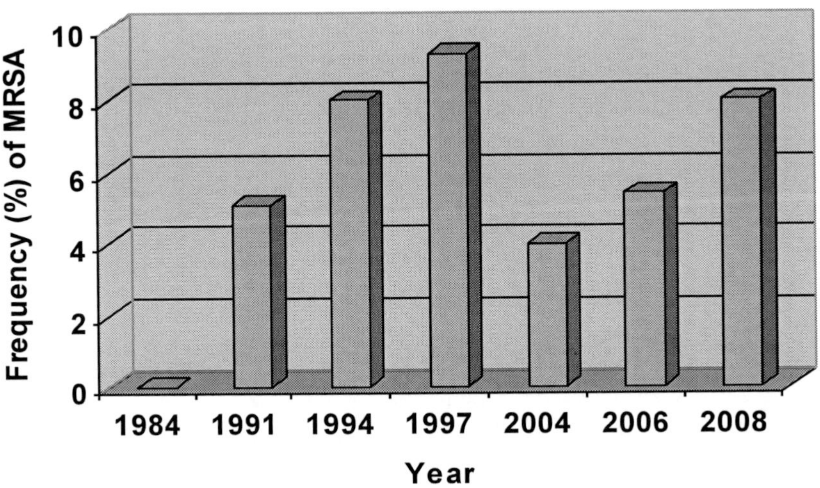

Figure 4. Chart showing the frequency of MRSA isolations (expressed as a percentage of Staphylococcus aureus isolates) at the University Hospital of the West Indies, Jamaica between 1984 and 2008.

Enterobacter spp. normally appear susceptible to third-generation cephalosporins in vitro, although they produce low levels of inducible chromosomal AmpC β-lactamase. However, mutation to constitutive hyperproduction of this β-lactamase is common, and results in complete resistance. This occurs in up to 20% of patients treated with third-generation cephalosporins (Chow *et al.*, 1991; Kaye *et al.*, 2001). In general, patients with cephalosporin-resistant *Enterobacter* infection have an increased risk of mortality compared with those with sensitive organisms (Chow et al., 1991). In a case control study, Cosgrove and colleagues (2002) showed that development of cephalosporin resistance during therapy was associated with significantly increased mortality (5-fold), hospital stay (1.5-fold), and hospital charges (1.5-fold). Taken overall, these results suggest that resistance to third-generation cephalosporins (which is nearly always associated with multiple antibiotic resistance) worsens the clinical outcome of serious infections with enterobacteria.

In Jamaica, a study of ESBL production in *K. pneumoniae* and *E. coli* at the UHWI between January and December 2002, found that 18.2% and 0% of *K. pneumoniae* and *E. coli* isolates, respectively were ESBL producers (Nicholson *et al.*, 2004a). The authors noted that infections with ESBL-producing organisms can pose a therapeutic challenge, leading to treatment failure if the wrong class of antibiotics is used. With increasing resistance to all classes of antibiotics, there is a narrowing of available treatment options. It is very important that these organisms be monitored and antibiotic policies as well as infection control policies be in place to curtail their spread.

4.3. *Pseudomonas aeruginosa*

P. aeruginosa causes about 10% of all hospital-acquired infection and is the third most common cause of hospital-acquired Gram-negative bacteraemia after *E. coli* and *K. pneumoniae*. *P. aeruginosa* is inherently resistant to most penicillins and cephalosporins. It is naturally susceptible to the aminoglycosides, the anti-pseudomonal penicillin piperacillin and the cephalosporin ceftazidime, the quinolones and carbapenems. However, acquired antibiotic resistance to all these agents is common, although most isolates remain susceptible to some of them.

In a study to assess the antibiotic resistance in clinical isolates of *P. aeruginosa* in Jamaica, Brown and Izundu (2004) noted that the aminoglycoside amikacin was the only antibiotic to which all isolates were susceptible, while all of the isolates were resistant to cefaclor, 96.1% were resistant to tetracycline and amoxicillin/clavulanic acid, 90.2% to ampicillin, 84.3% to chloramphenicol, 82.4% to nalidixic acid, 76.5% to kanamycin and 56.9% to trimethoprim/sulfamethoxazole. In addition, most of the isolates were from Kingston and St. Andrew and Manchester. Ten multi-drug resistant isolates were recovered (resistant to eight or more of the antibiotics). In 2005, a study in Kingston and St. Andrew (Finlayson and Brown, unpublished results) noted that 19% and 7% of the isolates were resistant to the aminoglycosides, amikacin and tobramycin, respectively. This contrasts with the results of the previously mentioned multi-parish study, where none and 25% of *P. aeruginosa* isolates were resistant to amikacin and tobramycin, respectively (Brown and Izundu, 2004). The problem of increasing aminoglycoside resistance is becoming a cause for concern as the results from study published a year later in 2005, conducted at the UHWI, found that 11% and 23% of *P. aeruginosa* isolates were resistant to amikacin and gentamicin (Tennant *et al.*, 2005; Figure 5). In Jamaica, amikacin and other aminoglycosides are among the main antibiotics administered for urinary tract infections (UTIs) and other infections including wounds and sepsis, and could be driving the increase observed.

Many of the aminoglycoside-resistant isolates were pigmented and were obtained from ear and respiratory samples, in contrast to the association elsewhere of these with outbreaks of UTIs (Keys and Washington, 1977). These isolates also had low levels of twitching motility, and lipase, DNase and protease activities, which suggest that they may not be as virulent as their aminoglycoside-susceptible counterparts (Khakoo and Kluge, 1978). It has been inferred that increased adherence of aminoglycoside-resistant strains to various cells (when compared to aminoglycoside-susceptible strains) result in these being excellent colonizers or epithelial surfaces. Further, in the absence of expression of virulence factors necessary for systemic invasion, the isolates may only promote superficial localized colonization and infections (Clark *et al.*, 1984).

The impact of drug resistance on the outcome of *P. aeruginosa* infection has been investigated in a few studies, but the results are not consistent. This may be in part because *P. aeruginosa* often colonises human mucosa and it may be difficult to distinguish colonisation from infection, especially in respiratory specimens. Furthermore, invasive disease and bacteraemia tend to occur in highly compromised patients with severe underlying disease, and may be a terminal event in patients dying from other causes. Outcome studies need to take these factors into account when analysing the effect of resistance in this organism.

Carmelli and colleagues (1999) studied the clinical consequences of the development of resistance during the course of a variety of *P. aeruginosa* infections. They reviewed resistance to four classes of anti-pseudomonal antibiotics: the penicillin piperacillin, the cephalosporin ceftazidime, the quinolone ciprofloxacin, and the carbapenem imipenem. Emergence of resistance during treatment was associated with a more than three-fold increase in mortality (27% compared with 7.6%), a ten-fold increase in secondary bacteraemia (14% vs. 1.4%), and a two-fold increase in hospital stay. The increased stay resulted in increased hospital charges. Resistance at baseline was not associated with any of these adverse outcomes. Other studies have found no significant relationship between adverse outcome and antibiotic resistance in *P. aeruginosa* causing bacteraemia (Hilf et al., 1989; Grisaru-Soen et al., 2000) or pneumonia (Paladino et al., 1999). In most cases the outcomes appeared to be determined primarily by the underlying disease of the patients.

Overall, these studies do not show that primary resistance in *P. aeruginosa* is independently associated with a poor outcome, perhaps because patients with serious *P. aeruginosa* infections usually have a poor prognosis due to other risk factors. Further work is needed to determine the relative contributions of antibiotic resistance and underlying disease to outcomes in these infections.

4.4. *Stenotrophomonas maltophilia*

Stenotrophomonas maltophilia is emerging worldwide as a nosocomial pathogen, and has been associated with certain risk factors and a wide range of infections. In recent years, a significant increase in the incidence of *Stenotrophomonas maltophilia* has occurred, particularly in immunocompromised individuals (Elting et al., 1990; Marshall et al., 1989; Morrison et al., 1986; Villarino et al., 1992). In addition to antimicrobial pressure, long-term hospitalization and catheterization are contributory factors to the increased *S.maltophilia* isolation rate evident throughout the country (Elting et al., 1990; Villarino et al., 1992). Often, recovery of *S.maltophilia* tends to be associated with colonization rather than true clinical infection (Laing et al., 1995; Vartivarian et al., 1994; Villarino et al., 1992), yet patients colonized with *S.maltophilia* are treated with antibiotics overextended periods, creating an opportunity for accelerated resistance development. With the exception of trimethoprim-sulfamethoxazole, many post-therapy isolates of *S.maltophilia* become resistant to therapeutic agents initially tested as susceptible by disk or microdilution methods (unpublished epidemiology records).

A retrospective study conducted between April 1997 and December 2000 by Nicholson et al. (2004b) in Jamaica to document the emergence of *S. maltophilia* at the UHWI, and to determine the incidence, distribution and risk factors associated with it, noted that 55% of cases came from the Intensive Care Unit (ICU). The authors noted that there was a slight increase in the prevalence of infection with increasing age, while the surgical service accounted for the largest number of isolates. Of the cases presented, 95.7% were exposed to a wide range of antibiotics and had some form of instrumentation. Underlying disease was found in 71.7% of the patients. *S maltophilia* was found most often in the sputum of ICU patients whereas it was most often isolated from wound swabs in the ward patients. The organism was isolated from blood more often in ICU patients (23.3%) than in ward patients (9.5%) and there was a 44% mortality rate among the cases in ICU compared with those on the wards (4.8%). More recently (2007-2008), Tennant (unpublished results) noted that most isolates of *S. maltophilia* were resistant to the carbapenems (90%) and cephalosporins, ceftriaxone and cefuroxime (94 and 88%, respectively). Frequencies of resistance to amikacin (49%) and gentamicin (45%) were high. However, these isolates appeared sensitive to co-trimoxazole and the fluoroquinolones (Figure 5).

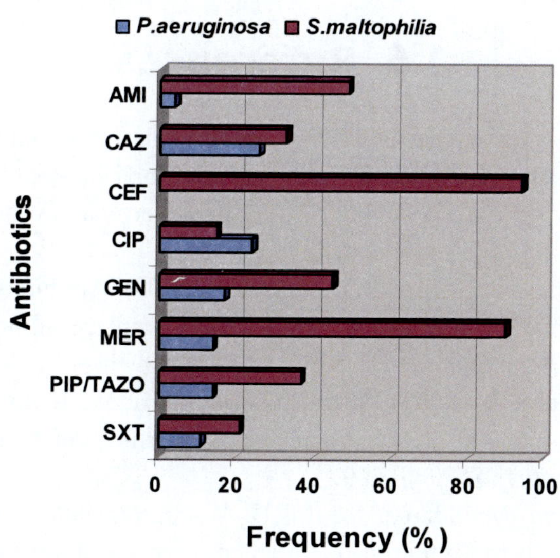

Figure 5. Bar chart showing the frequency of resistance among isolates of P. aeruginosa and S. maltophilia to particular antibiotics

Therapy for *S.maltophilia* is largely empiric; however, the need for effective therapy in significantly immunocompromised patients is critical. Given the rapid emergence of resistant *S. maltophilia* strains to all classes of bactericidal agents, it is unlikely that single-drug therapy will be effective in managing neutropenic patients with severe *S. maltophilia* infections. Present susceptibility methods may be able to detect high-level resistance but are inadequate in predicting true susceptibility and ultimately therapeutic efficacy. Until this information is available, in vitro susceptibility data for *S. maltophilia* should be cautiously interpreted.

5. Conclusion

Since antibiotic use became widespread about 50 years ago, bacteria have steadily and routinely developed resistance. Control of the emergence of resistance in Jamaica and elsewhere will depend on new approaches to prudent antibiotic use in hospitals and clinics, based in part on improved surveillance for MDR bacteria, de-escalation when appropriate, and on better systems to encourage staff adherence to contact isolation procedures. Equally important will be development of new drugs with narrower spectra of activity aimed at known and potentially new targets and the evolution of market conditions that favor their use. Multidrug resistance among certain important bacterial pathogens in Jamaica appear to be proportionately lower than in the developed countries, however, local research has shown an increasing trend. Much of the molecular assessment of multidrug resistance is still in its fledgling status, and further work will possibly demonstrate the significant role that plasmid-mediated genes and/or environmentally-disseminated genes play in the increasing trend observed in both hospital and community settings.

6. References

Aarestrup, FM; Lertworapreecha, M; Evans, MC; Bangtrakulnonth, A; Chalermchaikit, T; Hendriksen, RS; Wegener, HC (2003). Antimicrobial susceptibility and occurrence of resistance genes among *Salmonella enterica* serovar Weltevreden from different countries. *J Antimicrob Chemother 52*: 715–718.

Adhikari, RP; Kalpana, KC; Shears, P; Sharma, AP (2000). Antibiotic resistance conferred by conjugative plasmid in *Escherichia coli* isolated from community ponds of Katmandu Valley. *J Health Popul Nutr 18*:57-59.

Agersø, Y; Guardabassi, L (2005). Identification of Tet39, a novel class of tetracycline resistance determinant in *Acinetobacter* spp. of environmental and clinical origin. *J Antimicrob Chemother 55,* 566–569.

Arakawa, Y; Murakami, M; Suzuki, K; Ito, H; Wacharotayankun, R; Ohsuka, S; Kato, N; Ohta, M (1995). A novel integron-like element carrying the metallo-beta-lactamase gene blaIMP. *Antimicrob Agents Chemother 39,* 1612-1615.

Baraniak, A; Fiett, J; Mrowka, A; Walory, J; Hryniewicz, W; Gniadkowski, M (2005). Evolution of TEM-type extended-spectrum beta-lactamases in clinical *Enterobacteriaceae* strains in Poland. *Antimicrob Agents Chemother 49*, 1872-80.

Bartlett, JG (2004). Pocket Book of Infectious Disease Therapy, 12 edn. Baltimore: Lippincott Williams & Wilkins.

Bass, L; Liebert, CA; Lee, MD; Summers, AO; White, DG; Thayer, SG; Maurer, JJ. (1999). Incidence and characterization of integrons, genetic elements mediating multiple-drug resistance, in avian *Escherichia coli. Antimicrob Agents Chemother. 43*, 2925-2929.

Bennett, PM (1999). Integrons and gene cassettes: a genetic construction kit for bacteria. *J Antimicrob Chemother. 43*, 1-4.

Bodonaik, NC; King, SD; Narla, VR (1984). Antimicrobial resistance i n clinical isolates of Staphylococcus aureus at the University Hospital o f the West Indies. *West Indian Med J 33*, 8—13.

Bou, G; Cartelle, M; Tomas, M; Canle, D; Molina, F; Moure, R; Eiros, JM; Guerrero, A (2002). Identification and broad dissemination of the CTX-M-14 beta-lactamase in different *Escherichia coli* strains in the northwest area of Spain. *J Clin Microbiol. 40*, 4030-4036.

Branthwaite, A; Pechere, JC (1996). Pan-European survey of patients' attitudes to antibiotics and antibiotic use. *J. Int. Med. Res.* 24, 229-238.

Brigante, G; Luzzaro, F; Perilli, M; Lombardi, G; Coli, A; Rossolini, GM; Amicosante, G; Toniolo, A (2005). Evolution of CTX-M-type beta-lactamases in isolates of *Escherichia coli* infecting hospital and community patients. *Int J Antimicrob Agents. 25*, 157-162.

Brinas, L; Zarazaga, M; Saenz, Y; Ruiz-Larrea, F; Torres, C (2002). Beta-lactamases in ampicillin-resistant *Escherichia coli* isolates from foods, humans, and healthy animals. *Antimicrob Agents Chemother. 46*, 3156-3163.

Brown, PD; Izundu, A (2004). Antibiotic resistance in clinical isolates of *Pseudomonas aeruginosa* in Jamaica. *Rev. Panam. Salud Publica 16*, 125–130.

Brown, PD; Ngeno, C (2007). Antimicrobial resistance in clinical isolates of *Staphylococcus aureus* from hospital and community sources in southern Jamaica. *Internat. J. Infect. Dis. 11*, 220-225.

Brumfitt, W; Hamilton-Miller, J (1989). Methicillin-resistant *Staphylococcus aureus. N. Engl. J. Med. 320,* 1188–1196.

Butaye, P; Cloeckaert, A; Schwarz, S (2003). Mobile genes coding for efflux-mediated antimicrobial resistance in Gram-positive and Gram-negative bacteria. *Int J Antimicrob Agents 22*, 205–210.

Bywater, R; Deluyker, H; Deroover, E; de Jong, A; Marion, H; McConville, M; Rowan, T; Shryock, T; Shuster, D; Thomas, V; Valle, M; Walters, J (2004). A European survey of antimicrobial susceptibility among zoonotic and commensal bacteria isolated from food-producing animals. *J Antimicrob Chemother. 54*, 744-754.

Carattoli, A (2003). Plasmid-mediated antimicrobial resistance in *Salmonella enterica. Curr Issues Mol Biol. 5*, 113-122.

Carattoli, A; Bertini, A; Villa, L; Falbo, V; Hopkins, KL; Threlfall, EJ (2005). Identification of plasmids by PCR-based replicon typing. *J Microbiol Methods 63,* 219-228.

Carleton, HA; Diep, BA; Charlebois, ED; Sensabaugh, GF; Perderau-Remington, F (2004). Community-adapted methicillin-resistant *Staphylococcus aureus* (MRSA): population dynamics of an expanding community reservoir. *J. Infect. Dis. 190*, 1730–1738.

Carmelli, Y; Troilett, N; Karchmer, AW; Samore, MH (1999). Health and economic outcomes of antibiotic resistance in *Pseudomonas aeruginosa, Arch. Intern. Med. 159*, 1127–1132.

CDC (Centers for Disease Control and Prevention) (1997a). Reduced susceptibility of *Staphylococcus aureus* to vancomycin - Japan, 1996. *MMWR 46*, 624-626

CDC (Centers for Disease Control and Prevention) (1997b). *Staphylococcus aureus* with reduced susceptibility to vancomycin - United States, 1997. MMWR 46, 765-766.

CDC (Centers for Disease Control and Prevention) (2004). Vancomycin-resistant *Staphylococcus aureus*—New York, 2004, *MMWR 53*, 322–323.

Chang, CY; Chang, LL; Chang, YH; Lee, TM; Chang, SF (2000). Characterization of drug resistance gene cassettes associated with class 1 integrons in clinical isolates of *Escherichia coli* from Taiwan, ROC. *J Med Microbiol. 49(12),* 1097-1102.

Chaslus-Dancla, E; Gerbaud, G; Martel, JL; Lagorce, M; Lafont, JP; Courvalin, P (1987). Detection of a second mechanism of resistance to gentamicin in animal strains of *Escherichia coli. Antimicrob Agents Chemother. 31(8)*, 1274-1277.

Cheung, TK; Chu, YW; Chu, MY; Ma, CH; Yung, RW; Kam, KM (2005). Plasmid-mediated resistance to ciprofloxacin and cefotaxime in clinical isolates of *Salmonella enterica* serotype Enteritidis in Hong Kong. *J Antimicrob Chemother. 56(3)*, 586-589.

Chitnis, V; Chitnis, D; Patil, S; Kant, R (2000). Hospital effluent: a source of multiple drug-resistant bacteria. Current Science, 79, 989-991.

Choi, SM; Kim, SH; Kim, HJ; Lee,DG; Choi, JH; Yoo,JH; Kang, JH; Shin,WS; Kang, MW (2003). Multiplex PCR for the detection of genes encoding aminoglycoside modifying enzymes and methicillin resistance among *Staphylococcus species. J Korean Med Sci. 18(5)*, 631-636.

Chow, JW; Fine, MJ; Shlaes, DM; Quinn, JP; Hooper, DC; Johnson, MP; Ramphal, R; Wagener, MM; Miyashiro, DK; Yu, VL (1991). *Enterobacter* bacteremia clinical features and emergence of antibiotic resistance during therapy. *Ann. Intern. Med. 115*, 585–590.

Clark, RB; Janda, JM; Bottone, EJ (1984). Phenotypic factors correlated with the absence of virulence among gentamicin-resistant *Pseudomonas aeruginosa* strains. *J Clin Microbiol. 20*, 235-238

Cohen, ML (2000): Changing patterns of infectious disease. *Nature*, *406*:762-767.

Cosgrove, SE; Kaye, KS; Eliopoulous, GM; Carmeli, Y (2002). Health and economic outcomes of the emergence of third-generation cephalosporin resistance in *Enterobacter* species. *Arch. Intern. Med. 162*, 185–190.

Cosgrove, SE; Sakoulas, G; Perencevich, EN; Schwaber, MJ; Karchmer, AW; Carmeli, Y (2003). Comparison of mortality associated with methicillin-resistant and methicillin-susceptible *Staphylococcus aureus* bacteremia: a meta-analysis, *Clin. Infect. Dis. 36*, 53–59.

Dahlberg, C; Hermansson, M (1995). Abundance of Tn3, Tn21, and Tn501 transposase (tnpA) sequences in bacterial community DNA from marine environments. *Appl Environ Microbiol. 61(8)*, 3051-3056.

Doublet, B; Butaye, P; Imberechts, H; Boyd, D; Mulvey, MR; Chaslus-Dancla, E; Cloeckaert, A (2004). *Salmonella* genomic island 1 multidrug resistance gene clusters in *Salmonella enterica* serovar Agona isolated in Belgium in 1992 to 2002. *Antimicrob Agents Chemother 48*, 2510–7.

Du, B; Long, Y; Liu, H; Chen, D; Liu, D; Xu, Y; Xie, X (2002). Extended-spectrum beta-lactamase-producing *Escherichia coli* and *Klebsiella pneumoniae* bloodstream infection risk factors and clinical outcome. *Intensive Care Med. 28*, 1718–1723.

Duan, RS; Sit, TH; Wong, SS; Wong, RC; Chow, KH; Mak, GC; Yam, WC; Ng, LT; Yuen, KY; Ho, PL (2006). *Escherichia coli* producing CTX-M beta-lactamases in food animals in Hong Kong. *Microb Drug Resist. 12(2)*, 145-148.

Dugan, J; Rockey, DD; Jones, L; Andersen, AA (2004). Tetracycline resistance in *Chlamydia suis* mediated by genomic islands inserted into the chlamydial *inv*-like gene. *Antimicrob Agents Chemother 48*, 3989–3995.

EARSS (The European Antimicrobial Resistance Surveillance System) Annual Report (2001).

Eguia, JM; Chambers, HF (2003). Community-acquired methicillin resistant *Staphylococcus aureus*: epidemiology and potential virulence factors. *Curr. Infect. Dis. Rep. 5*, 459–466.

Engemann, JJ; Carmeli, Y; Cosgrove, SE; Fowler, VG; Bronstein, MZ; Trivette, SL; Briggs, JP; Sexton, DJ; Kaye, KS (2003). Adverse clinical and economic outcomes attributable to methicillin resistance among patients with *Staphylococcus aureus* surgical site infection. *Clin. Infect. Dis. 36*, 592–598.

Elting, LS; Khardori, N; Bodey, GP; Fainstein, V (1990). Nosocomial infection caused by *Xanthomonas maltophilia*: a case-control study of predisposing factors. *Infect. Control Hosp. Epidemiol. 11*, 134–138.

Fey, PD; Saı¨d-Salim, B; Rupp, ME; Hinrichs, SH; Boxrud, DJ; Davis, CC; Kreiswirth, BN; Schlievert, PM (2003). Comparative molecular analysis of community- or hospital-acquired methicillin-resistant *Staphylococcus aureus*. *Antimicrob. Agents Chemother. 47*, 196–203.

French, GL; Cheng, AF; Ling, JM; Mo, P; Donnan, S (1990). Hong Kong strains of methicillin-resistant and methicillin-sensitive *Staphylococcus aureus* have similar virulence. *J. Hosp. Infect. 15*, 117–125.

Furushita, M; Shiba, T; Maeda, T; Yahata, M; Kaneoka, A; Takahashi, Y; Torii, K; Hasegawa, T; Ohta, M (2003). Similarity of tetracycline resistance genes isolated from fish farm bacteria to those from clinical isolates. *Appl Environ Microbiol. 69*, 5336-5342.

Galland, JC; Hyatt, DR; Crupper, SS; Achelson, DW (2001). Prevalence, antibiotic susceptibility and diversity of *Escherichia coli* 0157:H7 isolates from a longitudinal study of beef cattle feedlots. *Appl Environ Microbiol 67*, 1619-1627.

Gaynes, RP; Cooksey, R; Thornsberry, C; Swenson, JM; Hughes, JM (1987). Mechanism of aminoglycoside resistance among beta-lactam-resistant *Escherichia coli* in the United States. *Diagn Microbiol Infect Dis. 7(1)*, 45-50.

Gebreyes, WA; Thakur, S (2005). Multidrug-resistant *Salmonella enterica* serovar Muenchen from pigs and humans and potential interserovar transfer of antimicrobial resistance. *Antimicrob Agents Chemother 49*: 503–11.

Goldstein, C; Lee, MD; Sanchez, S; Hudson, C; Phillips, B; Register, B; Grady, M; Liebert, C; Summers, AO; White, DG; Maurer, JJ (2001). Incidence of class 1 and 2 integrases in clinical and commensal bacteria from livestock, companion animals, and exotics. *Antimicrob Agents Chemother. 45(3)*, 723-726.

Goussard, S; Courvalin, P (1999). Updated sequence information for TEM beta-lactamase genes. *Antimicrob Agents Chemother. 43(2)*, 367-370.

Grape, M; Sundstrom, L; Kronvall, G (2003). Sulphonamide resistance gene *sul3* found in *Escherichia coli* isolates from human sources. *J Antimicrob Chemother. 52(6)*, 1022-1024.

Grisaru-Soen, G; Lerner-Geva, L; Keller, N; Berger, H; Passwell, JH; Barzilai, A (2000). *Pseudomonas aeruginosa* bacteremia in children analysis of trends in prevalence, antibiotic resistance and prognostic factors. *Pediatr. Infect. Dis. J. 19,* 959–963.

Guardabassi, L; Broennum, PT; Tanoe, R; Dalsgaard, A (2002). Dissemination of vancomycin-resistant enterococci harbouring *vanA* through industrial production of vancomycin. *Microb. Drug Resist. 8*, 401-406.

Guardabassi, L; Dijkshoorn, L; Collard, JM; Olsen, JE; Dalsgaard, A (2000). Distribution and in-vitro transfer of tetracycline resistance determinants in clinical and aquatic *Acinetobacter* strains. *J Med Microbiol 49,* 929–936.

Guardabassi, L; Olsen, JE; Dalsgaard, A (1998). Antibiotic resistance in *Acinetobacter* spp. isolated from sewers receiving waste effluent from a hospital and a pharmaceutical plant. *Appl. Environ. Microbiol. 64*, 3499-3502.

Guerra B, Soto SM, Argüelles JM, Mendoza MC (2001). Multidrug resistance is mediated by large plasmids carrying a class 1 integron in the emergent *Salmonella enterica* serotype [4,5,12:i:-]. *Antimicrob Agents Chemother 45,* 1305–1308.

Guerra, B; Soto, S; Helmuth, R; Mendoza, MC (2002). Characterization of a self-transferable plasmid from *Salmonella enterica* serotype Typhimurium clinical isolates carrying two integron-borne gene cassettes together with virulence and drug resistance genes. *Antimicrob Agents Chemother. 46(9),* 2977-81.

Guerra, B; Junker, E; Schroeter, A; Malorny, B; Lehmann, S; Helmuth, R (2003). Phenotypic and genotypic characterization of antimicrobial resistance in German *Escherichia coli* isolates from cattle, swine and poultry. *J Antimicrob Chemother 52,* 489–492.

Hall, RM; Stokes, HW (1990). The structure of a partial duplication in the integron of plasmid pDGO100. *Plasmid 23*, 76-79.

Hall, RM; Stokes, HW (1993).Integrons: novel DNA elements which capture genes by site-specific recombination. *Genetica 90(2-3)*, 115-132.

Hartman, AB; Essiet, II; Isenbarger, DW; Lindler, LE (2003). Epidemiology of tetracycline resistance determinants in *Shigella* spp. and enteroinvasive *Escherichia coli*: characterization and dissemination of *tet*(A)-1. *J Clin Microbiol 41,* 1023–1032.

Hasman, H; Mevius, D; Veldman, K; Olesen, I; Aarestrup, FM (2005). Beta-Lactamases among extended-spectrum beta-lactamase (ESBL)-resistant *Salmonella* from poultry, poultry products and human patients in The Netherlands. *J Antimicrob Chemother. 56(1)*, 115-121.

Hata, M; Suzuki, M; Matsumoto, M; Takahashi, M; Sato, K; Ibe, S; Sakae, K (2005). Cloning of a novel gene for quinolone resistance from a transferable plasmid in *Shigella flexneri* 2b. *Antimicrob Agents Chemother. 49(2)*, 801-803.

Hilf, M; Yu, VL; Sharp, J; Zuravleff, JJ; Korvick, JA; Muder, RR (1989). Antibiotic therapy for *Pseudomonas aeruginosa* bacteraemia outcome correlations in a prospective study of 200 patients. *Am. J. Med. 87*, 540–546.

Ho, BS; Hare, RS; Shaw, KJ; Miller, GH; Ng, MH (1993). Determination of aminoglycoside resistance mechanisms of *Enterobacteriaceae* isolated from a hospital in Hong Kong with antibiogram and genotyping. *J Antimicrob Chemother. 31(1)*, 174-176.

Horak, R; Kivisaar, M (1998). Expression of the transposase gene tnpA of Tn4652 is positively affected by integration host factor. *J Bacteriol. 180(11)*, 2822-2829.

Huys, G; D'Haene, K; Collard, JM; Swings, J (2004). Prevalence and molecular characterization of tetracycline resistance in *Enterococcus* isolates from food. *Appl Environ Microbiol 70,* 1555–1562.

Ito, T; Katayama, Y; Asada, K; Mori, N; Tsutsumimoto, K; Tiensasitorn, C; Hiramatsu, K (2001). Structural comparison of three types of staphylococcal cassette chromosome *mec* integrated in the chromosome in methicillin-resistant *Staphylococcus aureus*. *Antimicrob. Agents Chemother. 45*, 1323-1336.

Iwanaga, M; Toma, C; Miyazato, T; Insisiengmay, S; Nakasone, N; Ehara, M (2004). Antibiotic resistance conferred by a class I integron and SXT constin in *Vibrio cholerae* O1 strains isolated in Laos. *Antimicrob Agents Chemother 48,* 2364–2369.

Jacoby, GA; Chow, N; Waites, KB (2003). Prevalence of plasmid-mediated quinolone resistance. *Antimicrob Agents Chemother. 47(2)*, 559-562.

Jacoby, GA; Medeiros, AA (1991). More extended-spectrum beta-lactamases. *Antimicrob Agents Chemother. 35*, 1697–1704.

Jacoby, GA; Walsh, KE; Mills, DM; Walker, VJ; Oh, H; Robicsek, A; Hooper, DC (2006). *qnrB*, another plasmid-mediated gene for quinolone resistance. *Antimicrob Agents Chemother, 50(4)*, 1178-1182.

Jarlier, V; Nikaido, H (1994). Mycobacterial cell wall: structure and role in natural resistance to antibiotics. *FEMS Microbiol. Lett. 123*, 11-18.

Jeong, JY; Yoon, HJ; Kim, ES; Lee, Y; Choi, SH; Kim, NJ; Woo, JH; Kim, YS (2005). Detection of qnr in clinical isolates of *Escherichia coli* from Korea. *Antimicrob Agents Chemother. 49(6)*, 2522-2524.

Johnson, AP; Burns, L; Woodford, N; Threlfall, EJ; Naidoo, J; Cooke, EM; George, RC (1994). Gentamicin resistance in clinical isolates of *Escherichia coli* encoded by genes of veterinary origin. *J Med Microbiol. 40(3)*, 221-226.

Johnson, TJ; Wannemuehler, YM; Johnson, SJ; Logue, CM; White, DG; Doetkott, C; Nolan, LK (2007). Plasmid replicon typing of commensal and pathogenic *Escherichia coli* isolates. *Appl Environ Microbiol. 73(6)*, 1976-1983.

Kaye, KS; Cosgrove, S; Harris, A; Eliopoulos, GM; Carmeli, Y (2001). Risk factors for emergence of resistance to broad spectrum cephalosporins among *Enterobacter* species. *Antimicrob. Agents Chemother. 45*, 2628–2630.

Keys, TF; Washington, JF (1977): Gentamicin-resistant *Pseudomonas aeruginosa*: Mayo Clinic experience, 1970-1976. *Mayo Clin. Proc., 52*, 797-801.

Khakoo, RA; Kluge, RM (1978): Decreased virulence of gentamicin-resistant strains of *Pseudomonas aeruginosa* in a rat model. *J. Lab. Clin. Med. 91*, 96-103.

Kim, YK; Pai, H; Lee, HJ; Park, SE; Choi, EH; Kim, J; Kim, JH; Kim, EC (2002). Bloodstream infections by extended-spectrum beta-lactamase-producing *Escherichia coli* and *Klebsiella pneumoniae* in children epidemiology and clinical outcome. *Antimicrob. Agents Chemother. 46*, 1481–1491.

Kuehnert, MJ; Hill, HA; Kupronis, BA; Tokars, JI; Solomon, SL; Jernigan, DB (2005). Methicillin-resistant–*Staphylococcus aureus* hospitalizations, United States. *Emerg Infect Dis 11*. Available from http://www.cdc.gov/ncidod/EID/vol11no06/04-0831.htm

Kümmerer, K (2001). Pharmaceuticals in the environment: sources, fate, effects and risk. Springer, Heidelberg, Germany.

Kümmerer, K (2003). Significance of antibiotics in the environment. *J Antimicrob Chemother 52*, 5-7

Krémery Jr, V; Hanzen, H; Ciznar, P; Brezaniova, T (1997). Vancomycin-resistant *Staphylococcus aureus* in an immunocompromised child with Job's syndrome. *Antibiotic Chemother, 1*, 6.

Laing, FP; Ramotar, K; Read, RR; Alfieri, N; Kureishi, A; Henderson, EA; Louie, TJ (1995). Molecular epidemiology of *Xanthomonas maltophilia* colonization and infection in the hospital environment. *J. Clin. Microbiol. 33*, 513–518.

Lartigue, MF; Leflon-Guibout, V; Poirel, L; Nordmann, P; Nicolas-Chanoine, MH (2002). Promoters P3, Pa/Pb, P4, and P5 upstream from bla(TEM) genes and their relationship to beta-lactam resistance. *Antimicrob Agents Chemother. 46(12)*: 4035-4037.

Lautenbach, E; Patel, JB; Bilker, WB; Edelstein, PH; Fishman, NO (2001). Extended-spectrum beta-lactamase-producing *Escherichia coli* and *Klebsiella pneumoniae* risk factors for infection and impact of resistance on outcomes. *Clin. Infect. Dis. 32*, 1162–1171.

Leflon-Guibout, V; Heym, B; Nicolas-Chanoine, M (2000). Updated sequence information and proposed nomenclature for *bla*(TEM) genes and their promoters. *Antimicrob Agents Chemother. 44(11)*, 3232-4.

Levy, SB; FitzGerald, GB; Macone, AB (1976). Spread of antibiotic-resistant plasmids from chicken to chicken and from chicken to man. *Nature 260*, 40-42.

Li, XZ; Ma, D; Livermore, DM; Nikaido, H (1994). Role of efflux pump(s) in intrinsic resistance of *Pseudomonas aeruginosa*: active efflux as a contributing factor to beta-lactam resistance. *Antimicrob Agents Chemother. 38*, 1742-1752.

Liassine, N; Auckenthaler, R; Descombes, MC; Bes, M; Vandenesch, F; Etienne, J (2004). Community-acquired methicillin-resistant *Staphylococcus aureus* isolated in Switzerland contains the Panton-Valentine leukocidin or exfoliative toxin genes. *J. Clin. Microbiol. 42*, 825–826.

Liebert, CA; Hall, RM; Summers, AO (1999). Transposon Tn21, flagship of the floating genome. *Microbiol Mol Biol Rev. 63(3)*, 507-522.

Linton, AH; Howe, K; Bennett, PM; Richmond, MH; Whiteside, EJ (1977). The colonization of the human gut by antibiotic resistant *Escherichia coli* from chickens. *J Appl Bacteriol 43*, 465-469.

Liu, C; Chambers, HF (2004). *Staphylococcus aureus* with heterogeneous resistance to vancomycin epidemiology, clinical significance, and critical assessment of diagnostic methods. *Antimicrob. Agents Chemother. 47*, 3040–3045.

Lotsu, DK; Imamura, T; Takamine, F (1995). Current status of antimicrobial susceptibility in MRSA isolates typed by coagulase and phage typing in Okinawa. *Acta Med. Okayama 49,* 81-89.

Lu, K; Asano, R; Davies, J (2004). Antimicrobial resistance gene delivery in animal feeds. *Emerg Infect Dis. 10(4)*, 679-683.

Magnet, S; Smith, TA; Zheng, R; Nordmann, P; Blanchard, JS (2003). Aminoglycoside resistance resulting from tight drug binding to an altered aminoglycoside acetyltransferase. *Antimicrob Agents Chemother. 47(5)*, 1577-1583.

Manian, FA (2003). Asymptomatic nasal carriage of mupirocin-resistant *S. aureus* (MRSA) in a pet dog associated with MRSA infection in household contacts. *Clin. Infect. Dis. 36*, 26-28.

Marshall, WF; Keating,MR; Anhalt, JP; Steckelberg, JM (1989). *Xanthomonas maltophilia*: an emerging nosocomial pathogen. *Mayo Clin. Proc. 64*, 1097–1104.

Martinez-Martinez, L; Pascual, A; Garcia, I; Tran, J; Jacoby, GA (2003). Interaction of plasmid and host quinolone resistance. *J Antimicrob Chemother. 51(4)*, 1037-1039.

Martinez-Martinez, L; Pascual, A; Jacoby, GA (1998). Quinolone resistance from a transferable plasmid. *Lancet. 351(9105)*, 797-799.

May, J; Shannon, K; King A; French, GL (1998). Glycopeptide tolerance in *Staphylococcus aureus*. *J. Antimicrob. Chemother. 42*, 189–197.

Maynard, C; Bekal, S; Sanschagrin, F; Levesque, RC; Brousseau, R; Masson, L; Lariviere, S; Harel, J (2004). Heterogeneity among virulence and antimicrobial resistance gene profiles of extraintestinal *Escherichia coli* isolates of animal and human origin. *J Clin Microbiol. 42(12)*, 5444-5452.

Mazel, D (2004). Integrons and the origin of antibiotic resistance gene cassettes. *ASM News. 70(11)*, 520-525.

Mazel, D; Dychinco, B; Webb, VA; Davies, J (1998). A distinctive class of integron in the *Vibrio cholerae* genome. *Science. 280(5363)*, 605-608.

Meng, J; Zhao, S; Doyle, MP; Joseph, SW (1998). Antibiotic resistance of *Escherichia coli* 0157:H7 and 0157:H7NM isolated from animals, foods and humans. *J Food Prot 61*, 1511-1514.

Michel, M; Gutmann, L (1997). Methicillin-resistant *Staphylococcus aureus* and vancomycin-resistant enterococci: therapeutic realities and possibilities, *Lancet 349*, 1901–1906.

Miles, TD; McLaughlin, W; Brown, PD (2006). Antimicrobial resistance of Escherichia coli isolates from broiler chickens and humans. *BMC Veterinary Research, 2*:7

Morrison, AJ; Hoffman, KK; Wenzel, RP (1986). Associated mortality and clinical characteristics of nosocomial *Pseudomonas maltophilia* in a university hospital. *J Clin Microbiol. 24*, 52–55.

Naimi, TS; LeDell, KH; Como-Sabetti, K; Borchardt, SM; Boxrud, DJ; Etienne, J; Johnson, SK; Vandenesch, F; Fridkin, S; O'Boyle, C; Nanila, RN; Lynfield, R (2003). Comparison of community- and health care associated methicillin-resistant *Staphylococcus aureus* infection. *JAMA 290*, 2976–2984.

NNIS (National Nosocomial Infections Surveillance) (2002). System Report, data summary from January 1992 to June 2002, issued August 2002. *Am. J. Infect. Control 30*, 458–475.

Nazic, H; Poirel, L; Nordmann, P (2005). Further identification of plasmid-mediated quinolone resistance determinant in *Enterobacteriaceae* in Turkey. *Antimicrob Agents Chemother. 49(5)*, 2146-2147.

Nemec, A; Dolzani, L; Brisse, S; van den Broek, P; Dijkshoorn, L (2004). Diversity of aminoglycoside-resistance genes and their association with class 1 integrons among strains of pan-European *Acinetobacter baumannii* clones. *J Med Microbiol. 53*, 1233-1240.

Nicholson, AM; Gayle, P; Roye-Green, K (2004a). Extended spectrum beta-lactamase producing organisms at the University Hospital of the West Indies. *West Indian Med J. 53(2),* 104-108.

Nicholson, AM; Castle, D; Akpaka, P; Tennant, I; Nelson, M (2004b). The emergence of *Stenotrophomonas maltophilia* as a significant nosocomial pathogen at the University Hospital of the West Indies. *West Indian Med J. 53(1)*, 17-22.

Nordmann, P; Poirel, L (2005). Emergence of plasmid-mediated resistance to quinolones in *Enterobacteriaceae*. *J Antimicrob Chemother. 56(3)*, 463-469.

Paladino, JA; Sunderlin, JL, Forrest, A; Schentag, JJ (1999). Characterization of the onset and consequences of pneumonia due to fluoroquinolone-susceptible or -resistant *Pseudomonas aeruginosa*. *J. Antimicrob. Chemother. 52*, 457–463.

Paterson, DL; Bonomo, RA (2005). Extended-spectrum beta-lactamases: a clinical update. *Clin Microbiol Rev. 18(4)*, 657-686.

Pechère, JC; Cenedese, C; Müller, O; Perez-Gorricho, B; Ripoll, M; Rossi, A; Stahl, JP; Stahlmann, R; Tramarin, A (2002). Attitudinal classification of patients receiving antibiotic treatment for mild respiratory tract infections. *Int. J. Antimicrob. Agents 20*, 399-406.

Peña, C; Pujol, M; Ardanuy, C; Ricart, A; Pallarés, R; Liñares, J; Ariza, J; Gudiol, F (2001). An outbreak of hospital-acquired *Klebsiella pneumoniae* bacteraemia, including strains producing extended-spectrum beta-lactamase, *J. Hosp. Infect. 47*, 53–59.

Perreten, V; Boerlin, P (2003). A new sulfonamide resistance gene (*sul3*) in *Escherichia coli* is widespread in the pig population of Switzerland. *Antimicrobial Agents and Chemotherapy 47*, 1169–1172.

Petersen, A; Dalsgaard, A (2003). Species composition and antimicrobial resistance genes of *Enterococcus* spp, isolated from integrated and traditional fish farms in Thailand. *Environ Microbiol 5*, 395–402.

Phillips, I; Casewell, M; Cox, T; De Groot, B; Friis, C; Jones, R; Nightingale, C; Preston, R; Waddell, J (2004). Does the use of antibiotics in food animals pose a risk to human health? A critical review of published data. *J Antimicrob Chemother. 53*, 28-52.

Pitout, JD; Gregson, DB; Church, DL; Elsayed, S; Laupland, KB (2005). Community-wide outbreaks of clonally related CTX-M-14 beta-lactamase-producing *Escherichia coli* strains in the Calgary health region. *J Clin Microbiol. 43(6)*, 2844-2849.

Poirel, L; Rodriguez-Martinez, JM; Mammeri, H; Liard, A; Nordmann, P (2005a). Origin of plasmid-mediated quinolone resistance determinant QnrA. *Antimicrob Agents Chemother. 49(8)*, 3523-3525.

Poirel, L; Van De Loo, M; Mammeri, H; Nordmann, P (2005b). Association of plasmid-mediated quinolone resistance with extended-spectrum beta-lactamase VEB-1. *Antimicrob Agents Chemother. 49(7)*, 3091-3094.

Poppe, C; Ziebell, K; Martin, L; Allen, K (2002). Diversity in antimicrobial resistance and other characteristics among *Salmonella typhimurium* DT104 isolates. *Microb Drug Resist 8*, 107–122.

Poyart, C;,Jardy, L; Quesne, G; Berche, P; Trieu-Cuot, P (2003). Genetic basis of antibiotic resistance in *Streptococcus agalactiae* strains isolated in a French hospital. *Antimicrob Agents Chemother 47*, 794–797.

Rådström, P; Swedberg, G; Sköld, O (1991). Genetic analyses of sulfonamide resistance and its dissemination in gram-negative bacteria illustrate new aspects of R plasmid evolution. *Antimicrob Agents Chemother 35* , 1840–1848.

Randall, LP; Cooles, SW; Osborn, MK; Piddock, LJ; Woodward, MJ (2004). Antibiotic resistance genes, integrons and multiple antibiotic resistance in thirty-five serotypes of *Salmonella enterica* isolated from humans and animals in the UK. *J Antimicrob Chemother 53*, 208–216.

Reyes, A; Bello, H; Domínguez, M; Mella, S; Zemelman, R; González, G (2003). Prevalence and types of class 1 integrons in aminoglycoside-resistant *Enterobacteriaceae* from several Chilean hospitals. *J Antimicrob Chemother. 51(2)*, 317-321.

Roberts, MC (2003). Tetracycline therapy: update. *Clin Infect Dis 36*: 462–467.

Roberts, MC (2005). Update on acquired tetracycline resistance genes. *FEMS Microbiol Lett 245*, 195–203

Robicsek, A; Sahm, DF; Strahilevitz, J; Jacoby, GA; Hooper, DC (2005). Broader distribution of plasmid-mediated quinolone resistance in the United States. *Antimicrob Agents Chemother. 49(7)*, 3001-3003.

Robicsek, A; Jacoby, GA; Hooper, DC (2006). The worldwide emergence of plasmid-mediated quinolone resistance. *Lancet Infect Dis, 6(10),* 629-640.

Rodriguez-Avial, I; Rodriguez-Avial, C; Culebras, E; Picazo, JJ (2003). Distribution of tetracycline resistance genes *tet*(M), *tet*(O), *tet*(L) and *tet*(K) in blood isolates of viridans group streptococci harbouring *erm*(B) and *mef*(A) genes. Susceptibility to quinupristin/dalfopristin and linezolid. *Int J Antimicrob Agents 21*, 536–541.

Rodriguez-Martinez, JM; Pascual, A; Garcia, I; Martinez-Martinez, L (2003). Detection of the plasmid-mediated quinolone resistance determinant *qnr* among clinical isolates of *Klebsiella pneumoniae* producing AmpC-type beta-lactamase. *J Antimicrob Chemother. 52(4)*, 703-706.

Rowe-Magnus, DA; Guerout, AM; Mazel, D (1999). Super-integrons. *Res Microbiol. 150*, 641-651.

Rysz, M; Alvarez, PJJ (2004). Amplification and attenuation of tetracycline resistance in soil bacteria: aquifer column experiments. *Water Res 38*, 3705-3712.

Saenz, Y; Brinas, L; Dominguez, E; Ruiz, J; Zarazaga, M; Vila, J; Torres, C (2004). Mechanisms of resistance in multiple-antibiotic-resistant *Escherichia coli* strains of human, animal, and food origins. *Antimicrob Agents Chemother. 48(10)*, 3996-4001.

Salyers, AA (1995). Antibiotic resistance transfer in the mammalian intestinal tract: implications for human health, food safety and biotechnology. R.G. Landes Company, Springer. 42-163.

Sayah, RS; Kaneene, JB; Johnson, Y; Miller, R (2005). Patterns of antimicrobial resistance observed in *Escherichia coli* isolates obtained from domestic- and wild-animal fecal samples, human septage, and surface water. *Appl Environ Microbiol 71*, 1394-1404.

Schroeder, CM; Zhao, C; DebRoy, C; Torcolini, J; Zhao, J; White, DG (2002). Antimicrobial resistance of *Escherichia coli* O157: H7 isolated from humans, cattle, swine and food. *Appl Environ Microbiol 68*, 576-581.

Sekiguchi, J; Fujino, T; Saruta, K; Konosaki, H; Nishimura, H; Kawana, A; Kudo, K; Kondo, T; Yazaki, Y; Kuratsuji, T; Yoshikura, H; Kirikae, T (2004). Prevalence of erythromycin-, tetracycline-, and aminoglycoside-resistance genes in methicillin resistant *Staphylococcus aureus* in hospitals in Tokyo and Kumamoto. *Jpn J Infect Dis 57*, 74–77.

Shannon, KP; French, GL (2004). Increasing resistance to antimicrobial agents of Gram-negative organisms isolated at a London teaching hospital, 1995–2000. *J. Antimicrob. Chemother. 53*, 818–825.

Shanson, DC (1981). Antibiotic resistance in *Staphylococcus aureus*, *J. Hosp. Infect. 2*, 11–36.

Shaw, KJ; Rather, PN; Hare, RS; Miller, GH (1993). Molecular genetics of aminoglycoside resistance genes and familial relationships of the aminoglycoside-modifying enzymes. *Microbiol Rev. 57(1)*, 138-163.

Sköld, O (2000). Sulfonamide resistance: mechanisms and trends. *Drug Resist Updat. 3(3)*, 155-160.

Sköld, O (2001). Resistance to trimethoprim and sulfonamides. *Vet Res 32*, 261-273.

Smith, DL; Harris, AD; Johnson, JA; Silbergeld, EK; Morris, JG (2002). Animal antibiotic use has an early but important impact on the emergence of antibiotic resistance in human commensal bacteria. *Proc Natl Acad Sci USA. 99*, 6434-9.

Solberg, OD; Ajiboye, RM; Riley, LW (2006). Origin of class 1 and 2 integrons and gene cassettes in a population-based sample of uropathogenic *Escherichia coli*. *J Clin Microbiol. 44(4)*, 1347-1351.

Stapleton, P; Wu, PJ; King, A; Shannon, K; French, G; Phillips, I (1995). Incidence and mechanisms of resistance to the combination of amoxicillin and clavulanic acid in *Escherichia coli*. *Antimicrob. Agents Chemother. 39*, 2478–2483.

Stokes, HW; Tomaras, C; Parsons, Y; Hall, RM (1993). The partial 3'-conserved segment duplications in the integrons In6 from pSa and In7 from pDGO100 have a common origin. *Plasmid 30(1)*, 39-50.

Strommenger, B; Kettlitz, C; Werner, G; Witte, W (2003). Multiplex PCR assay for simultaneous detection of nine clinically relevant antibiotic resistance genes in *Staphylococcus aureus*. *J Clin Microbiol 41*, 4089–4094.

Swartz, MN (1994). Hospital-acquired infections: Diseases with increasingly limited therapies *Proc. Natl. Acad. Sci. USA 91*, 2420-2427

Swedberg G; Sköld O (1980). Characterization of different plasmid-borne dihydropteroate synthases mediating bacterial resistance to sulfonamides. *J Bacteriol 142(1)*, 1-7.

Swedberg G; Sköld O (1983). Plasmid-borne sulfonamide resistance determinants studied by restriction enzyme analysis. *J Bacteriol 153(3)*, 1228-1237.

Tennant, I; Harding; H; Nelson, M; Roye-Green, K (2005). Microbial isolates from patients in an intensive care unit, and associated risk factors. *West Indian Med. J. 54*, 225-231.

Tiemersma, EW; Bronzwaer, S; Lyytikainen, O; Degener, JE; Schrijnemakers, P; Bruinsma, N; Monen, J; Witte, W; Grundmann, H; European Antimicrobial Resistance Surveillance System Participants (2004). Methicillin-resistant *Staphylococcus aureus* in Europe, 1999-2002, *Emerg. Infect. Dis. 5*, 34–36.

Toleman, MA; Bennett, P M; Walsh, TR (2006). ISCR elements: Novel gene capturing systems of the 21st Century? *Microbiol. Mol. Biol. Rev. 70*, 296-316.

Toro, CS; Farfán, M; Contreras, I; Flores, O; Navarro, N; Mora, GC; Prado, V (2005). Genetic analysis of antibiotic resistance determinants in multidrug-resistant *Shigella* strains isolated from Chilean children. *Epidemiol Infect 133*, 81–86.

Tran, JH; Jacoby, GA (2002). Mechanism of plasmid-mediated quinolone resistance. *Proc Natl Acad Sci USA. 99,* 5638-5642.

Tran, JH; Jacoby, GA; Hooper, DC (2005). Interaction of the plasmid-encoded quinolone resistance protein Qnr with *Escherichia coli* DNA gyrase. *Antimicrob Agents Chemother, 49(1)*, 118-125.

Vakulenko, SB; Mobashery, S (2003). Versatility of aminoglycosides and prospects for their future. *Clin Microbiol Rev. 16(3)*, 430-450.

van den Bogaard, AE; London, N; Driessen, C; Stobberingh, EE (2001). Antibiotic resistance of faecal *Escherichia coli* in poultry, poultry farmers and poultry slaughterers. *J Antimicrob Chemother. 47(6)*, 763-771.

Vanhoof, R; Content, J; Van Bossuyt, E; Dewit, L; Hannecart-Pokorni, E (1992). Identification of the aadB gene coding for the aminoglycoside- 2''-O-nucleotidyltransferase, ANT(2''), by means of the polymerase chain reaction. *J Antimicrob Chemother. 29(4)*, 365-374.

Vartivarian, SE; Konstantinos, KA; Palacios, JA; Manning Jr, JT; Anaissie, EJ (1994). Mucocutaneous and soft tissue infections caused by *Xanthomonas maltophilia*. *Ann. Intern. Med. 121*, 969–973.

Villarino, ME; Stevens,LE; Schwable,B; Mayers,G; Miller,Jm; Burke,JP; Jarvis, WR (1992). Risk factors for epidemic *Xanthomonas maltophilia* infections/colonizations in the intensive care unit patient. *Infect. Control Hosp. Epidemiol.13*, 201–206.

Viveiros, M; Leandro, C; Amaral, L (2003). Mycobacterial efflux pumps and chemotherapeutic implications. *Int J Antimicrob Agents 22*, 274–278.

Vliegenthart, JS; Ketelaar-van Gaalen, PA; van de Klundert, JA (1991). Nucleotide sequence of the aacC3 gene, a gentamicin resistance determinant encoding aminoglycoside-(3)-N-acetyltransferase III expressed in *Pseudomonas aeruginosa* but not in *Escherichia coli*. *Antimicrob Agents Chemother. 35(5)*, 892-897.

Wang, M; Sahm, DF; Jacoby, GA; Hooper, DC (2004a). Emerging plasmid-mediated quinolone resistance associated with the *qnr* gene in *Klebsiella pneumoniae* clinical isolates in the United States. *Antimicrob Agents Chemother. 48(4)*, 1295-1299.

Wang, M; Sahm, DF; Jacoby, GA; Zhang, Y; Hooper, DC (2004b). Activities of newer quinolones against *Escherichia coli* and *Klebsiella pneumoniae* containing the plasmid-mediated quinolone resistance determinant qnr. *Antimicrob Agents Chemother. 48(4)*:1400-1401.

Wang, M; Tran, JH; Jacoby, GA; Zhang, Y; Wang, F; Hooper, DC (2003). Plasmid-mediated quinolone resistance in clinical isolates of *Escherichia coli* from Shanghai, China. *Antimicrob Agents Chemother. 47(7)*, 2242-2248.

Ward, E; Grinsted, J (1987). The nucleotide sequence of the tnpA gene of Tn21. *Nucleic Acids Res. 15(4)*:1799-1806.

Watanabe, T; Fukasawa, T (1960). Episome mediated transfer of drug resistance in *Enterobacteriaceae. J Bacteriol. 81*, 669-678.

White, PA; McIver, CJ; Rawlinson, WD (2001). Integrons and gene cassettes in the enterobacteriaceae. *Antimicrob Agents Chemother. 45*, 2658-2661.

Wilcox, M; Nathwani, D; Dryden, M (2004). Linezolid compared with teicoplanin for the treatment of suspected or proven gram-positive infections. *J. Antimicrob. Chemother. 53*, 335–344.

Wunderink, RG; Rello, J; Cammarata, SK; Croos-Dabrera, RV; Kollef, MH (2003). Linezolid vs. vancomycin: analysis of two double-blind studies of patients with methicillin-resistant *Staphylococcus aureus* nosocomial pneumonia, *Chest 124*, 1789–1797.

Wu, JJ; Ko, WC; Tsai, SH; Yan, JJ (2007). Prevalence of plasmid-mediated quinolone resistance determinants QnrA, QnrB, and QnrS among clinical isolates of *Enterobacter cloacae* in a Taiwanese hospital. *Antimicrob Agents Chemother, 51(4)*, 1223-1227.

Wu, PJ; Shannon, K; Phillips, I (1992). β-Lactamases and susceptibility to β-lactam antibiotics in *Escherichia coli. J. Antimicrob. Chemother. 30*, 868–871.

Yang, H; Chen, S; White, DG; Zhao, S; McDermott, P; Walker, R; Meng, J (2004). Characterization of multiple-antimicrobial-resistant *Escherichia coli* isolates from diseased chickens and swine in China. *J Clin Microbiol. 42(8)*, 3483-3489.

Zhang, H; Shi, L; Li, L; Guo, S; Zhang, X; Yamasaki, S; Miyoshi, S; Shinoda, S (2004). Identification and characterization of class 1 integron resistance gene cassettes among *Salmonella* strains isolated from healthy humans in China. *Microbiol Immunol. 48(9)*:639-645.

Zuhlsdorf, MT; Wiedemann, B (1992). Tn21-specific structures in gram-negative bacteria from clinical isolates. *Antimicrob Agents Chemother. 36(9)*, 1915-1921.

In: Multiple Drug Resistance
Editors: A. Meszaros, G. Balogh, pp. 99-128

ISBN: 978-1-60741-595-4

Chapter IV

Herb-Drug Interactions and Implication in Drug Monitoring

***Ping Li*[1*] *and Shu-Feng Zhou*[2**]**
[1]Key Laboratory of Modern Chinese Medicines, China Pharmaceutical University, Ministry of Education, No. 24, Tongjia Lane, Nanjing 210009, China.
[2]School of Health Sciences, RMIT University, Victoria 3083, Australia.

Abstract

By searching the literature, it was found that a total of 32 drugs interact with herbal medicines in humans. These drugs mainly include anticoagulants (warfarin, aspirin and phenprocoumon), sedatives and antidepressants (midazolam, alprazolam and amitriptyline), oral contraceptives, anti-HIV agents (indinavir, ritonavir and saquinavir), a cardiovascular drug (digoxin), immunosuppressants (cyclosporine and tacrolimus) and anticancer drugs (imatinib and irinotecan). Most of them are substrates for cytochrome P450s (CYPs) and/or P-glycoprotein (P-gp) and many of which have narrow therapeutic indices. However, several drugs including acetaminophen, carbamazepine, mycophenolic acid, and pravastatin did not interact with herbs. Both pharmacokinetic (e.g., induction of hepatic CYPs and intestinal P-gp) and/or pharmacodynamic mechanisms (e.g., synergistic or antagonistic interaction on the same drug target) may be involved in herb-drug interactions, leading to altered drug clearance, response and toxicity. Toxicity arising from herb-drug interactions may be minor, moderate, or even fatal, depending on a number of factors associated with the patients, herbs and drugs. Predicting drug-herb interactions, timely identification of drugs that interact with herbs and therapeutic drug monitoring may minimize toxic drug-herb interactions. Predicting pharmacokinetic herb-drug interactions is likely if one follows the pharmacokinetic principles and utilizes proper models that are used for predicting drug-drug interactions. Identification of drugs that interact with herbs can be incorporated into the early stages of drug development.

* Corresponding author: Tel: +86 25 95391244; Fax: +86 25 85322747., E-mail: liping2004@126.com or lipingli@public1.ptt.js.cn.
** Tel: +61 3 9925 7794; Fax: +61 3 9925 7178., Email:_shufeng.zhou@rmit.edu.au.

More studies are needed and new approaches are required to minimize toxicity arising from herb-drug interactions.

Keywords: herb-drug interaction; cytochrome P450; P-glycoprotein; drug monitoring.

1. Introduction

Herbal products are becoming popular as alternative medicines in the Western world and an estimated one-third of adults in the developed countries use herbal medicines. There are about 11,000 species of herbal plants for medicinal use and about 500 species of them are commonly used in Traditional Chinese Medicine. The World Health Organization (WHO) defines herbal supplements as "Finished, labelled medicinal products that contain active ingredients from aerial or underground parts of plants, or other plant material, or combinations thereof, whether crude state or as other preparations" [1]. These herbs are often coadministered with therapeutic drugs, raising the potential of herb-drug interactions. There are an increased number of reports on herb-drug interactions, although many of them are from case reports and limited clinical observations [2].

Herb-drug interactions may be significantly under-reported and underestimated, and probably more frequently than drug-drug interactions. Potential interaction of herbal medicines with drugs is a major safety concern, especially, for drugs with narrow therapeutic indices (e.g., warfarin and digoxin), and may lead to severe adverse reactions that are sometimes life-threatening. Due to the potential clinical outcomes of herb-drug interactions, there is a strong necessity to characterize, analyse and predict these interactions. Here, the common pharmacological properties of drugs that have been reported to interact with herbs are discussed in this paper. This may provide a strategy for predicting a drug's potential for interaction with herbs and for designing new drugs that do not interact with herbs.

2. Properties of Drugs that Interact or do not Interact with Herbs

2.1. Drugs Reported to Interact with Herbs

The author has reviewed the literature to identify reported interactions between herbal medicines and prescribed drugs in humans. Literature searches were performed using the following databases: Medline (via Pubmed), Biological Abstracts, Cochrane Library, and Embase (all from their inception to November 2008). In addition, a number of Chinese journals related to herbal studies were hand-searched from the first publication date onwards. All human *in vivo* studies relating to herb-drug interactions were included, whereas data from animal and *in vitro* drug interaction studies were excluded except for those exploring mechanisms for herb-drug interactions. Human studies included case reports, case series, clinical trials or other types of studies.

As shown in **Table 1**, a total of 32 drugs have been found to interact with herbal medicines in humans. These drugs mainly include anticoagulants (warfarin, aspirin and phenprocoumon), sedatives and antidepressants (midazolam, alprazolam and amitriptyline), anti-HIV agents (indinavir, ritonavir and saquinavir), oral contraceptives, cardiovascular drug (digoxin), immunosuppressants (cyclosporine and tacrolimus) and anticancer drugs (imatinib and irinotecan). Most of them are chronically used by oral route, or in combination with other drugs.

Many of these drugs including warfarin, digoxin, cyclosporine and theophylline have narrow therapeutic indices. Warfarin (*Coumadin*) is one of the most frequently prescribed drugs used to prevent blood clotting. There are some reports of interactions between warfarin and herbs such as St John's wort, danshen [3], Dong quai [4], ginseng [5], and ginkgo [6, 7]. Ginkgo may interact with warfarin, as a few case reports link concomitant use of ginkgo and warfarin with the development of intracerebral haemorrhage [8]. However, ginkgoes interfere with platelet function, and have been associated with bleeding even in the absence of warfarin or other anticoagulant treatments [9]. It is not known whether there are any pharmacokinetic interactions between ginkgo and warfarin, but rat studies have indicated that the pharmacokinetics of warfarin are not altered after a single or multiple doses of ginseng [10]. Moreover, some herbs such as Dong quai contain coumarins, which may augment the effects of a coumarin-derived anticoagulant [9].

Most drugs in Table 1 are extensively metabolized by cytochrome P450s (CYPs), in particular, CYP3A4. For example, warfarin is extensively metabolized by CYP1A2, 3A4, and 2C9, thus the efficacy of warfarin may be affected when metabolism of warfarin (in particular S-enantiomer) is altered by coadministered herbs [11]. Among CYPs, the subfamily CYP3A is responsible for the metabolism of about 60% of the currently known therapeutic drugs [12-16]. CYP3A subfamily in humans includes CYP3A4, 3A5, 3A7 [16], and 3A43 [17]. CYP3A4 has the highest abundance in the human liver (~40%) and metabolizes more than 50% of the clinically used drugs [13, 18], whereas polymorphic CYP3A5 accounts for 5–50% of total CYP3A abundance [19, 20] and is present in an appreciable amount in about 25% of the adult population [21].

Not surprisingly, many drugs in Table 1 are also substrates for P-glycoprotein (P-gp). P-gp (MDR1/ABCB1) is a 170 kDa plasma glycoprotein encoded by the human *MDR1* gene, belonging to the ATP-binding cassette family of transporters [22-24]. P-gp is expressed constitutively in a number of normal tissues and is found at high levels on the apical surfaces of epithelial cells in the liver (bile canaliculi), kidney (proximal tubule), pancreas (pancreatic ductal cell), small intestine and colon (columnar mucosal cell) and adrenal gland [25, 26]. Moreover, P-gp is present at high levels in the blood-brain barrier, limiting the penetration of a number of drugs into the brain [27-29]. P-gp in the intestine, liver and kidney may play an important role in the absorption, distribution, or excretion of drugs [24, 30-33]. It has been shown that the oral absorption and brain penetration of P-gp substrates are significantly lower in normal mice compared with $mdr1a^{-/-}$ mice [34]. P-gp is subject to induction and inhibition by a number of herbal components [35].

2.2. Drugs Reported Not to Interact with Herbs

On the other hand, clinical studies have indicated that several drugs including acetaminophen, carbamazepine, mycophenolic acid, digoxin, warfarin and pravastatin did not interact with concomitant herbs (Table 2). Among these drugs, only digoxin and pravastatin are P-gp substrates. Acetaminophen and mycophenolic acid undergo extensive Phase II (conjugation) metabolism, while carbamazepine and pravastatin are mainly metabolized by CYPs. Carbamazepine has inducing effects on multiple CYP enzymes [36], but it is not a substrate of P-gp [37]. It appears that when a drug is mainly metabolized by Phase II reaction and is not a P-gp substrate, its potential for herbal interaction is reduced.

3. Potential Mechanisms for Herb-Drug Interactions

For most reported herb-drug interactions, the mechanisms are unknown. However, it is suggested that both pharmacokinetic and pharmacodynamic components of drugs can be altered by coadministered herbs [11].

3.1. Pharmacokinetic Mechanisms

Pharmacokinetic herb-drug interactions are caused due to altered absorption, metabolism, distribution and excretion of drugs. The underlying mechanisms for the altered drug concentrations by concomitant herbal medicines are always to be determined, but the induction or inhibition of hepatic and intestinal CYPs and P-gp have been suggested [38-43]. The CYP superfamily may be particularly vulnerable to modulation by the multiple active constituents of herbs, as it is well known that the CYPs are subject to induction and inhibition by exposure to a wide variety of xenobiotics.

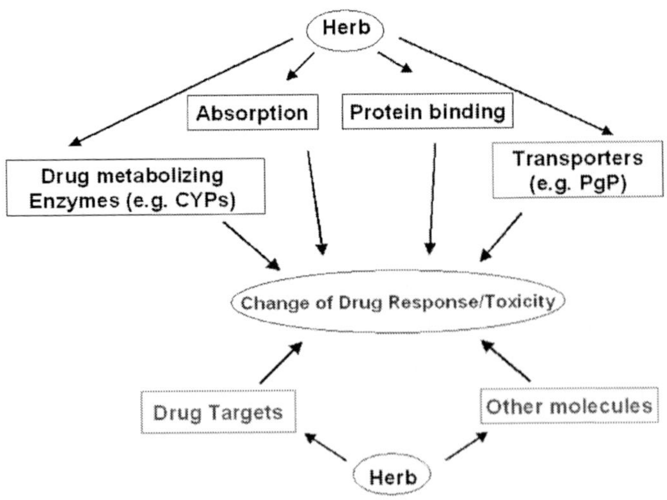

Figure 1. Pharmacokinetic and pharmacodynamic mechanisms for herb-drug interactions.

A number of herbs may be inducers or inhibitors of intestinal and hepatic CYPs, leading to altered drug metabolism and clearance [43]. For example, In vitro studies have demonstrated that St John's wort extract was a potent inducer of CYP2B6 and 3A4, and the responsible component was hyperforin [44-46]. St John's wort extracts have also been reported to inhibit the activities of recombinant CYP1A2, 2C9, 2C19, 2D6, and 3A4 [47]. Animal studies also indicate that St John's wort is a potent modulator of various CYP enzymes using probe drugs. Administration of St John's wort extract (140 or 280 mg/kg/day) to the mouse for 3 weeks resulted in a 2-fold increase in both the CYP3A and 2E1 activities [48], and the administration of St John's wort extract to rats resulted in a significant increase in hepatic CYP3A4 protein expression [49]. In addition, St John's wort is an inducer of CYP3A4 as indicated by increased urinary 6β-hydroxycortisol/cortisol ratio [50]. Clinical studies using a probe drug cocktail indicated that long-term (2 weeks) St John's wort administration in humans significantly induced intestinal and hepatic CYP3A4, but did not alter the CYP2C9, 1A2, or 2D6 activities when probe substrates were used [50]. *In vitro* studies have shown that hyperforin was a potent ligand (K_i = 27 nM) for the pregnane X receptor [44], which is an orphan nuclear receptor regulating expression of CYP2B6 and 3A4 [46, 49]. However, treatment of low-dose of St John's wort (240 mg/day) for 10 days did not affect the pharmacokinetics of alprazolam, caffeine, tolbutamide, and digoxin in healthy subjects [51]. In vitro studies indicated that garlic constituents modulated various CYP enzymes. Extracts from fresh and aged garlic inhibited CYP3A4 in human liver microsomes [52]. A number of garlic preparations (aged, odourless, oil, freeze-dried) and 3 varieties of fresh garlic bulbs (common, Elephant and Chinese) have been examined for their potential to alter cDNA-expressed human CYP2C9,, 2C19, 2D6, 3A4, 3A5 and 3A7 activities using an in vitro fluorometric microtiter plate assay [52]. In vivo studies in the mouse indicated that garlic administration increased CYP2E1 and 1A2 levels, although it did not change the total content of hepatic CYP [53].

Herbs may inhibit CYPs by three mechanisms: competitive inhibition, non-competitive inhibition, and mechanism-based inhibition [43]. Mutual competitive inhibition may occur between herbal constituent and drug, which are often metabolised by the same CYP enzyme. For example, diallyl sulfide from garlic is a competitive inhibitor of CYP2E1 [54]. Non-competitive inhibition is caused by the binding of herbal constituents containing electrophilic groups (e.g. imidazole or hydrazine group) to the haem portion of the CYP molecule. For example, piperine inhibited arylhydrocarbon hydroxylase (CYP1A) and 7-ethoxycourmarin deethylase (CYP2A) by non-competitive mechanism [55]. Hyperforin present in St John's wort is a potent non-competitive inhibitor of CYP2D6 activity [47]. The mechanism-based inhibition of CYP is due to the formation of a complex between herbal metabolite with CYP. Diallyl sulfone is a suicide inhibitor of CYP2E1 by forming complex, leading to autocatalytic destruction of CYP2E1 [56].

Herbs can also modulate the expression and activity of P-gp [35]. Several studies also indicate that St Johns wort induce intestinal P-gp *in vitro* and *in vivo* [49, 57, 58]. Treatment of LS-180 intestinal carcinoma cells with St John's wort or hypericin at 3-300 μM caused 4-to 7-fold increase in the expression of P-gp [58]. Cells chronically treated with St John's wort had decreased accumulation of rhodamine 123. The administration of St John's wort extract to rats for 14 days resulted in a 3.8-fold increase of intestinal P-gp expression [49]. Oral administration of St John's wort for 14 days in healthy volunteers resulted in a 1.4-fold increase in P-gp expression [49]. The probe substrates of P-gp, fexofenadine and cyclosporine were found to have increased clearance in healthy subjects treated with St John's wort [59]. Moreover, chronic treatment with St John's wort (16 associated with enhanced drug efflux function resulting in reduced intracellular accumulation of rhodamine. In addition, ginsenosides Rg_1, Re, Rc, and Rd were found to have a moderate inhibitory effect on P-gp [60].

Herbs are often given orally and thus herbal constituents may modulate gastrointestinal pH and motility. Due to high concentrations in the gut lumen, herbal constituents are likely to exert a major effect on intestinal enterocytes. These cells represent the first cell lining limiting entry of orally administered drugs into the body. Both P-gp and CYP3A4 are expressed at high levels in the villus tip of enterocytes, the primary site of absorption for orally administered drugs. The interplay of both intestinal P-gp and CYP3A4 determines bioavailability of many drugs such as cyclosporine [61], midazolam [62], HIV protease inhibitors [63], verapamil [64], digoxin [65], and talinolol [66]. Thus, the modulation of intestinal P-gp and CYP3A represents an important mechanism for the enhanced or reduced bioavailability of coadministered drugs.

Since most CYPs are polymorphic, pharmacogenetic study may play a role in herb-drug interactions. In a recent clinical study involving 18 healthy Chinese subjects, treatment of *G. biloba* (140 mg, bid) for 12 days significantly decreased the plasma concentrations of omeprazole and its sulfone conjugate, while 5-hydroxyomeprazole level was significantly increased [67]. A significant decrease in the ratio of omeprazole AUC to 5-hydroxyomeprazole was observed in poor and extensive metabolizers with regard to *CYP2C19* genotype, with the decrease be greater in poor metabolizers than extensive metabolizers [67]. No significant changes in the AUC ratios of omeprazole to its sulfone were observed. These results indicate that ginkgo is able to induce CYP2C19 and thus enhance omeprazole hydroxylation in a *CYP2C19* genotype-dependent manner. Thus, cautions should be taken when patients concomitantly take ginkgo and CYP2C19 substrates.

Another study in healthy volunteers investigated both short- and long-term effects of St John's wort on the pharmacokinetics of the antifungal voriconazole, which is metabolized by CYP3A4, 2C9 and 2C19 [68]. In this controlled, open-label study, single oral doses of 400 mg voriconazole were administered to 16 healthy men stratified for *CYP2C19* genotype before and on day 1 and day 15 of concomitant St John's wort intake (300 mg LI 160 3 times daily). During the initial 10 hours of the first day of St John's wort administration, the area under the plasma concentration-time curve (AUC) of voriconazole was increased by 22% compared with control, whereas the AUC was reduced by 59% after 15 days of St John's wort intake, with a corresponding increase in oral voriconazole clearance (CL/F) by 144% [68]. The baseline CL/F of voriconazole and the absolute increase in CL/F were smaller in carriers of 1 or 2 deficient *CYP2C19*2* alleles compared with wild-type individuals. These results indicate that coadministration of SJW results in a short-term but clinically irrelevant increase followed by a prolonged extensive reduction in voriconazole exposure. *CYP2C19* wild-type individuals are at highest risk for potential voriconazole treatment failure in patients on St John's wort.

Detailed pharmacogenetic studies are needed to explore the role of mutations in genes encoding CYPs and P-gp in the drug-herb interactions. In particular, for drugs that have narrow therapeutic indices, there is great potential for pharmacogenetics to characterize the drug-herb interactions. The findings would provide insights into genetic factors influencing drug-herb interactions.

3.2. Pharmacodynamic Mechanisms

Combined use of herbs with drugs may mimic, increase, or reduce the effects of either component, resulting in clinically important herb-drug interactions [6, 7, 69, 70]. Synergistic or additive therapeutic effects may lead to unfavourable toxicities and complicate the dosing regimen of long-term medications, while antagonistic interactions will result in decreased efficacy and therapeutic failure. The synergistic or antagonistic effects often result from the competitive or complementary effect of the drug and the combined herbal constituents on the same drug target.

There was a one-case report of interaction between kava and alprazolam that may have caused a semicomatose state in a 54-year old man [71]. The patient was taking cimetidine, alprazolam and terazosin with self-medicated kava for 3 days prior to hospitalization. The authors suggested that both kavalactones and alprazolam had additive effects, since both act on the same γ-aminobutyric acid (GABA) receptors [72, 73]. A 80-year old women with Alzheimer's disease fell into coma when taking a low dose of the atypical antidepressant, trazodone, and ginkgo [74]. The mechanism is unclear, but it may be associated with enhanced GABA-related neuronal activity in the brain by ginkgo. Furthermore, cases have been reported where the combination of St John's wort and selective serotonin re-uptake inhibitors (e.g. sertraline and nefazodone) caused symptoms characteristic of central serotonergic syndrome [75-79], in particular in the elderly. This syndrome is characterized by confusion, agitation, hyperreflexia, shivering or tremor, diaphoresis, nausea, diarrhea, lack of co-ordination, fever, coma, flushing or rhabdomyolysis [80]. This may be due to that St John's wort inhibited rat vesicular uptake of monamines including serotonin, dopamine and norepinephrine [81, 82].

4. Clinical Outcomes of Drug-Herb Interactions

4.1. Altered Drug Pharmacokinetics

Herbs that could modulate intestinal or hepatic CYPs or P-gp may lead to changes in drug pharmacokinetic parameters such as the AUC and maximum plasma concentration (C_{max}), which are related to drug efficiency and toxicity [2]. Many commonly used herbs have been shown to modulate the plasma clearance of important therapeutic drugs. Clinical studies has documented that St John's wort reduced the plasma the area of the plasma concentration-time curve (AUC) of cyclosporin [83, 84], amitriptyline [85], digoxin [86], indinavir [87], nevirapine [88], oral contraceptives [89], warfarin [89], phenprocoumon [90], theophylline [91], and simivastatin [92]; garlic supplement decreased the plasma AUC and maximum plasma concentration (C_{max}) of the protease inhibitor saquinavir [93]; piperine increased C_{max} and AUC of phenytoin [94], propranolol, and theophylline [95]; and glycyrrhizin from Licorice increased the plasma AUC of prednisolone.

4.2. Altered Drug Efficacy

Drug efficacy may be changed when combined with herbs. For example, a few case reports of interactions between cyclosporine and St John's wort had been published [96-99]. The published cases concerned patients who received transplantation of heart, liver, kidney and pancreas. Decreased blood trough concentrations of cyclosporine had been observed and this was associated with transplant graft rejection observed in all of these cases.

The altered drug response of herb-drug interactions depends on factors that are related to coadministered drugs (dose, dosing regimen, administration route, pharmacokinetic and therapeutic range), herbs (species, dose, dosing regimen, and administration route) and patients (genetic polymorphism, age, gender and pathological conditions) [100]. Generally, a doubling or more in drug plasma concentration/AUC has the potential for enhanced drug effects and/or appearance of adverse effects. However, less marked changes may still be clinically important for drugs with a steep concentration-response relationship or a narrow therapeutic index. In most cases, the extent of herb-drug interaction varies markedly among individuals, depending on interindividual differences in drug metabolizing enzymes (in particular CYP3A4) and transporters (e.g. PgP), existing medical condition, age and other factors [35, 43].

4.3. Toxicity Concerns

A major safety concern is potential interactions of herbal products with prescribed drugs. This issue is especially important with respect to drugs with narrow therapeutic indexes (e.g. warfarin and digoxin) [101]. This may lead to adverse reactions that are sometimes life-threatening or lethal [102]. For example, when St John's wort was combined with oral contraceptives (ethinylestradiol/desogestrel), loperamide, or selective serotonin-reuptake inhibitors (sertaline, paroxetine, nefazodone), it caused intermenstrual bleeding, delirium, or mild serotonin syndrome, respectively [69, 103, 104]. Ginseng induced mania when used concomitantly with phenelzine [105]. Ginkgo raised blood pressure when combined with a thiazide diuretic and coma when combined with trazodone [74, 106]. Garlic produced hypoglycaemia when taken with chlorpropamide. Kava caused a semicomatose state when given concomitantly with alprazolam [71].

5. Strategy for Eliminating Toxicity Arising from Drug-Herb Interactions

5.1. Predicting Herb-Drug Interactions

There is of importance for the prediction of herb-drug metabolic interactions, as toxic or fatal herb-drug interaction may be avoided. It may be necessary to assess the clinical risks by predicting qualitatively and quantitatively drug–herb interactions. A simple qualitative prediction of the potential for herbal interaction may be made based on the properties of drugs. For example, if a drug is a substrate for CYP3A4 and P-gp, its potential for herbal interaction would be increased. Generally, it can be anticipated that a herb such as St John's wort containing potent CYP3A4/P-gp inducers would decrease the bioavailability of coadministered drugs that are primarily metabolized by CYP3A4, due to intestinal and/or hepatic induction of CYP3A4 and P-gp.

However, the quantitative prediction of drug-herb interactions would be difficult. Unlike the prediction of metabolic drug-drug interactions where there have been a number of successes with those drugs mainly metabolized by CYPs [107], the prediction of herb-drug metabolic interaction appears difficult due to the following reasons: a) herb preparations may contain multiple CYP-modulating constituents, with unknown amounts and inhibition/induction potency for CYPs; b) the inhibitor/induction of CYP by herbs may by temporally distinguishable, depending on the herb's dosing, administration route and tissues; c) many herbs are used chronically; d) marked variability in the contents of herbal constituents [108]; and e) drug-related factors such as inappropriate design of *in vitro* experiments; presence of extra-hepatic metabolism; and active transport in liver. In addition, the *in vitro* scaling of kinetic and inhibition data from human tissues is more complex, particularly as the metabolism of many drugs by CYP3A4, which metabolize >50% therapeutic drugs, was inconsistent with classical Michaelis-Menten kinetic models [109, 110].

To obtain successful prediction for herb-drug metabolic interactions, the following basic criteria should be met before quantitative correlations of *in vivo* pharmacokinetic data obtained from *in vitro* metabolic inhibition data based on *in vitro* models such as hepatic microsomes and hepatocytes [47, 111]: a) drug clearance must be primarily through metabolism; b) drug is not subject to substantial conjugation or other non-CYP metabolism; c) the liver is the primary organ of metabolic clearance; and d) the compound does not possess physiochemical properties that are associated with absorption problems (i.e. limited solubility, low intestinal permeability). The following factors determine the degree of change in plasma concentration at steady-state (C_{ss}) and AUC caused by the herb-drug interaction in vivo [111, 112]:

- The route of administration (intravenous or oral, i.e., whether the drug undergoes first-pass metabolism).
- Fraction (f_h) of hepatic clearance (CL_h) in total clearance (CL_{tot}).
- Fraction (f_m) of the metabolic process subject to inhibition in CL_h.
- Unbound concentration of the inhibitory herbal component ([I]) around the CYP and inhibition constant (K_i).
- Plasma unbound concentration [S] of the drug subject to inhibition. Michaelis-Menten constant (K_m) for the drug subject to inhibition.

The effects of inhibition of drug metabolism on in vivo pharmacokinetics are highly variable and depend on a number of factors associated with the drug and combined herb (dose and the route of administration) and patients. Generally, the extent of inhibition (R, %) of drug metabolism by herbal constituents depends on the inhibition mechanism when the substrate concentration [S] is high. For example, the R value of a particular metabolic pathway by a competitive inhibitor from co-administered herb can be calculated by Eq. 1 [109, 110, 113]:

$$R\,(\%) = \frac{[I]}{[I] + K_i \times (1 + [S]/K_m)} \times 100 \quad \text{(Eq.1)}$$

where [S] and [I] are the maximal unbound substrate and inhibitor concentration respectively; K_i, the inhibitory constant; and K_m, Michaelis-Menten constant. When multiple inhibitory herbal constituents are involved, R is calculated by Eq. 2:

$$R\,(\%) = \sum_{i=1}^{n} \left[\frac{[I_i]}{[I_i] + K_{i(i)} \times (1 + [S]/K_m)} \times 100 \right] \quad \text{(Eq. 2)}$$

In clinical situations, [S] is often much lower than K_m, then R is expressed by Eq.3, independent of the inhibition nature, except for the uncompetitive inhibition [114]:

$$R\,(\%) = \frac{1}{1 + K_i/[I]} \times 100 \quad \text{(Eq.3)}$$

From Eq. 3, given that both f_h and $f_m \rightarrow 1$, and f_u remains unchanged, it is clear that the AUC ratio ($\frac{AUC'}{AUC}$, the ratio of AUC in the presence of inhibitor over that in the absence of inhibitor) is calculated by

$$\text{AUC ratio} = \frac{AUC'}{AUC} = \frac{CL_{int}}{CL_{int}'} = 1 + [I]/K_i \quad \text{(Eq.4)}$$

where CL_{int} is the intrinsic clearance inhibited by the inhibiting constituent; ' represents the value after alteration by herb-drug interaction. Since herbs usually contain multiple inhibitory constituents, an herb-drug interaction *in vivo* is considered likely if the following is true:

$$\text{AUC ratio} = 1 + \sum_{i=1}^{n} \left[[I_i]/K_{i(i)} \right] \quad \text{(Eq.5)}$$

where $[I_i]$ is the maximal unbound inhibitor concentration of each inhibitory constituent, $K_{i(i)}$, the inhibition constant for each constituent, n, the number of inhibitory constituents in the herb.

The expected AUC ratio in steady-state concentration or the AUC by an inhibiting constituent is dependent on the route of administration, as this will determine if the drug undergoes first pass in the liver and/or the gut [109, 110, 115]. If drugs are administered by i.v. bolus, AUC ratio can be calculated by Eq. 6:

$$\text{AUC ratio} = \frac{AUC'}{AUC} = \frac{C_{ss}'}{C_{ss}} = \frac{CL_{tot}}{CL_{tot}'} = \frac{CL_h/f_h}{CL_h' + CL_h/f_h - CL_h} = \frac{1}{f_h \times CL_h'/CL_h + 1 - f_h} \quad \text{(Eq. 6)}$$

where f_h is the fraction of hepatic clearance in total clearance; CL_h is the hepatic clearance; and ' represents the value after alteration by drug interaction.

For high clearance drugs administered by i.v. bolus, CL_h is rate-limited by the flow rate. When the altered CL_h remains rate-limited by the flow rate, then $CL_h = CL_h'$, i.e. AUC ratio = 1, AUC is not altered. However, this is not true when the inhibition is extensive that CL_h is not limited by the flow rate. However, for a low clearance drug administered by i.v., AUC ratio is given by Eq. 7.

$$\text{AUC ratio} = \frac{1}{f_h \times f_m \times CL_{\text{int}}'/CL_{\text{int}} + 1 - f_h \times f_m} \qquad \text{(Eq. 7)}$$

where CL_{int} is the intrinsic clearance inhibited by the inhibiting constituent; ' represents the value after alteration by herb-drug interaction; and f_m is the fraction of the specific metabolic pathway in hepatic clearance. In the clinical settings, [S] is often much lower than K_m, then AUC ratio is given by the following equation [109, 110]:

$$\text{AUC ratio} = \frac{1}{f_h \times f_m \times \left\{\frac{1}{(1+[I]/K_i)}\right\} + 1 - f_h \times f_m} \qquad \text{(Eq.8)}$$

Obviously, the AUC ratio is determined by K_i, [I], f_h, and f_m, but not by K_m or [S]. It should be noted that multiple inhibitory herbal constituents are always involved in the inhibition of the same metabolic pathway of a drug, thus AUC ratio is calculated by Eq. 9.

$$\text{AUC ratio} = \frac{1}{\sum_{i=1}^{n}\left[f_h \times f_m \times \left\{\frac{1}{(1+[I]/K_i)}\right\} + 1 - f_h \times f_m\right]} \qquad \text{(Eq. 9)}$$

The change in AUC_{po} after a single oral administration and that in C_{ss} after repeated oral administration can be expressed by the following equation, if the dose and administration interval is constant.

$$\text{AUC ratio} = \frac{1}{[f_h \times CL_h'/CL_h + 1 - f_h] \times \frac{F_h}{F_h'}} \qquad \text{(Eq. 10)}$$

where F_h is hepatic availability, ' represents the value after alteration by herb-drug interaction. Since the first-pass hepatic availability is close to unity for low clearance drugs, Eq.9 & 10 are also valid for low clearance drug by oral route. However, for high clearance drug by oral route, the AUC ratio is given by Eq. 11, if the dose and administration interval is constant:

$$\text{AUC ratio} = \frac{1}{f_m \times \left\{\frac{1}{(1+[I]/K_i)}\right\} + 1 - f_m} \quad \text{(Eq. 11)}$$

When the herb contains multiple inhibitory constituents for CYP enzymes, AUC ratio is calculated by Eq. 12.

$$\text{AUC ratio} = \frac{1}{\sum_{i=1}^{n}\left[f_m \times \left\{\frac{1}{(1+[I]/K_i)}\right\} + 1 - f_m\right]} \quad \text{(Eq.12)}$$

Obviously, it is necessary to know the values of K_i, [I], f_h, f_m, and n to predict *in vivo* metabolic herb-drug interactions [109, 110]. The values of f_h and f_m can be determined from the urinary recovery of the parent molecule and each metabolite. K_i can be estimated by *in vitro* inhibition studies using liver microsomes, hepatocytes and cDNA-expressed microsomes. However, the determination of these parameters is difficult for herbs which often contain multiple components and low plasma levels are reached when administered.

The observed $[I_i]$, K_i and estimated AUC ratio for St John's wort, ginkgo and milk thistle are shown in

Table 3. The expected AUC ratio was mainly dependent on [I], K_i, f_h, number of inhibitory herbal constituents (n) and f_m. As shown in Figure 2 for Eq.5, herb-drug interactions would be with low risk if $\sum_{i=1}^{n}\left[[I_i]/K_{i(i)}\right]$ is less than 0.1, medium risk if it is between 0.1-1.0, and high risk if it is greater than 1.

Table 4 shows the estimated AUC ratio (based on Eq.5) with regard to a CYP enzyme inhibited by individual herbal constituents using St John's wort, ginkgo and milk thistle as examples. It appeared that St John's wort might cause medium to high risk for metabolic interactions with drugs that are primarily metabolized by CYP1A2, 2C9, 2D6 or 3A4, whereas both ginkgo and milk thistle would just cause low risk for metabolic interactions with drugs that are mainly eliminated by these enzymes, with an exception for CYP3A4 by milk thistle (AUC ratio = 1.47).

The AUC ratio due to herb-drug combination can be estimated using Eq. 9. Coadministration of St John's wort was expected to significantly increase the AUC values of most CYP3A4 substrates such as carbamazepine, cyclosporine A, indinavir, midazolam and tacrolimus, but it would not remarkably change the AUC of caffeine, theophylline (both CYP1A2 substrates) and dextromethorphan (CYP2D6 substrate). Digoxin, a minimally metabolized drug by CYP3A4, would not interact with gingko due to metabolic interaction. However, these predictions did not fall into reasonable ranges except for theophylline (estimated vs observed AUC ratio: 1.07:1.00). Indeed, coadministered St John's wort significantly reduced AUC values of most combined CYP3A4 substrate drugs in humans [116], indicating the induction of CYP3A4 and/or PgP. St John's wort caused no change of

AUC for carbamazepine in humans. These findings reflect the difficulties and complexity when predicting herb-drug interactions.

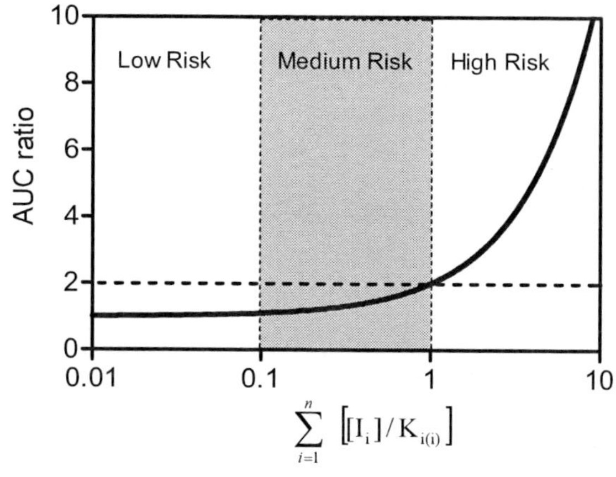

Figure 2. Quantitative prediction of herb-drug interaction based on inhibitor concentration ($[I_i]$) and inhibition constant (K_i).

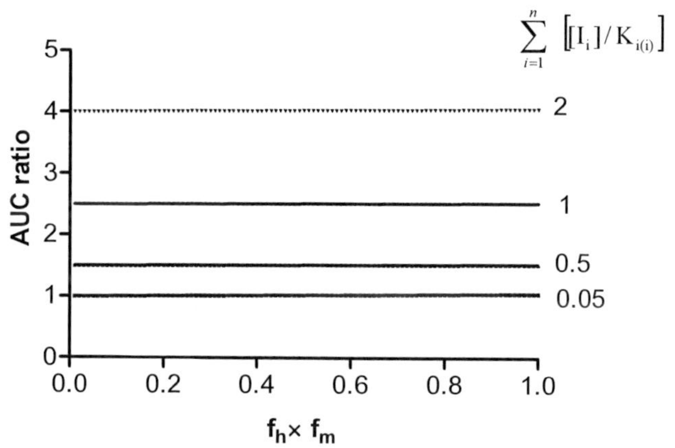

Figure 3. Effect of hepatic (f_h) and metabolic fraction (f_m) on the AUC ratio.

The effects of coadministered herb on drugs depend on a number of factors associated with the herb, drug and the patient. For high clearance drugs (e.g. imipramine and propranolol), their CL_h is rate-limited by the hepatic blood flow rate (Q) but insensitive to changes in protein binding and enzyme activity. When $f_u \times CL_{int} >> Q$, $CL_h = Q$. Thus the change of $f_h \times f_m$ had minor influence on AUC ratio when $\sum_{i=1}^{n} [[I_i]/K_{i(i)}]$ values were fixed (Figure 2). For low clearance drugs such as diazepam and tolbutamide, hepatic metabolism often constitutes the major pathway of their elimination and CL_h of these drugs is mainly affected by changes in their binding to plasma proteins (but not affected by hepatic blood flow). Thus, the f_m values (usually > 0.75) of these drugs did not significantly affect the AUC ratio.

5.2. Timely Identification of Drugs that Interact with Herbs

To avoid or minimize toxic drug-herb interactions, it is important to identify drugs that can interact with herbs using proper in vitro and in vivo models in the early stages of drug development. This information is useful for providing warning and proper advices to patients in clinical practice. The identification of drugs causing drug-herb interactions and the mechanisms involved are important in term of rational use of therapeutic drugs. As in vitro drug-drug and drug-CYP interaction studies have been incorporated into drug development, studies on herb-drug, herb-CYP and herb-P-gp interactions should also be included. The application of high throughput approaches to the study of drug-herb, herb-CYP and herb-P-gp interactions is becoming possible. If potential toxic drug-herb interactions have been observed, the combined use of related drugs and herbs should be generally avoided. In some cases where the avoidance is difficult, proper dose adjustment or alternative drugs may be needed.

5.3. Therapeutic Drug Monitoring

Monitoring plasma concentrations of concurrently administered drugs that are CYP3A4 substrates and/or have narrow therapeutic indices and observing for signs of clinical toxicity are necessary. Due to frequent pharmacokinetic drug-herb interactions by modulating CYPs and P-gp, monitoring of plasma concentrations of drugs with narrow therapeutic indices are always important in patients also taking herbs. This will allow early identification of potential drug-herb interactions and subsequent toxicities. For example, when HIV protease inhibitors are used in combination with Milk thistle, therapeutic drug monitoring is always necessary. Herbal components may also behave as mechanism-based CYP3A4 inhibitors. Treatment of milk thistle at 175 mg (equivalent to silymarin 153 mg) 3 times per day for 3 weeks caused a 9% and 25% reduction in the AUC and mean trough level of indinavir, respectively (C8, the concentration at 8 hours) in healthy volunteers [117]. Therefore, monitoring of plasma indinavir concentrations is required when the patients also take Milk thistle.

Caution should be taken when drugs are used in combination with herbs, particularly when for drugs narrow therapeutic indices. In some instances, if the combination cannot be avoided, proper dose adjustment or alternative drugs may be needed. For example, St John's wort reduces the plasma concentrations of cyclosporine and may result in organ rejection. Such interactions will require an increased dose of cyclosporine.

6. Conclusions and Future Perspectives

Both pharmacokinetic and/or pharmacodynamic mechanisms may be involved in drug-herb interactions, leading of altered drug clearance, response and toxicity. A major safety concern is potential interactions of herbal products with drugs. This issue is especially important with respect to drugs with narrow therapeutic indexes (e.g., warfarin and digoxin).

This may lead to adverse reactions that are sometimes lethal. The clinical consequences of herb-drug interactions depend on factors that are related to drug, herb and patient.

High throughput screening assays may represent a useful strategy for the study of drug-herb interactions. They are capable of handling the great number of herbal constituents (e.g., a single herb usually contains dozens of constituents), and have the ability to provide in vitro inhibition data as a criterion for monitoring herb-drug metabolic interactions involving human drug metabolizing enzymes (in particular the CYPs) and/or P-gp. For example, a high throughput screening procedure has been validated to assess the effects of dietary and herbal flavonoids on human CYP1A1 expression using HepG2 cells expressing this enzyme [118]. The application of genomic and proteomic approaches to the study of drug-herb interactions, as well as the use of heterogeneous expression systems (e.g., for CYP3A4 or P-gp), has the potential to lead to a more effective screen due to a high-throughput capacity. *In silico* approaches also represent a useful tool for the study of herb-CYP interactions as demonstrated by hyperforin of St John's wort. Recently, the crystal structure of PXR has been elucidated, and four hydrophobic regions and one hydrogen bond acceptor have been identified, allowing molecules of differing sizes to bind in multiple orientations [119]. More possible ligands of PXR arising from herbal products are expected to be identified with this model.

For new drug application, its potential for CYP interactions is needed by the FDA and subsequently *in vitro* drug-drug and drug-CYP interaction studies have been incorporated into drug development. Given that herb-drug interactions in humans are increasingly reported and fatal events are highly possible, studies on drug-herb, herb-CYP and herb-P-gp interactions should also be included and implemented at the early stage of drug development. With the current techniques, it is increasingly possible to identify drugs that are highly likely to interact with herbs. By screening drug candidates for possible interactions with CYPs and P-gp, it is possible to identify and eliminate such chemicals at an early stage of development.

Clinicians should adopt proper strategies to minimize toxic drug-herb interactions. Early identification of drugs that interact with herbs and the mechanism involved is important. Identification of drugs that interact with herbs can be incorporated into the early stages of drug development. If these drugs have to be used in combination with the herbs in some instances, rational use of such drugs becomes necessary, including the use of a safe drug combination regimen, dose adjustment, and discontinuation of therapy when toxic drug-herb interactions occur. When herbs are combined with drugs with narrow therapeutic indices, the monitoring of plasma drug concentrations and observing of potential toxicities should be conducted. Predicting the risks for potential herb-drug interactions following proper pharmacokinetic principles that are used for predicting drug-drug interactions and in vitro–in vivo extrapolation is likely.

Table 1. Drugs that have been reported to interact with herbs in humans

Drugs	CYP(s) substrate	P-gp substrate	Interacting herb	Study type & subject No.	Outcomes of interaction	Possible mechanism	References
Alprazolam	3A4	–	SJW	BAC; 7 HV	↓AUC by 41%, $t_{1/2}$ by 24%; ↑ C_{max} by 15% ($P > 0.05$)	Minor induction of CYP3A4	[120]
Amitriptyline	2C19, 2D6, 3A4	–	SJW	Open BAC; 12 PTS	↓AUC (amitriptyline) by 22% and nortriptyline by 41%	Induction of CYP3A	[85]
Aspirin	–	–	Ginkgo	Case report	Spontaneous hyphema	Additive effect	[121]
Cyclosporine	3A4	+	SJW	Case report & series; 88 PT	↓blood concentration and rejection events	Induction of enzyme and P-gp	[84, 89, 96, 99, 122-126]
			SJW	BAC; 11 PTS	↓AUC by 46%, C_{max} by 42%, C_{trough} by 41%, altered metabolite profiles	Induction of enzyme and P-gp	[127]
Dextromethorphan	2D6	–	SJW	BAC	⇔dextromethorphan metabolic ratio		[120]
Digoxin	–	+	SJW	Placebo-controlled parallel study; 25 HV	↓AUC by 25%, C_{max} by 33%, C_{trough} by 26%,	P-gp induction	[86]
			Ginkgo	Open crossover; 8 HV	↑AUC by 21.9%, ⇔C_{max} and $t_{1/2}$	Modulation of P-gp?	[128]
			Siberian ginseng	Case report; 1 PT	↑digoxin concentration	Interference with assay	[129]
Fexofenadine	–	+	SJW	Open BAC; 12 HV	↓C_{max} by 45% and oral CL by 20% (single dose of herb)	P-gp inhibition	[130]
Imatinib	3A4	+	SJW	Open crossover; 10 HV	↓AUC by 32%, C_{max} by 29%	CYP3A induction	[131]
			SJW	Open fixed-sequence; 12 HV	↓AUC by 30%, ↑CL by 42%	CYP3A induction	[132]
Indinavir	3A4	+	SJW	BAC; 8 HV	↓AUC by 57%, C_{trough} by 81%	Enzyme induction	[87]
			Milk Thistle	Open crossover, 10 HV	↓AUC by 9%, ↓ trough level (C_8) by 25%	Modulation of CYP3A and P-gp	[117]
Irinotecan	3A4 (minor)	+	SJW	Open BAC; 5 PTS	↓SN-38 by 42%, ↓myelosuppression	Modulation of P-gp?	[133]
Loperamide	Unknown	Unknown	SJW	Case report; 1PT	Acute delirium episode	MAO inhibition	[134]

Table 1. (Continued)

Drugs	CYP(s) substrate	P-gp substrate	Interacting herb	Study type & subject No.	Outcomes of interaction	Possible mechanism	References
Levodopa			Kava	Case report	↑ "off" period	Unknown	[135]
Methadone	3A4, 2C8, 2D6	Unknown	SJW	Case series; 4 PTS	↓C_{trough} by 47%	Enzyme induction	[136]
Midazolam	3A4	–	SJW	BAC; 12 HV	↑oral CL by 108.9% and ↓oral bioavailability by 39.3%; ↓20% of AUC (i.v.)	Induction of CYP3A4	[137]
			SJW	BAC; 21 HV	↑1.5-fold (i.v.) and 2.7-fold (oral) of CL.	Induction of CYP3A4	[59]
Nefazodone	3A4	Unknown	SJW	Case report; 1PT	Nausea, vomiting, headache	Additive effect on serotonin uptake inhibition, enzyme inhibition?	[75]
Nevirapine	2B6, 3A4	–	SJW	Case report; 1 PT	↑CL	Induction of Enzyme and P-gp	[88]
Omeprazole	2C19, 3A4	–	SJW	12 HV, crossover			[138]
Paroxetine	2D6	Unknown	SJW	Case report; 1 PT	Nausea, weakness, lethargy	Additive effect on serotonin uptake inhibition, enzyme inhibition?	[76]
Oral contraceptives	3A4	Unknown	SJW	Single-blind sequential, 16 HV	↓13-15% in norethindrone and ethinyl estradiol levels. ↑breakthrough bleeding	Enzyme induction	[139]
Phenprocoumon	Unknown	Unknown	SJW	Single-blind, placebo-controlled, crossover; 10 HV	↓AUC by 17.4%	Enzyme induction?	[90]
Procyclidine	–	–	Betel nut	Case reports	Severe extrapyramidal symptoms (rigidity, tremor, bradykinesis)	Antagonism of procyclidine by arecoline	[140]
Propranolol	1A2	–	Piperine	Open crossover; 6 HV	time to C_{max}, ↑C_{max} and AUC	CYP1A2 inhibition	[95]

Table 1. (Continued)

Drugs	CYP(s) substrate	P-gp substrate	Interacting herb	Study type & subject No.	Outcomes of interaction	Possible mechanism	References
Ritonavir			Garlic	Open crossover, 10 HV	↓AUC by 17%, ⇔C_{max}	Minor induction of CYP3A4 and P-gp	[141]
Saquinavir			Garlic	Open crossover, 10 HV	↓AUC by 51%, ↓C_{8h} by 49%, ↓C_{max} by 54%	Induction of CYP3A4 and P-gp	[93]
Sertraline	2B6, 2C9, 2C19, 2D6, 3A4	Unknown	SJW	Case series; 5 PTS	Nausea, vomiting, anxiety, confusion, restlessness, manic episode	Additive effect on serotonin uptake inhibition, enzyme inhibition?	[75, 77]
Simvastatin	3A4	+	SJW	Double-blind, crossover; 16 HV	↓C_{max} & AUC of simvastatin hydroxy acid	Induction of enzyme and PgP	[92]
Tacrolimus	3A4	+	SJW	BAC; 10 PTS	↓AUC by 57.8%	Induction of enzyme and PgP	[142]
Theophylline	1A2	–	Piperine	Open crossover; 6 HV	↑C_{max}, $t_{1/2}$, AUC	Inihhition of enzymes	[95]
			SJW	Case report; 1 PT	↓blood level	Enzyme induction	[91]
Tolbutamide	2C9	–	SJW	BAC; 12 HV	⇔AUC, CL, C_{max}, V_d, $t_{1/2\beta}$, ↑hypoglycemia episode	Additive effect?	[137]
Trazodone			Ginkgo	Case report	Coma	Unknown	[74]
Voriconazole	3A4, 2C9, 2C19	Unknown	SJW	Controlled, open-label, 16 HV	↓AUC by 59%; ↑oral CL by 144%	Enzyme induction	[68]
Warfarin	2C9	–	SJW	Case series; 7PTS	↓INR	Enzyme induction	[89]
			Garlic	Case report; 1 PT	↑INR and clotting time	Additive effect	[143]
			Donggui	Case reports; 2 PTS	↑INR and bruise	Herb as COX inhibitor	[144, 145]
			Ginkgo	Case report; 1 PT	PT16.9, PTT35.5, left parietal hemorrhage	Additive effect	[146]
			Ginseng	Case report; 1 PT	↓INR to 1.5	Additive effect	[5]
			Danshen	Case reports; 3 PTS	↑INR	Additive effect	[144, 147, 148]

AUC = area under the plasma concentration-time curve; BAC = before and after comparison; C_{max} = maximum plasma concentration; CL = clearance; HV = Healthy volunteers; INR = internationally normalized ratio; MAO = Monoamine oxidase; PTS = Patients; SJW = St John's wort; $t_{1/2\beta}$ = elimination half-life; TDM = therapeutic drug monitoring. ↑ = Increase; ↓ = Decrease; ⇔ = Unchanged.

Table 2. Drugs lacking interaction with herbs in humans

Drugs	CYP(s) substrate	P-gp substrate	Study type & subject No.	Concomitant herbs	References
Acetaminophen	1A2, 3E1	–	BAC, 16 HV	Garlic	[149]
Carbamazepine	3A4, 2C8	–	Open BAC; 8 HV	SJW	[150]
Digoxin	–	+	Crossover, 8HV	Hawthorn	[151]
Mycophenolic acid	–	–	BAC, 10 PTS	SJW	[142]
Pravastatin	3A4	+	Double-blind crossover, 16 HV	SJW	[92]
Warfarin	2C9	–	Open label, three-way crossover, 12 HV	Ginkgo or ginger	[152]

Table 3. The $[I_i]$, K_i and AUC ratio for St John's wort, ginkgo and milk thistle

Herb	CYP inhibited	Major constituent	$[I_i]$ (μM)	K_i (μM)	$\sum_{i=1}^{n}[[I_i]/K_{i(i)}]$	Estimated AUC ratio (R)	Risk of herb-drug interaction
St John's wort	CYP1A2	I3,II8-Biapigenin	0.05	0.95	0.11	1.11	Medium
		Quercetin	0.2	3.3			
	CYP2C9	Hyperforin	1.0	1.8	0.66	1.66	Medium
		Hypericin	0.15	1.4			
	CYP2D6	Hyperforin	0.15	1.5	0.18	1.18	Medium
		I3,II8-Biapigenin	0.05	2.3			
		Hypericin	0.15	2.6			
	CYP3A4	Hyperforin	1.0	0.49	3.39	4.39	High
		I3,II8-Biapigenin	0.05	0.038			
		Hypericin	0.15	4.2			
Ginkgo	CYP1A2	Ginkgolide A	0.08	2.4	0.04	1.04	Low
		Ginkgolide B	0.01	2.4			
	CYP2C9	Ginkgolide A	0.08	0.9	0.09	1.09	Low
		Ginkgolide B	0.01	1.2			
	CYP2C19	Ginkgolide A	0.08	2.1	0.04	1.04	Low
		Ginkgolide B	0.01	2.2			
	CYP2D6	Ginkgolide A	0.08	3.9	0.02	1.02	Low
		Ginkgolide B	0.01	5.2			

Table 3. (Continued)

Herb	CYP inhibited	Major constituent	$[I_i]$ (μM)	K_i (μM)	$\sum_{i=1}^{n}[[I_i]/K_{i(i)}]$	Estimated AUC ratio (R)	Risk of herb-drug interaction
	CYP3A4	Ginkgolide A	0.08	3.2	0.03	1.03	Low
		Ginkgolide B	0.01	3.4			
Milk thistle	CYP2E1	Silybin	2.1	28.7	0.08	1.08	Low
		Silydianin	0.2	65.8			
		Silycristin	0.1	36			
	CYP3A4	Silybin	2.1	4.9	0.47	1.47	Medium
		Silydianin	0.2	8.1			
		Silycristin	0.1	6.5			

aAUC ratio was estimated using equation 5.

bData for St John's wort are from Obach et al. 2000 [47]; Biber et al. 1998 [153] and Brockmoller et al., 1997 [154]. Data for Ginkgo are from Mauri et al. 2001[155] and Zou et al. 2002 [156]. Data for milk thistle are from Weyhenmeyer et al. 1992 [157] and Zuber et al. 2002 [158].

Table 4. Predicted metabolic herb-drug interactions

Herb + Drug	$\sum_{i=1}^{n}[[I_i]/K_{i(i)}]$	Major CYP involved	f_h	f_m	Estimated AUC ratio	Observed AUC ratio	Ref.
St John's wort							
Caffeine	0.11	1A2	0.95	0.79	1.08	0.80	[159]
Carbamazepine	3.39	3A4	0.80	0.65	1.97	0.99	[150]
Cyclosporine A	3.39	3A4	0.94	0.76	2.63	0.54	[127]
Indinavir	3.39	3A4	0.85	0.70	2.20	0.43	[87]
Dextromethorphan	0.18	2D6	0.88	0.82	1.13	0.8	[159]
Midazolam	3.39	3A4	0.88	0.75	2.42	0.50-0.80	[59, 137]
Tacrolimus	3.39	3A4	0.86	0.70	2.22	0.42-0.65	[142, 160]
Theophylline	0.11	1A2	0.84	0.69	1.06	1.00	[161]
Ginkgo							
Digoxin	0.03	3A4	0.10	0.05	1.02	1.20	[150]
Milk thistle							
Indinavir	0.47	3A4	0.85	0.70	1.24	0.91	[117]

aAUC ratio was estimated using equation 9.

Abbreviations

AUC	area under the plasma concentration-time curve
CL	total body clearance
CL_h	hepatic clearance
C_{max}	maximum plasma concentration
C_{ss},	plasma concentration at steady-state
CNS	central nervous system

CYP	cytochrome P450
γ-aminobutyric acid	GABA
IC_{50}	concentration inhibiting 50% of the effect
K_i	inhibition constant
K_m,	Michaelis-Menten constant
PgP	P-glycoprotein
INR	internationally normalized ratio
$t_{1/2\beta}$	elimination half-life.

References

[1] WHO. World Health Organization Program on Traditional Medicines: Guidelines for the assessment of herbal medicines. Geneva: *World Health Organization*, 1991.

[2] Hu, Z; Yang, X; Ho, PC; Chan, SY; Heng, PW; Chan, E; et al. Herb-drug interactions: a literature review. *Drugs*, 2005, 65, 1239-82.

[3] Tam, LS; Chan, TYK; Leung, WK; Critchley, JAJH. Warfarin Interactions with Chinese traditional medicines: danshen and methyl salicylate medicated oil. *Aust NZ J Med*, 1995, 25, 258.

[4] Page, RL; 2nd, Lawrence, JD. Potentiation of warfarin by dong quai. *Pharmacotherapy*, 1999, 19, 870-6.

[5] Janetzky, K; Morreale, AP. Probable interaction between warfarin and ginseng. *Am J Health-Syst Pharm*, 1997, 54, 692-3.

[6] Fugh-Berman, A. Herb-drug interactions. *Lancet*, 2000, 355, 134-8.

[7] Fugh-Berman, A; Ernst, E. Herb-drug interactions: review and assessment of report reliability. *Br J Clin Pharmacol*, 2001, 52, 587-95.

[8] Vaes, LP; Chyka, PA. Interactions of warfarin with garlic, ginger, ginkgo, or ginseng: nature of the evidence. *Ann Pharmacother*, 2000, 34, 1478-82.

[9] Chan, TY. Interaction between warfarin and danshen (*Salvia miltiorrhiza*). *Ann Pharmacother*, 2001, 35, 501-4.

[10] Zhu, M; Chan, KW; Ng, LS; Chang, Q; Chang, S; Li, RC. Possible influences of ginseng on the pharmacokinetics and pharmacodynamics of warfarin in rats. *J Pharm Pharmacol*, 1999, 51, 175-80.

[11] Kaminsky, LS; Zhang, ZY. Human P450 metabolism of warfarin. *Pharmacol Ther*, 1997, 73, 67-74.

[12] Rendic, S. Summary of information on human CYP enzymes: Human P450 metabolism data. *Drug Metab Rev.*, 2002, 34, 83-448.

[13] Rendic, S; Di Carlo, FJ. Human cytochrome P450 enzyme: a status report summarizing their reactions, substrates, induction, and inhibitors. *Drug Metab Rev.*, 1997, 29, 413-580.

[14] Wormhoudt, LW; Commandeur, JNM; Vermeulen, NPE. Genetic polymorphisms of human N-acetyltransferase, cytochrome P450, glutathione-S-Transferase, and epoxide hydrolase enzymes: relevance to xenobiotic metabolism and toxicity. *Crit Rev Toxicol*, 1999, 29, 59-124.

[15] Rodrigues, AD; Rushmore, TH. Cytochrome P450 pharmacogenetics in drug development: In vitro studies and clinical consequences. *Curr Drug Metab*, 2002, 3, 289-309.

[16] Nelson, DR; Koymans, L; Kamataki, T; Stegeman, JJ; Feyereisen, R; Waxman, DJ; et al. P450 superfamily: update on new sequences, gene mapping, accession numbers and nomenclature. *Pharmacogenetics*, 1996, 6, 1-42.

[17] Domanski, TL; Finta, C; Halpert, JR; Zaphiropoulos, PG. cDNA cloning and initial characterization of CYP3A43, a novel human cytochrome P450. *Mol Pharmacol*, 2001, 59, 386-92.

[18] Shimada, T; Yamazaki, H; Mimura, M; Inui, Y; Guengerich, FP. Interindividual variations in human liver cytochrome P450 enzymes involved in the oxidation of drugs, carcinogens and toxic chemicals. *J Pharmacol Exp Ther*, 1994, 270, 414-23.

[19] Kuehl, P; Zhang, J; Lin, Y; Lamba, J; Assem, M; Schuetz, J; et al. Sequence diversity in CYP3A promoters and characterization of the genetic basis of polymorphic CYP3A5 expression. *Nat Genet*, 2001, 27, 383-91.

[20] Westlind-Johnsson, A; Malmebo, S; Johansson, A; Otter, C; Andersson, TB; Johansson, I; et al. Comparative analysis of cyp3a expression in human liver suggests only a minor role for cyp3a5 in drug metabolism. *Drug Metab Dispos*, 2003, 31, 755-61.

[21] Wrighton, SA; Brian, WR; Sari, MA; Iwasaki, M; Guengerich, FP; Raucy, JL; et al. Studies on the expression and metabolic capabilities of human liver cytochrome P450IIIA5 (HLp3). *Mol Pharmacol*, 1990, 38, 207-13.

[22] Schinkel, AH; Jonker, JW. Mammalian drug efflux transporters of the ATP binding cassette (ABC) family: an overview. *Adv Drug Deliv Rev.*, 2003, 55, 3-29.

[23] Borst, P; Elferink, RO. Mammalian ABC transporters in health and disease. *Annu Rev Biochem*, 2002, 71, 537-92.

[24] Ambudkar, SV; Dey, S; Hrycyna, CA; Ramachandra, M; Pastan, I; Gottesman, MM. Biochemical, cellular, and pharmacological aspects of the multidrug transporter. *Annu Rev Pharmacol Toxico*l, 1999, 39, 361-98.

[25] Gottesman, MM; Pastan, I. Biochemistry of multidrug resistance mediated by the multidrug transporter. *Annu Rev Biochem*, 1993, 62, 385-427.

[26] Chen, CJ; Chin, JE; Ueda, K; Clark, DP; Pastan, I; Gottesman, MM; et al. Internal duplication and homology with bacterial transport proteins in mdr1 (P-glycoprotein) gene from multidrug-resistant human cells. *Cell*, 1996, 47, 381-9.

[27] Sun, H; Dai, H; Shaik, N; Elmquist, WF. Drug efflux transporters in the CNS. *Adv Drug Deliv Rev.*, 2003, 55, 83-105.

[28] Demeule, M; Regina, A; Jodoin, J; Laplante, A; Dagenais, C; Berthelet, F; et al. Drug transport to the brain: key roles for the efflux pump P-glycoprotein in the blood-brain barrier. *Vascul Pharmacol*, 2002, 38, 339-48.

[29] Schinkel, AH. The physiological function of drug-transporting P-glycoproteins. *Semin Cancer Biol.*, 1997, 8, 161-70.

[30] Yu, DK. The contribution of P-glycoprotein to pharmacokinetic drug-drug interactions. *J Clin Pharmacol*, 1999, 39, 1203-11.

[31] Lin, JH; Yamazaki, M. Role of P-glycoprotein in pharmacokinetics: clinical implications. *Clin Pharmacokinet*, 2003, 41, 59-98.

[32] Bodo, A; Bakos, E; Szeri, F; Varadi, A; Sarkadi, B. The role of multidrug transporters in drug availability, metabolism and toxicity. *Toxicol Lett*, 2003, 140-141, 133-43.

[33] Ayrton, A; Morgan, P. Role of transport proteins in drug absorption, distribution and excretion. *Xenobiotica*, 2001, 31, 469-97.

[34] Schinkel, AH. Pharmacological insights from P-glycoprotein knockout mice. *Int J Clin Pharmacol Ther*, 1998, 36, 9-13.

[35] Zhou, S; Lim, LY; Chowbay, B. Herbal modulation of P-glycoprotein. *Drug Metab Rev.*, 2004, 36, 57-104.

[36] Tateishi, T; Asoh, M; Nakura, H; Watanabe, M; Tanaka, M; Kumai, T; et al. Carbamazepine induces multiple cytochrome P450 subfamilies in rats. *Chem-Biol Interact*, 1999, 117, 257-68.

[37] Owen, A; Pirmohamed, M; Tettey, JN; Morgan, P; Chadwick, D; Park, BK. Carbamazepine is not a substrate for P-glycoprotein. *Br J Clin Pharmacol*, 2001, 51, 345-9.

[38] Wilkinson, GR. The effects of diet, aging and disease-states on presystemic elimination and oral drug bioavailability in humans. *Adv Drug Deliver Rev.*, 1997, 27, 129-59.

[39] Evans, AM. Influence of dietary components on the gastrointestinal metabolism and transport of drugs. *Ther Drug Monit*, 2000, 22, 131-6.

[40] Ioannides, C. Pharmacokinetic interactions between herbal remedies and medicinal drugs. *Xenobiotica*, 2002, 32, 451-78.

[41] Zhou, SF; Gao, YH; Wen, QJ; Huang, M; Xu, AL; Paxton, JW. Interactions of herbs with cytochrome P450. *Drug Metab Rev.*, 2003, 35, 35-98.

[42] Walter-Sack, I; Klotz, U. Influence of diet and nutritional status on drug metabolism. *Clin Pharmacokinet*, 1996, 31, 47-64.

[43] Zhou, S; Gao, Y; Jiang, W; Huang, M; Xu, A; Paxton, JW. Interactions of herbs with cytochrome P450. *Drug Metab Rev.*, 2003, 35, 35-98.

[44] Moore, LB; Goodwin, B; Jones, SA; Wisely, GB; Serabjit-Singh, CJ; Willson, TM. St. John's wort induces hepatic drug metabolism through activation of the pregnane X receptor. *Proc Natl Acad Sci USA*, 2000, 97, 7500-2.

[45] Goodwin, B; Moore, LB; Stoltz, CM; McKee, DD; Kliewer, SA. Regulation of the human CYP2B6 gene by the nuclear pregnane X receptor. *Mol Pharmacol*, 2001, 60, 427-31.

[46] Wentworth, JM; Agostini, M; Love, J; Schwabe, JW; Chatterjee, VK. St John's wort, a herbal antidepressant, activates the steroid X receptor. *J Endocrinol*, 2000, 166, R11-6.

[47] Obach, RS. Inhibition of human cytochrome P450 enzymes by constituents of St. John's Wort, an herbal preparation used in the treatment of depression. *J Pharmacol Exp Ther*, 2000, 294, 88-95.

[48] Bray, BJ; Perry, NB; Menkes, DB; Rosengren, RJ. St. John's wort extract induces CYP3A and CYP2E1 in the Swiss Webster mouse. *Toxicol Sci.*, 2002, 66, 27-33.

[49] Durr, D; Stieger, B; Kullak-Ublick, GA; Rentsch, KM; Steinert, HC; Meier, PJ; et al. St John's wort induces intestinal P-glycoprotein/MDR1 and intestinal and hepatic CYP3A4. *Clin Pharmacol Ther*, 2000, 68, 598-604.

[50] Roby, CA; Anderson, GD; Kantor, E; Dryer, DA; Burstein, AH. St John's Wort: effect on CYP3A4 activity. *Clin Pharmacol Ther*, 2000, 67, 451-7.

[51] Arold, G; Donath, F; Maurer, A; Diefenbach, K; Bauer, S; Henneicke-von Zepelin, HH; et al. No relevant interaction with alprazolam, caffeine, tolbutamide, and digoxin by treatment with a low-hyperforin St John's wort extract. *Planta Med*, 2005, 71, 331-7.

[52] Foster, BC; Foster, MS; Vandenhoek, S; Krantis, A; Budzinski, JW; Arnason, JT; et al. An in vitro evaluation of human cytochrome P450 3A4 and P-glycoprotein inhibition by garlic. *J Pharm Pharm Sci.*, 2001, 4, 176-84.

[53] Kishimoto, R; Ueda, M; Yoshinaga, H; Goda, K; Park, SS. Combined effects of ethanol and garlic on hepatic ethanol metabolism in mice. *J Nutr Sci Vitaminol*, 1999, 45, 275-86.

[54] Teyssier, C; Guenot, L; Suschetet, M; Siess, MH. Metabolism of diallyl disulfide by human liver microsomal cytochromes P-450 and flavin-containing monooxygenases. *Drug Metab Dispos*, 1999, 27, 835-41.

[55] Dalvi, RR; Dalvi, PS. Comparison of the effects of piperine administered intragastrically and intraperitoneally on the liver and liver mixed-function oxidases in rats. *Drug Metab Drug Interact*, 1991, 9, 23-30.

[56] Jin, JX; Baillie, TA. Metabolism of the chemoprotective agent diallyl sulfide to glutathione conjugates in rats. *Chem Res Toxicol*, 1997, 10, 318-27.

[57] Hennessy, M; Kelleher, D; Spiers, JP; Barry, M; Kavanagh, P; Back, D; et al. St John's Wort increases expression of P-glycoprotein: implications for drug interactions. *Br J Clin Pharmacol*, 2002, 53, 75-82.

[58] Perloff, MD; von Moltke, LL; Stormer, E; Shader, RI; Greenblatt, DJ. Saint John's wort: an in vitro analysis of P-glycoprotein induction due to extended exposure. *Br J Pharmacol*, 2001, 134, 1601-8.

[59] Dresser, GK; Schwarz, UI; Wilkinson, GR; Kim, RB. Coordinate induction of both cytochrome P4503A and MDR1 by St John's wort in healthy subjects. *Clin Pharmacol Ther*, 2003, 73, 41-50.

[60] Molnar, J; Szabo, D; Pusztai, R; Mucsi, I; Berek, L; I. Ocsovszki; et al. Membrane associated antitumor effects of crocine-, ginsenoside- and cannabinoid derivatives. *Anticancer Res.*, 2000, 20, 861-7.

[61] Kolars, JC; Awni, WM; Merion, RM; Watkins, PB. First-pass metabolism of cyclosporin by the gut. *Lancet*, 1991, 338, 1488-90.

[62] Paine, MF; Shen, DD; Kunze, KL; Perkins, JD; Marsh, CL; McVicar, JP; et al. First-pass metabolism of midazolam by the human intestine. *Clin Pharmacol Ther*, 1996, 60, 14-24.

[63] Kim, RB; Fromm, MF; Wandel, C; Leake, B; Wood, AJ; Roden, DM; et al. The drug transporter P-glycoprotein limits oral absorption and brain entry of HIV-1 protease inhibitors. *J Clin Invest*, 1998, 101, 289-94.

[64] Fromm, MF; Busse, D; Kroemer, HK; Eichelbaum, M. Differential induction of prehepatic and hepatic metabolism of verapamil by rifampin. *Hepatology*, 1996, 24, 796-801.

[65] Greiner, B; Eichelbaum, M; Fritz, P; Kreichgauer, HP; von Richter, O; Zundler, J; et al. The role of intestinal P-glycoprotein in the interaction of digoxin and rifampin. *J Clin Invest*, 1999, 104, 147-53.

[66] Westphal, K; Weinbrenner, A; Zschiesche, M; Franke, G; Knoke, M; Oertel, R; et al. Induction of P-glycoprotein by rifampin increases intestinal secretion of talinolol in human beings: a new type of drug/drug interaction. *Clin Pharmacol Ther*, 2000, 68, 345-55.

[67] Yin, OQ; Tomlinson, B; Waye, MM; Chow, AH; Chow, MS. Pharmacogenetics and herb-drug interactions: experience with Ginkgo biloba and omeprazole. *Pharmacogenetics*, 2004, 14, 841-50.

[68] Rengelshausen, J; Banfield, M; Riedel, KD; Burhenne, J; Weiss, J; Thomsen, T; et al. Opposite effects of short-term and long-term St John's wort intake on voriconazole pharmacokinetics. *Clin Pharmacol Ther*, 2005, 78, 25-33.

[69] Izzo, AA; Ernst, E. Interactions between herbal medicines and prescribed drugs - A systematic review. *Drugs*, 2001, 61, 2163-75.

[70] Fugh-Berman, A. Herbal medicinals: selected clinical considerations, focusing on known or potential drug-herb interactions. *Arch Intern Med*, 1999, 159, 1957-8.

[71] Almeida, JC; Grimsley, EW. Coma from the health food store: interaction between Kava and alprazolam. Ann Intern Med, 1996, 125, 940-1.

[72] Yuan, CS; Dey, L; Wang, A; Mehendale, S; Xie, JT; Aung, HH; et al. Kavalactones and dihydrokavain modulate GABAergic activity in a rat gastric-brainstem preparation. *Planta Med*, 2002, 68, 1092-6.

[73] Jussofie, A; Schmiz, A; Hiemke, C. Kavapyrone enriched extract from Piper methysticum as modulator of the GABA binding site in different regions of rat brain. *Psychopharmacology (Berl)*, 1994, 116, 469-74.

[74] Galluzzi, S; Zanetti, O; Binetti, G; Trabucchi, M; Frisoni, GB. Coma in a patient with Alzheimer's disease taking low dose trazodone and *Ginkgo biloba*. *J Neurol Neurosurg Psychiatr*, 2000, 68, 679-80.

[75] Lantz, MS; Buchalter, E; Giambanco, V. St. John's wort and antidepressant drug interactions in the elderly. *J Geriatr Psychiatr Neurol*, 1999, 12, 7-10.

[76] Gordon, JB. SSRIs and St.John's Wort: possible toxicity? *Am Fam Physician*, 1998, 57, 950.

[77] Barbenel, DM; Yusufi, B; O'Shea, D; Bench, CJ. Mania in a patient receiving testosterone replacement postorchidectomy taking St John's wort and sertraline. *J Psychopharmacol*, 2000, 14, 84-6.

[78] Spinella, M; Eaton, LA. Hypomania induced by herbal and pharmaceutical psychotropic medicines following mild traumatic brain injury. *Brain Inj.*, 2002, 16, 359-67.

[79] Dannawi, M. Possible serotonin syndrome after combination of buspirone and St John's Wort. *J Psychopharmacol*, 2002, 16, 401.

[80] Cookson, J. Side-effects of antidepressants. *Br J Psychiatry*, 1993, 163, 20-4.

[81] Roz, N; Mazur, Y; Hirshfeld, A; Rehavi, M. Inhibition of vesicular uptake of monoamines by hyperforin. *Life Sci.*, 2002, 71, 2227-37.

[82] Wonnemann, M; Singer, A; Siebert, B; Muller, WE. Evaluation of synaptosomal uptake inhibition of most relevant constituents of St. John's wort. *Pharmacopsychiatry*, 2001, 34, S148-51.

[83] Moschella, C; Jaber, BL. Interaction between cyclosporine and *Hypericum perforatum* (St. John's wort) after organ transplantation. *Am J Kidney Dis.*, 2001, 38, 1105-7.

[84] Breidenbach, T; Kliem, V; Burg, M; Radermacher, J; Hoffmann, MW; Klempnauer, J. Profound drop of cyclosporin A whole blood trough levels caused by St. John's wort (*Hypericum perforatum*). *Transplantation*, 2000, 69, 2229-30.

[85] Johne, A; Schmider, J; Brockmoller, J; Stadelmann, AM; Stormer, E; Bauer, S; et al. Decreased plasma levels of amitriptyline and its metabolites on comedication with an extract from St. John's Wort (*Hypericum perforatum*). *J Clin Psychopharmacol*, 2002, 22, 46-54.

[86] Johne, A; Brockmoller, J; Bauer, S; Maurer, A; Langheinrich, M; Roots, I. Pharmacokinetic interaction of digoxin with an herbal extract from St John's wort (*Hypericum perforatum*). *Clin Pharmacol Ther*, 1999, 66, 338-45.

[87] Piscitelli, SC; Burstein, AH; Chaitt, D; Alfaro, RM; Falloon, J. Indinavir concentrations and St John's wort. *Lancet*, 2000, 355, 547-8.

[88] de Maat, MM; Hoetelmans, RM; Mathot, RA; van Gorp, EC; Meenhorst, PL; Mulder JW; et al. Drug interaction between St John's wort and nevirapine. *AIDS*, 2001, 15, 420-1.

[89] Yue, QY; Bergquist, C; Gerden, B. Safety of St John's wort (*Hypericum perforatum*). *Lancet*, 2000, 355, 548-9.

[90] Maurer, A; Johne, A; Bauer, S. Interaction of St. John's wort extract with phenprocoumon. *Eur J Clin Pharmacol*, 1999, 55, A22.

[91] Nebel, A; Schneider, BJ; Baker, RK; Kroll, DJ. Potential metabolic interaction between St. John's wort and theophylline. *Ann Pharmacother*, 1999, 33, 502.

[92] Sugimoto, K; Ohmori, M; Tsuruoka, S; Nishiki, K; Kawaguchi, A; Harada, K; et al. Different effects of St John's Wort on the pharmacokinetics of simvastatin and pravastatin. *Clin Pharmacol Ther*, 2001, 70, 518-24.

[93] Piscitelli, SC; Burstein, AH; Welden, N; Gallicano, KD; Falloon, J. The effect of garlic supplements on the pharmacokinetics of saquinavir. *Clin Infect Dis.*, 2001, 34, 234-8.

[94] Bano, G; Amla, V; Raina, RK; Zutshi, U; Chopra, CL. The effect of piperine on pharmacokinetics of phenytoin in healthy volunteers. *Planta Med*, 1987, 53, 568-9.

[95] Bano, G; Raina, RK; Zutshi, U; Bedi, KL; Johri, RK; Sharma, SC. Effect of piperine on bioavailability and pharmacokinetics of propranolol and theophylline in healthy volunteers. *Eur J Clin Pharmacol*, 1991, 41, 615-7.

[96] Ruschitzka, F; Meier, PJ; Turina, M; Luscher, TF; Noll, G. Acute heart transplant rejection due to Saint John's wort. *Lancet*, 2000, 355, 548-9.

[97] Barone, GW; Gurley, BJ; Ketel, BL; Lightfoot, ML; Abul-Ezz, SR. Drug interaction between St. John's wort and cyclosporine. *Ann Pharmacother*, 2000, 34, 1013-6.

[98] Mai, I; Kruger, H; Budde, K; Johne, A; Brockmoller, J; Neumayer, HH; et al. Hazardous pharmacokinetic interaction of Saint John's wort (*Hypericum perforatum*) with the immunosuppressant cyclosporin. *Int J Clin Pharmacol Ther*, 2000, 38, 500-2.

[99] Karliova, M; Treichel, U; Malago, M; Frilling, A; Gerken, G; Broelsch, CE. Interaction of *Hypericum perforatum* (St. John's wort) with cyclosporin A metabolism in a patient after liver transplantation. *J Hepatol*, 2000, 33, 853-5.

[100] Dresser, GK; Spence, JD; Bailey, DG. Pharmacokinetic-pharmacodynamic consequences and clinical relevance of cytochrome P450 3A4 inhibition. *Clin Pharmacokinet*, 2000, 38, 41-57.

[101] Heck, AM; DeWitt, BA; Lukes, AL. Potential interactions between alternative therapies and warfarin. *Am J Health-System Pharm*, 2000, 57, 1221-7.

[102] Elvin-Lewis, M. Should we be concerned about herbal remedies. *J Ethnopharmacol*, 2001, 75, 141-64.

[103] Ingram, KD; Dragosavac, GB; Benner, KG; Flora, KD. Risks of drug interactions with St John's Wort. *Am J Gastroenterol*, 2000, 95, 3323-4.

[104] Biffignandi, PM; Bilia, AR. The growing knowledge of St. John's wort (*Hypericum perforatum* L) drug interactions and their clinical significance. *Curr Ther Res.*, 2000, 61, 389-94.

[105] Jones, BD; Runikis, AM. Interaction of ginseng with phenelzine. *J Clin Psychopharmacol*, 1987, 7, 201-2.

[106] Izzo, AA; Capasso, R; Pinto, L; Di Carlo, G; Mascolo, N; Capasso, F. Effect of vanilloid drugs on gastrointestinal transit in mice. *Br J Pharmacol*, 2001, 132, 1411-6.

[107] Houston, JB. Utility of in vitro drug metabolism data in predicting in vivo metabolic clearance. *Biochem Pharmacol*, 1994, 47, 1469-79.

[108] Bergonzi, MC; Bilia, AR; Gallori, S; Guerrini, D; Vincieri, FF. Variability in the content of the constituents of *Hypericum perforatum* L. and some commercial extracts. *Drug Dev Ind Pharm*, 2001, 27, 491-7.

[109] Lin, JH. Applications and limitations of interspecies scaling and in vitro extrapolation in pharmacokinetics. *Drug Metab Dispos*, 1998, 26, 1202-12.

[110] Houston, JB; Kenworthy, KE. In vitro-in vivo scaling of CYP kinetic data not consistent with the classical Michaelis-Menten model. *Drug Metab Dispos*, 2000, 28, 246-54.

[111] Zhou, S; Huang, M; Xu, A; Yang, H; Duan, W; Paxton, JW. Prediction of herb-drug metabolic interactions: a simulation study. *Phytother Res.*, 2005, 19, 464-71.

[112] Zhou, S; Chan, E; Li, SC; Huang, M; Chen, X; Li, X; et al. Predicting pharmacokinetic herb-drug interactions. *Drug Metabol Drug Interact*, 2004, 20, 143-58.

[113] von Moltke, LL; Greenblatt, DJ; Schmider, J; Wright, CE; Harmatz, JS; Shader, RI. In vitro approaches to predicting drug interactions in vivo. *Biochem Pharmacol*, 1998, 55, 113-22.

[114] Tucker, GT. The rational selection of drug interaction studies: implications of recent advances in drug metabolism. *Int J Clin Pharmacol Ther Toxicol*, 1992, 30, 550-3.

[115] Ito, K; Iwatsubo, T; Kanamitsu, S; Ueda, K; Suzuki, H; Sugiyama, Y. Prediction of pharmacokinetic alterations caused by drug-drug interactions: metabolic interaction in the liver. *Pharmacol Rev.*, 1998, 50, 387-411.

[116] Zhou, SF; Chan, E; Pan, SQ; Huang, M; Lee, EJD. Pharmacokinetic interactions of drugs with St John's wort. *J Psychopharmacol*, 2004, 18, 269-83.

[117] Piscitelli, SC; Formentini, E; Burstein, AH; Alfaro, R; Jagannatha, S; Falloon, J. Effect of milk thistle on the pharmacokinetics of indinavir in healthy volunteers. *Pharmacotherapy*, 2002, 22, 551-6.

[118] Allen, SW; Mueller, L; Williams, SN; Quattrochi, LC; Raucy, J. The use of a high-volume screening procedure to assess the effects of dietary flavonoids on human CYP1A1 expression. *Drug Metab Dispos*, 2001, 29, 1074-9.

[119] Ekins, S; Schuetz, E. The PXR crystal structure: the end of the beginning. *Trend Pharmacol Sci.*, 2002, 23, 49-50.

[120] Markowitz, JS; DeVane, CL; Boulton, DW; Carson, SW; Nahas, Z; Risch, SC. Effect of St. John's wort (*Hypericum perforatum*) on cytochrome P-450 2D6 and 3A4 activity in healthy volunteers. *Life Sci.*, 2000, 66, PL133-PL9.

[121] Rosenblatt, M; Mindel, J. Spontaneous hyphema associated with ingestion of *Ginkgo biloba* extract. *N Engl J Med*, 1997, 336, 1108.

[122] Rey, JM; Walter, G. *Hypericum perforatum* (St John's wort) in depression: pest or blessing? *Med J Aust.*, 1998, 169, 583-6.

[123] Bon, S; Hartmann, K; Kubn, M. Johanniskraut: ein enzyminduktor? *Schweitzer Apothekerzeitung*, 1999, 137, 535-6.

[124] Breidenbach, T; Hoffmann, MW; Becker, T; Schlitt, H; Klempnauer, J. Drug interaction of St John's wort with cyclosporin. *Lancet*, 2000, 355, 1912.

[125] Roots, I; Johne, A; Maurer, A. Arzneimittel interaktionen von hypericum-extract. In: Roots I, Kemper FH; editors. *Proc Germ Soc Pharmacol. Berlin:* Conference *Organising Committer,* 2000, 16-7.

[126] Barone, GW; Gurley, BJ; Ketel, BL; Abul-Ezz, SR. Herbal supplements: a potential for drug interactions in transplant recipients. *Transplantation*, 2001, 71, 239-41.

[127] Bauer, S; Stormer, E; Johne, A; Kruger, H; Budde, K; Neumayer, HH; et al. Alterations in cyclosporin A pharmacokinetics and metabolism during treatment with St John's wort in renal transplant patients. *Br J Clin Pharmacol*, 2003, 55, 203-11.

[128] Mauro, VF; Mauro, LS; Kleshinski, JF; Khuder, SA; Wang, Y; Erhardt, PW. Impact of ginkgo biloba on the pharmacokinetics of digoxin. *Am J Ther*, 2003, 10, 247-51.

[129] McRae, S. Elevated serum digoxin levels in a patient taking digoxin and Siberian ginseng. *Can Med Assoc J*, 1996, 155, 293-5.

[130] Wang, ZQ; Hamman, MA; Huang, SM; Lesko, LJ; Hall, SD. Effect of St John's wort on the pharmacokinetics of fexofenadine. *Clin Pharmacol Ther*, 2002, 71, 414-20.

[131] Smith, P. The influence of St. John's wort on the pharmacokinetics and protein binding of imatinib mesylate. *Pharmacotherapy*, 2004, 24, 1508-14.

[132] Frye, RF; Fitzgerald, SM; Lagattuta, TF; Hruska, MW; Egorin, MJ. Effect of St John's wort on imatinib mesylate pharmacokinetics. *Clin Pharmacol Ther*, 2004, 76, 323-9.

[133] Mathijssen, RH; Verweij, J; de Bruijn, P; Loos, WJ; Sparreboom, A. Effects of St. John's wort on irinotecan metabolism. *J Natl Cancer Inst.*, 2002, 94, 1247-9.

[134] Khawaja, IS; Marotta, RF; Lippmann, S. Herbal medicines as a factor in delirium. *Psychiatr Serv.*, 1999, 50, 969-70.

[135] Schelosky, L; Raffauf, C; Jendroska, K; Poewe, W. Kava and dopamine antagonism. *J Neurol Neurosurg Psychiatry*, 1995, 58, 639-40.

[136] Eich-Hochli, D; Oppliger, R; Golay, KP; Baumann, P; Eap, CB. Methadone maintenance treatment and St. John's wort - A case report. *Pharmacopsychiatry*, 2003, 36, 35-7.

[137] Wang, ZQ; Gorski, C; Hamman, MA; Huang, SM; Lesko, LJ; Hall, SD. The effects of St John's wort (*Hypericum perforatum*) on human cytochrome P450 activity. *Clin Pharmacol Ther*, 2001, 70, 317-26.

[138] Wang, LS, Zhou, G; Zhu, B; Wu, J; Wang, JG; Abd El-Aty, AM; et al. St John's wort induces both cytochrome P450 3A4-catalyzed sulfoxidation and 2C19-dependent hydroxylation of omeprazole. *Clin Pharmacol Ther*, 2004, 75, 191-7.

[139] Murphy, PA; Kern, SE; Stanczyk, FZ; Westhoff, CL. Interaction of St. John's Wort with oral contraceptives: effects on the pharmacokinetics of norethindrone and ethinyl estradiol, ovarian activity and breakthrough bleeding. *Contraception*, 2005, 71, 402-8.

[140] Deahl, M. Betel nut-induced extrapyramidal syndrome: an unusual drug interaction. *Mov Disord*, 1989, 4, 330-2.

[141] Gallicano, K; Foster, B; Choudhri, S. Effect of short-term administration of garlic supplements on single-dose ritonavir pharmacokinetics in healthy volunteers. *Br J Clin Pharmacol*, 2003, 55, 199-202.

[142] Mai, I; Stormer, E; Bauer, S; Kruger, H; Budde, K; Roots, I. Impact of St John's wort treatment on the pharmacokinetics of tacrolimus and mycophenolic acid in renal transplant patients. *Nephrol Dial Transplant*, 2003, 18, 819-22.

[143] Sunter, WH. Warfarin and garlic. *Pharm J*, 1991, 246, 772.

[144] Page, RL; 2nd.; Lawrence, JD. Potentiation of warfarin by dong quai. *Pharmacotherapy*, 1999, 19, 870-6.

[145] Ellis, GR; Stephens, MR. Untitled (photograph and brief case report). *Br Med J*, 1999, 319, 650.

[146] Mathews, MK. Association of *Ginkgo biloba* with intracerebral haemorrhage. *Neurology*, 1998, 50, 1933.

[147] Yu, CM; Chan, JC; Sanderson, JE. Chinese herbs and warfarin potentiation by 'danshen'. *J Int Med*, 1997, 241, 337-9.

[148] Shaw, D; Leon, C; Kolev, S; Murray, V. Traditional remedies and food supplements. A 5-year toxicological study (1991-1995). *Drug Saf*, 1997, 17, 342-56.

[149] Gwilt, PR; Lear, CL; Tempero, MA; Birt, DD; Grandjean, AC; Ruddon, RW; et al. The effect of garlic extract on human metabolism of acetaminophen. *Cancer Epidemiol Biomarkers Prev.*, 1994, 3, 155-60.

[150] Burstein, AH; Horton, RL; Dunn, T; Alfaro, RM; Piscitelli, SC; Theodore, W. Lack of effect of St John's Wort on carbamazepine pharmacokinetics in healthy volunteers. *Clin Pharmacol Ther*, 2000, 68, 605-12.

[151] Tankanow, R; Tamer, HR; Streetman, DS; Smith, SG; Welton, JL; Annesley, T; et al. Interaction study between digoxin and a preparation of hawthorn (Crataegus oxyacantha). *J Clin Pharmacol*, 2003, 43, 637-42.

[152] Jiang, X; Williams, KM; Liauw, WS; Ammit, AJ; Roufogalis, BD; Duke, CC; et al. Effect of ginkgo and ginger on the pharmacokinetics and pharmacodynamics of warfarin in healthy subjects. *Br J Clin Pharmacol*, 2005, 59, 425-32.

[153] Biber, A; Fischer, H; Romer, A; Chatterjee, SS. Oral bioavailability of hyperforin from hypericum extracts in rats and human volunteers. *Pharmacopsychiatry*, 1998, 31, 36-43.

[154] Brockmoller, J; Reum, T; Bauer, S; Kerb, R; Hubner, WD; Roots, I. Hypericin and pseudohypericin: pharmacokinetics and effects on photosensitivity in humans. *Pharmacopsychiatry*, 1997, 30, 94-101.

[155] Mauri, P; Simonetti, P; Gardana, C; Minoggio, M; Morazzoni, P; Bombardelli, E; et al. Liquid chromatography/atmospheric pressure chemical ionization mass spectrometry of terpene lactones in plasma of volunteers dosed with Ginkgo biloba L. extracts. *Rapid Commun Mass Spectrometr*, 2001, 15, 929-34.

[156] Zou, L; Harkey, MR; Henderson, GL. Effects of herbal components on cDNA-expressed cytochrome P450 enzyme catalytic activity. *Life Sci.*, 2002, 71, 1579-89.

[157] Weyhenmeyer, R; Mascher, H; Birkmayer, J. Study on dose-linearity of the pharmacokinetics of silibinin diastereomers using a new stereospecific assay. *Int J Clin Pharmacol Ther Toxicol*, 1992, 30, 134-41.

[158] Zuber, R; Modriansky, M; Dvorak, Z; Rohovsky, P; Ulrichova, J; Simanek, V; et al. Effect of silybin and its congeners on human liver microsomal cytochrome P450 activities. *Phytother Res.*, 2002, 16, 632-8.

[159] Wenk, M; Todesco, L; Krahenbuhl, S. Effect of St John's wort on the activities of CYP1A2, CYP3A4, CYP2D6, N-acetyltransferase 2, and xanthine oxidase in healthy males and females. *Br J Clin Pharmacol*, 2004, 57, 495-9.

[160] Hebert, MF; Park, JM; Chen, YL; Akhtar, S; Larson, AM. Effects of St. John's wort (*Hypericum perforatum*) on tacrolimus pharmacokinetics in healthy volunteers. *J Clin Pharmacol*, 2004, 44, 89-94.

[161] Morimoto, T; Kotegawa, T; Tsutsumi, K; Ohtani, Y; Imai, H; Nakano, S. Effect of St. John's wort on the pharmacokinetics of theophylline in healthy volunteers. *J Clin Pharmacol*, 2004, 44, 95-101.

In: Multiple Drug Resistance
Editors: A. Meszaros, G. Balogh, pp. 129-152

ISBN: 978-1-60741-595-4

Chapter V

Cell Membranes, Cytosolic pH and Drug Transport in Cancer and MDR: Physics, Biochemistry and Molecular Biology

Cyril Rauch[1*], Adam Blanchard[1], Eleanor Wood[1], Eleanor Dillon[1], Miriam L. Wahl[2] and Salvador Harguindey[2]

[1]School of Veterinary Medicine and Science, University of Nottingham, College Road, Sutton Bonington, LE12 5RD, UK.

[2]Institute of Clinical Biology and Metabolism, c) Postas 13, 01004 Vitoria, Spain.

Abstract

Pleiotropic resistance (or multidrug resistance, or MDR) to anticancer drugs in malignant diseases takes place either primarily or secondarily in the treatment of cancer. The first report suggesting that MDR could be the result of active drug extrusion was published in 1973 by Dano [1]. A few years later, P-glycoprotein (Pgp) was identified by Juliano and Ling as a membrane protein that actively extrudes membrane embedded drugs. Biochemistry is a "science of contacts" between at least two biochemical elements (e.g. a drug and a transporter). These elements have to interact in order for a reaction to occur (e.g. drug extrusion). Taking into account that drugs do not necessarily incorporate into the membrane in the vicinity of a drug transporter, these transporters have been thought to exhibit a "vacuum cleaner" like-activity on membrane embedded drugs. Accordingly, understanding this activity is essential; as the movement of membrane embedded drugs, or otherwise, movement of the transporters must occur if extrusion is to take place. These activities should be considered as targets for anticancer drugs. Drug movement occurs by lateral diffusion (Brownian movement) in the membrane and the physical conditions required for drug extrusion by membrane transporters is known as the "2D random walk" theory. A deeper understanding is now possible, because there is enough literature enabling understanding of: (a) why the membrane is central to Pgp-

* Corresponding author: Email: Cyril.rauch@nottingham.ac.uk, Tel: 0044 (0)115 9516451, Fax: 0044 (0)1115 95 16 440.

mediated drug extrusion; (b) why the drug's molecular weight is an essential determinant in MDR, and; (c) why an alkaline cytosolic pH is essential in MDR.

After recalling the importance of pH in many aspects of cancer, including MDR, we will focus on the reason why a better understanding of the "vacuum cleaner" hypothesis is needed to clarify the subsequent processes involved in MDR. This will lead us to consider the cell membrane's mechanical properties and cytosolic pH alkalinization as important factors in the etiopathogenesis and understanding of MDR.

Introduction

A. The Role of pH in Cancer and MDR: An Overview

It appears that we have now reached a deadlock in cancer chemotherapy [2]. This seems to be related to the fact that most of the antitumor agents used in the clinical situation are based upon the old "anti DNA" paradigm which, over the last 60 years, has attempted to induce an antitumor effect by targeting DNA synthesis or cell division and proliferation. It has recently been proposed that the modest progress achieved in this area, and the lack of selectivity of current antitumor agents, suggests that the "anti DNA" framework is either conceptually poor or at least too simplistic for such a complex disease [2]. Some of these authors have proposed that the limitations of the present-day approaches can be responsible for the fact that some therapies can even exacerbate the original malignant phenotype, induce suppression of apoptosis and negatively affect the progression of the disease [2-4]. As an alternative to this approach, a proton-related mechanism underlying the initiation and progression of the neoplastic process has recently been described [5-8].

This model is based upon the fact that regardless of their origin and genetic background, all cancer cells and tissues have a pivotal energetic and homeostatic disturbance of their metabolism that is completely different to all normal tissues: an aberrant regulation of hydrogen ion dynamics that leads to a reversal of the pH gradient in cancer cells and tissues [5-8]. This causes an interstitial acid microenvironment secondary to an initial, specific and etiopathogenic intracellular alkalosis, which is the opposite of the normal pH gradient. This specific abnormality of cancer cells and tissues, called "proton reversal or H^+-reversal, is increasingly considered to be one of the most differential hallmarks of cancer [7, 9]. It is remarkable that at the intracellular level, an elevated intracellular pH (pH_i) plays a direct and specific role in transformation and tumor development [6-8, 10, 11].

The basic abnormality in the relationship between intracellular and extracellular dynamics of the hydrogen ion allows for the creation of a unifying view of several of the most important aspects of cancer research. These include diverse topics such as etiopathogenesis, cancer cell metabolism and neovascularisation, and multiple drug resistance (MDR), selective apoptosis, the metastatic process, cancer chemotherapy and even the spontaneous regression of cancer (SRC) [5, 7, 12, 13]. There is now ample data demonstrating that this reversed proton gradient is driven by a variety of proton (export) extrusion mechanisms that underlie the initiation and progression of the neoplastic process, as well as resistance to treatment [14]. This means that therapeutic targeting of the transporters that are more active in cancer cells could be selective for malignancy. These findings are likely to lead to the development of more specific and less toxic therapeutic measures for malignant diseases.

B. pH_i and Multiple Drug Resistance (MDR) to Anticancer Drugs

A direct cause and effect relationship between the degree of MDR and the elevation of tumor pH_i has been reported by several laboratories [15-22]. The following conclusions can be reached based on the following lines of experimental evidence:

1. A failure to induce intracellular acidification and reverse the altered and specific proton reversal of cancer tissues has been proposed to be the main factor underlying drug resistance, and including resistance to the induction of therapeutic apoptosis, in both highly alkaline cancer cells and in malignant cells with a normal or slightly elevated pH_i, [23-27].
2. The alkalinity characteristic of many, or possibly all, kinds of malignant cells is also known to decrease the retention of anticancer drugs such as vinblastine, adriamycin, cisplatin, paclitaxel, and campthothecin [20, 27-34].
3. In a parallel manner, the accumulation of some drugs in the cytosol increases with cellular acidification and decreases with an alkaline shift. This feature is mediated by overexpression of the Na^+/H^+ antiporter, or other proton transporters [21, 35, 36].

To exemplify points 1, 2 and 3, one of the most representative and seminal findings in this area has been the observation that pH alkalization from pH_i 7.0 to pH_i 7.4 triggers a ~2000-fold increase in adriamycin resistance in human lung cancer cells [15]. This level of resistance can be reversed by cellular acidification via administration of verapamil [15]. In parallel studies, the intracellular concentration of adriamycin was shown to be increased by more than 100-fold after inducing cellular acidification, an acid-base energetic change that behaves on its own as a "chemosensitizing agent" [18].

4. At the same time, no matter how paradoxical it may seem, some drugs, mainly weak bases, can be sequestered away from the cytosol within highly acidic organelles, such as lysosomes, endosomes, and the Golgi network of otherwise alkalinized cells, and in this way are inactivated (the so called protonation effect or ion trapping effect) [23, 29, 37, 38].
5. There is a large body of work suggesting that the main function of P-glycoprotein (P-gp) is to catalyze ATP-dependent proton extrusion. P-gp expressing cells exhibit cytoplasmatic alkalinization [22, 39]. In addition, the overexpression of specific H^+-ATPases leads to a increase in pH_i which has a positive correlation with drug resistance [21, 32, 33, 40], and inhibition of apoptosis [29, 41]. In support of these observations, specific inhibitors of H^+-ATPase, like Bafilomyicin A_1, induce the intracellular accumulation of drugs by inhibiting their efflux via an acidifying mechanism [40, 42-44].

6. Furthermore, extracellular acidity, secondary to intracellular alkalinization and H^+-reversal, has a positive effect on P-glycoprotein expression and also decreases the cytotoxicity of some chemotherapeutic drugs [45-47].
7. Lastly, findings directly relating cytosolic alkalinization with abnormalities in membrane depolarization in MDR-positive drug resistant cancer cells have been published [18, 24, 28, 35, 48, 49]. The energetic alterations of cell membrane depolarization, low transmembrane potential, pH_i elevations and the perturbations in cellular ion transport are considered to be responsible for most of the characteristics of multidrug-resistant cells.

In conclusion, a large set of available data in the literature indicates that any mechanism that leads to an elevation of pH_i, either through overexpression/activation of the NHE1 following activation of Na^+-K^+-ATPase [6, 50]; via hyperactivity of vacuolar H^+-ATPases, or by other mechanisms contribute to the onset and/or maintenance of MDR, which inhibits tumor cell death induced by anticancer drugs [3, 18, 21, 36, 51-56].

C. Weighing the Role of Drug Handling and Extrusion by Transporters against Changes in Cytosolic pH

There have also been reports suggesting that pH changes, either extracellular or intracellular, may have no significant effect on drug extrusion by P-glycoprotein [57-59]. However, it has been widely accepted that Pgp is a transporter that binds to and extrudes drugs.

These two hypotheses describing MDR may appear to be deadlocked. On one hand, it is argued that cytosolic pH alkalinization is central to MDR and can be mediated by Pgp expression levels. On the other hand, it is suggested that drugs are directly extruded by Pgp-like transporters. Although these hypotheses are different, they are not necessarily mutually exclusive. It is possible to envisage MDR as resulting from a drug handling mechanism *and* a high cytosolic pH. It follows that the contribution of each of these two processes could be measured and their respective involvement in MDR could be elucidated.

This exercise would be possible if the "vacuum cleaner" hypothesis that has been invoked to explain how drugs interact with transporters prior to extrusion is re-examined.

D. The "Vacuum Cleaner" Hypothesis: A Model in Need of Clarification

Pgp-like transporters are presumed to impair the intracellular accumulation of drugs by extruding them at a rapid rate from the plasma membrane inner leaflet, even before they reach the cytosol [60-70]. Although the function whereby these transporters extrude drugs from the inner leaflet is well defined once a drug binds to a Pgp-like transporter, a further hypothesis is usually invoked, namely, that these transporters act as "vacuum cleaners" that vacuum membrane-embedded drugs. This assumption is usually invoked as therapeutic drugs partition efficiently into cellular membranes and their insertion into membranes is widespread. Therefore, there is no reason to conceive of why a drug should insert itself into the membrane in the vicinity of a transporter. It follows that the efficiency of Pgp-like transporters to mediate MDR should rely on the transporters' ability to extrude drugs, and also fundamentally, on the transport of drugs from their initial incorporation in plasma membranes to the transporters *prior* to extrusion. Given this naïve standpoint, it was suggested that MDR results from different and synergic processes.

Impeding the activity of transporters in order to increase the intracellular accumulation of drugs, is possible by the use of drug resistance modulators. Although some modulators alter the activity of certain transporters through direct physical interactions [71, 72], modulators are also commonly known to affect the membrane's biophysical properties, and thus permeability to drugs [73-78]. These data indicate that specific cellular membrane biophysical properties and Pgp-like transporters are fundamental in the pathogenesis of MDR.

Transbilayer movement of drugs is not spontaneous; it occurs via lateral diffusion. The lateral diffusion of drugs might explain how they come to interact with transporters. The longer the diffusive lateral path, the higher the probability of a drug binding to a transporter. However, as the binding of drugs mediated by Pgp-like transporters takes place in the inner leaflet, it follows that part of the activation energy needed for a drug to traverse the membrane completely resides within this leaflet. Thus, drugs are prevented from moving in the reverse direction, and are extruded.

The ability of a drug to traverse the cell membrane has been shown to be dependent on specific biophysical properties of lipid bilayers. One of these is fluidity, which refers to the packing of lipids within a layer. Parameters include surface pressure and surface tension. Accordingly, changes have been noted regarding the cellular membrane of MDR cells. In particular, higher rates of endocytosis have been measured [79, 80]. It is worth noting that the local membrane budding which leads to membrane vesiculation and controls the kinetics of endocytosis has been associated with an endogenous higher compression of the cellular membrane inner leaflet [81-84]. Thus, a possible mechanism involved in the membrane barrier of MDR cells that could play a role in the inner leaflet, may be linked to membrane endocytosis itself and also may be related to the membranes' mechanical properties.

Given the need to add additional dimensions to the "vacuum cleaner" model, it was decided to address theoretically, whether it can be further developed by exploring additional factors related to the membrane physical properties, endocytosis, and the relationship between intracellular and extracellular pH.

I. The Physical Biology of MDR

A. The Role of Physical, Chemical, and Mechanical Factors Affecting the Transverse Movement of Drugs Across the Cell Membrane

Once they are incorporated into cellular membranes, studies have demonstrated that classical anticancer drugs that have an affinity with Pgp-like transporters, have a relatively slow transbilayer diffusion ~10s [85]. With a membrane thickness ~5nm, an apparent diffusion coefficient through biomembranes ~$10^{-6}\mu m^2/s$ can be obtained. However, based on the Stokes-Einstein relation, these therapeutics have a diffusion coefficient in water of ~$10^2\mu m^2/s$ [86, 87], which gives a ratio in the diffusion coefficients of eight orders of magnitude. Such a difference can be explained either by the intrinsic membrane viscosity and/or a membrane activation energy needed for a drug to traverse the membrane. In this context, it can be demonstrated that the connection that exists between the activation energy needed to cross the plasma membrane and the drug residency time is:

$$t_0 \cong \frac{h^2}{2D}\left[\frac{1}{h}\int_0^h e^{\left[U(x)-U_{out}^0\right]/k_BT}dx\right] \quad (1)$$

where t_0 is the drug residency time in the membrane, D is the average value of the membrane diffusion coefficient, h is the membrane thickness, k_B is Boltzmann's constant, T is the abolsute temperature, and U_{out}^0 is the drug's energy in the outer leaflet and within the membrane (Figure 1B). $U(x)$ is usually a very complex function of the set of interactions between a drug and the membrane components, which varies over the membrane thickness. Initially in the outer leaflet, in order to traverse the bilayer, the drug must transfer its hydrophilic (polar) part into the hydrophobic core of the membrane [88], and compensate the potential difference in surface tensions existing between leaflets (Figure 1A). This will inevitably increase the drug's energy. One will assume that both the drug's dehydration energy, ΔG, and the outer and inner leaflets surface tension , σ_{out} and σ_{in} respectively, are constant, i.e. are average values over the membrane thickness. Under these conditions, the above formula can be reduced to:

$$t_0 \cong \frac{h^2}{4D}e^{\Delta G/k_BT}\left(1+e^{-a\Delta\sigma/k_BT}\right) \quad (2)$$

where $\Delta\sigma = (\sigma_{in} - \sigma_{out})$ corresponds to the difference in surface tensions between the inner and outer leaflet respectively and a is the drug's cross section area once intercalated in the cell membrane. The difference in surface tensions has been shown to be the causation of membrane budding leading to the creation of intracellular vesicles of radius R, written under the form $R = -8k_c/h\Delta\sigma$, where k_c is the bending modulus of the membrane (Figure 1A) [84]. Thus, Eq.6 can also be rewritten as:

$$t_0 \cong \frac{h^2}{4D} e^{\frac{\Delta G}{k_B T}} \left(1 + e^{8 \frac{k_c a}{k_B T h R}} \right) \tag{3}$$

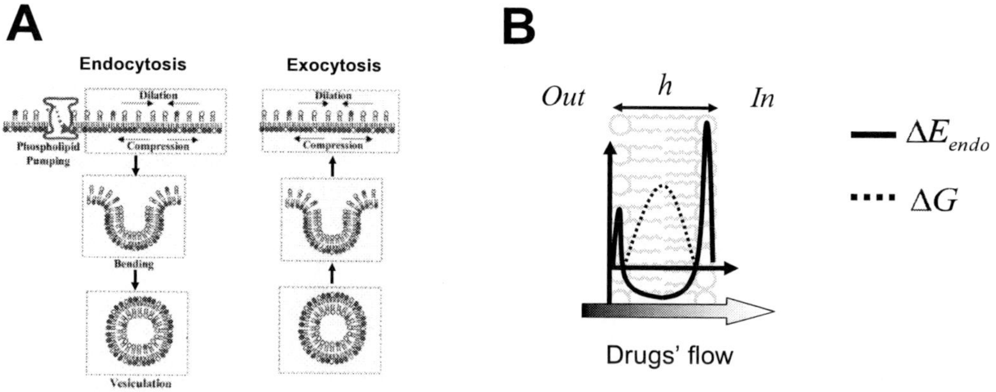

Figure 1: (A) The lipid number asymmetry induced fluid phase endocytosis (FPE) model: Sketch representing the current model that has been applied in living cells linking FPE and the membrane phospholipid number asymmetry thought to be maintained by aminophospholipid translocase. In the left panel, the translocation of lipids into the inner leaflet (shaded heads) induces a differential lipid packing between leaflets (namely a difference in surface tensions) leading to membrane bending and vesiculation [83, 84]. Note that the membrane recycling that occurs in cells (right panel), i.e. the exocytosis of vesicles with a size similar to endocytic vesicles, also allows the maintenance of the lipid asymmetry at the level of the plasmalemma. The relationship existing between the lipid number asymmetry and the vesicle radius is given by $R = -8k_c / h\Delta\sigma$ or equivalently $R = 4k_c / hK \cdot 1/(\delta N / N_0)$, where k_c, K, h, $\Delta\sigma$ and $\delta N / N_0$ are the membrane bending modulus, membrane elastic modulus, membrane thickness, difference in surface tensions and the lipid number asymmetry between leaflets. Accordingly, the lipid number asymmetry has been experimentally deduced from studies on drug sensitive cells (K562) with a value $\delta N / N_0 = 2 \pm 0.5\%$ providing a ~35nm vesicle radius [84]. **(B)** Representation of the different energy barriers involved when a drug traverses the bilayer cellular membrane. Two leaflets have been represented with an inner leaflet containing more phospholipids related to the increase in the difference in surface tensions. Energy profiles (noted U(x) in the text) of both surface tension in leaflets (solid curve) and hydrophobic core of membrane (dashed curve) are involved in providing a penalty energy with regard to the transbilayer movement of drugs.

It is worth noting that the latter equation contains three physical parameters that are likely to be involved in affecting the transverse movement of drugs. The first one already mentioned is the membrane viscosity (hidden in the diffusion coefficient), the second one has a physico-chemical origin and is classically related to the drug dehydration energy, and the last one, related to the difference in surface tension, states that specific mechanical constraints exist when drugs cross the cell membrane and that these constraints are directly related to membrane endocytosis (Figure 1A&B).

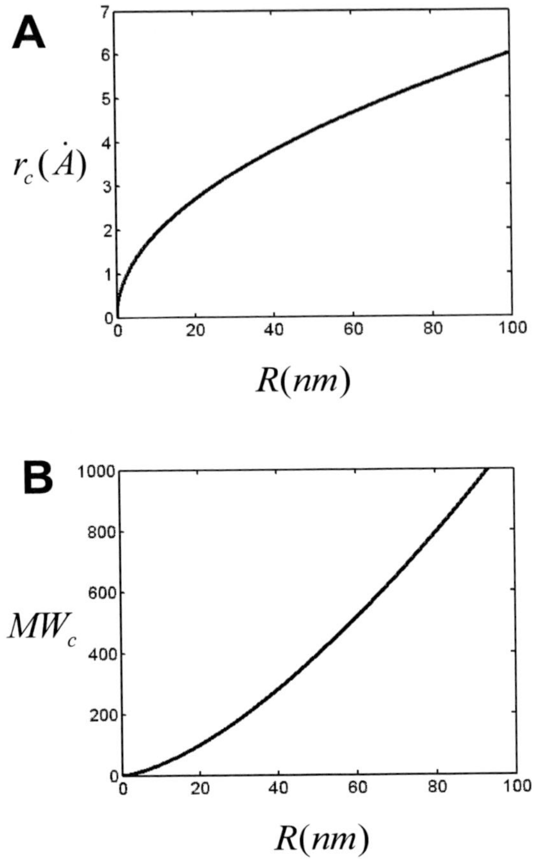

Figure 2: (A) Relationship existing between the drugs' Van der Waals radius, $r_c(\dot{A})$ and their ability to bypass the membrane barrier as a function of vesicular radius, $R(nm)$ (i.e. function of the difference in surface tension), scaling as $r_c \sim R^{1/2}$ [exactly: $r_c \cong 0.6\ R^{1/2}$]. (B) Relation existing between the drugs' MW and their ability to bypass the membrane barrier as a function of vesicles radius $R(nm)$, scaling as $MW_c \sim r_c^3 \sim R^{3/2}$ [exactly: $MW_c = 4\pi r_c^3/3 \cong 1.1\ R^{3/2}$].

From Eq.3, it follows that the time required for the transbilayer movement of drugs is a function of the cross sectional area of the drug which is expected to become involved in MDR if $a > a_c = hRk_BT/8k_c$, where a_c indicates a critical cross sectional area beyond which the difference in surface tensions is likely to affect its transbilayer movement (namely beyond which the exponential function will be numerically high). A numerical value of a_c can be determined; considering a membrane thickness $h \sim 5nm$, a vesicle radius $R \sim 35nm$ determined for drug sensitive cells [84] and a membrane bending modulus, $k_c \sim 2.10^{-19}J$ [89], it follows $a_c \sim 0.4nm^2$ at 37°C (Figure 2A). Assuming legitimately that the MW of the drug is proportional to its Van der Waals volume (expressed in $\dot{A}^3$), a critical MW can also be deduced $MW_c = (4/3\sqrt{\pi})(hRk_BT/8k_c)^{3/2} \sim 240$ (Figure 2B), providing a law with regard to the drug size (or MW) selectivity on its permeation across the cell membrane. As endocytosis is altered in drug resistant cells and the kinetics of endocytosis is inversely proportional to vesicle radius [83], it follows that the mechanical interaction between a drug and the membrane can be re-written as:

$$8k_c a / hRk_B T = 8k_c a / hR_0 k_B T \cdot R_0 / R = a / a_c \cdot k / k_0 = (MW / MW_c)^{2/3} \cdot k / k_0 \quad (4)$$

where R_0, k_0 and R, k are the vesicle radius and the rate of endocytosis when cells are sensitive (subscript "0") and resistant to drugs respectively. Finally, the drug residency time can be rewritten as:

$$t_0 \cong \frac{h^2}{4D} e^{\frac{\Delta G}{k_B T}} \left(1 + e^{\frac{k}{k_{0c}} \left(\frac{MW}{MW_c} \right)^{2/3}} \right) \quad (5)$$

Since the membrane barrier energy will prolong the turnover time of the drugs in the membrane, the drugs are expected to diffuse laterally, which may in turn increase the probability that they bind to and are extruded by a Pgp-like transporter.

So far we have determined how the duration of time of drugs are in the cell membrane can be affected by the membrane's physical properties. We need now to determine how the duration of time within the membrane will favor interaction with drug transporters.

B. The Critical Relationship between The Two Dimensional (2D) Random Walk Of Membrane –Embedded Drugs and Pgp-Like Transporter Surface Density in Mediating MDR

The previous section may be summarized as follows: (i) the number of Pgps on the cellular surface of MDR cells remains globally constant; (ii) due to their large transmembrane structure the lateral diffusion time of Pgp-like transporters can be considered negligible when compared to the lateral diffusion time of drugs; and (iii) the number of drugs in the membrane and the outward pumping kinetics are respectively low and fast enough, such that the probability of two drugs interacting with a given transporter at the same time is negligible.

As a result, transporters can be considered as static with a probability of presence on the cellular surface given by $\rho_{Pgp} = N_{Pgp} S_{Pgp} / S_{cell}$, where N_{Pgp}, S_{Pgp} and S_{cell} represent the number of transporters, the cross section area of transporters and the cellular surface, respectively. During its time within the cellular membrane, a drug is expected to follow a 2D random walk, with a formal condition restricted to time scales greater than the single transverse diffusion time, i.e. $h^2 / 4D$. Consequently, the number of steps performed is $K = t_0 / (h^2 / 4D)$. Nonetheless, the probability of a drug and a transporter meeting will depend on non recurring walks and for a number of steps large enough (i.e. $t_0 > h^2 / 4D$) it is possible to demonstrate that the probability of the event "drug meeting a Pgp" in the membrane, p_{Pgp}, is [90]:

$$p_{Pgp} \cong \rho_{Pgp} \pi \, e^{\frac{\Delta G}{k_B T}\left(1+e^{\frac{k}{k_0}\cdot\left(\frac{MW}{MW_c}\right)^{2/3}}\right)} \Bigg/ \ln\left[e^{\frac{\Delta G}{k_B T}\left(1+e^{\frac{k}{k_0}\left(\frac{MW}{MW_c}\right)^{2/3}}\right)}\right] \tag{6}$$

However, meeting a Pgp is not enough and Pgp-mediated drug extrusion requires the location of the drug in the inner leaflet of the plasma membrane. For that the probability that a drug enters the inner leaflet can be approached by Maxwell-Boltzmann's distribution, written as:

$$\int_{\Delta G}^{+\infty} e^{-E/k_B T} dE \Bigg/ \int_{0}^{+\infty} e^{-E/k_B T} dE = e^{-\Delta G/k_B T} \tag{7}$$

Assuming that when entering the inner leaflet and meeting a transporter a drug is extruded. The probability, $\widetilde{p}_{Pgp}$, that a drug is effectively expelled from the membrane by a transporter becomes finally:

$$\widetilde{p}_{Pgp} \cong e^{-\frac{\Delta G}{k_B T}} p_{Pgp} \tag{8}$$

From the later equation, it follows that a membrane-embedded drug will inevitably meet a drug transporter only if $\widetilde{p}_{Pgp} = 1$. With this condition and by using Eq.6, it is thus possible to determine the critical surface density of transporters ρ^c_{Pgp} to generate MDR:

$$\rho^c_{Pgp} = 1/\pi \cdot \ln\left[e^{\frac{\Delta G}{k_B T}\left(1+e^{\frac{k}{k_0}\cdot\left(\frac{MW}{MW_c}\right)^{2/3}}\right)}\right] \Bigg/ \left(1+e^{\frac{k}{k_0}\cdot\left(\frac{MW}{MW_c}\right)^{2/3}}\right) \tag{9}$$

It is worth noting that when the mechanical effect becomes dominant, namely when the drug MW is large (MW>240) or when the kinetics of endocytosis is steadily increased as cells become resistant to drugs, then the surface density of Pgp-like transporters needed to trigger drug resistance is predicted to be low. Formally, this regime is best described by

$$\rho^c_{Pgp} \sim e^{-\frac{k}{k_0}\cdot\left(\frac{MW}{MW_c}\right)^{2/3}}$$

Doxorubicin with a MW of 545 can be used as an example. Assuming that the kinetics of endocytosis is increased 4-fold in the MDR state (which remains a realistic value, reviewed in [79, 91, 92]), it follows that the surface density of Pgp required would only represent ~0.1% of the cellular surface area. This means that as the kinetics of endocytosis increases then the number of P-gp transporter with a drug handling activity required decreases in an exponential way. Thus, if the main activity of P-gp is to handle drugs, then most of them would be functionally ineffective.

Given that MDR assays measure the effective dose (ED), defined as the ability of drugs to kill 50% of a cell population (that is related to drug influx), we need to model how P-gp transporter and endocytosis interact to affect drug influx.

C. Determination of the Drug Influx into MDR Cells

The ability of any classical drug to kill a cell is dependent on its ability to cross the membrane. The drug's influx is modulated both by their slow transbilayer movement and the presence of Pgp-like transporters. In this context, the probability per unit of time that a drug escapes the membrane to go into the cytoplasm, noted r_{MDR}, can be expressed as the probability that a drug is not extruded by Pgp, i.e. $1-\tilde{p}_{Pgp}$ (Eq.8), divided by the drug residency time within the membrane t_0 (Eq.5), which using Eq.9 leads to:

$$r_{MDR} = \frac{e^{-\left(\frac{\Delta G}{k_B T}+\frac{k}{k_0}\cdot\left(\frac{MW}{MW_c}\right)^{2/3}\right)}}{h^2/4D}\left(1-\frac{\rho_{Pgp}}{\rho_{Pgp}^c}\right) \tag{10}$$

Assuming that the membrane diffusion coefficient remains identical between drug sensitive and resistant cells, Eq.10 can also be used to describe the escape rate of a drug from the membrane of sensitive cells, noted as $r_{non-MDR}$, by posing $\rho_{Pgp}=0$ and $k=k_0$. Thus, the ratio between escape rates in drug resistant and sensitive cells can therefore be deduced:

$$\frac{r_{MDR}}{r_{non-MDR}} \cong e^{-\left(\frac{MW}{MW_c}\right)^{2/3}\cdot\left(\frac{k}{k_0}-1\right)}\left(1-\frac{\rho_{Pgp}}{\rho_{Pgp}^c}\right) \tag{11}$$

Eq.11 shows that although the inhibition of the transmembrane flow of drugs going into the cellular cytoplasm can be linearly performed through the expression of Pgp-like transporters, i.e. when $\rho_{Pgp}=\rho_{Pgp}^c$, the transmembrane flow of drugs can also be reduced exponentially as a function of the kinetics of endocytosis.

Finally, by taking the logarithm of Eq.11 it emerges a universal power law (i.e. 2/3) that describes the drug/membrane mechanical interaction, and is directly related to the MW of the drug used:

$$\ln\left(r_{MDR} / r_{non-MDR}\right) \cong -\left(MW / MW_c\right)^{2/3} \cdot \left(k / k_0 - 1\right) + \ln\left(1 - \rho_{Pgp} / \rho_{Pgp}^{c}\right) \tag{12}$$

The right member of Eq.12 is a function of three parameters. These parameters are never measured simultaneously in MDR studies. However, what has been measured is the relationship between MDR levels and the drug MW. Eq.12 demonstrates that if the theory presented here is correct, then the ability of drugs to cross the cell membrane should follow a power law that is a function of their MW. Thus, it should be possible to test the validity of the theory proposed.

II. The Role of Drug Size in MDR

Bielder and Riehm's Seminal 1970's Study: Proof That the Membrane's Mechanical Properties Are Central to MDR

Eq.9 explains MDR when both drug properties (MW and dehydration energy) and transporter surface density are fixed. A problem immediately arises when cross resistance to drugs is taken into consideration. In this case the theoretical relationship discussed above (Eq.9) may not be verified. In particular, the surface density of transporters may not be adequate to expel another drug with different physical properties. The latter scenario would be the case if a smaller drug (i.e. a drug with a lower MW) than the one used to select the resistant phenotype is used, as it would cross the membrane more easily, which would decrease the probability of interaction between a drug and a transporter. If this scenario occurs, the theory suggests that the influx of drugs into the cytosol would be chiefly dependent on the mechanical interaction between the difference in surface tension and the MW/volume of drugs (see the exponential dependency in Eq.11).

The theory suggested in the last paragraph should be able to predict the levels of cross resistance to drugs observed; at least by giving the "power law" of the relationship between the MDR levels and the MW/volume of drugs; at best by matching published data on the subject.

The role of drug sizes involved in MDR was initially discovered in 1970 [93] and confirmed later [94]. The authors of this seminal study generated a drug resistant cell line (DC3F lung-derived cell line) and studied the concept of cross resistance. As a first step they generated a resistant cell line by selective incubation with actinomycin D (MW=1255) for several months, which led to expression of Pgp transporters [95]. As a second step they measured cross resistance levels using several other drugs (MW<1255). They looked at how both resistant and sensitive cell lines would respond to various drugs.

As they used smaller drugs, the main expected effect opposing drug entry should be driven by the drug/membrane mechanical interaction (and not transporters). In this case, the amount of a drug entering cells should follow:

$$\ln\left(r_{MDR} / r_{non-MDR}\right) \cong -\left(MW / MW_c\right)^{2/3} \cdot \left(k / k_0 - 1\right) \tag{13}$$

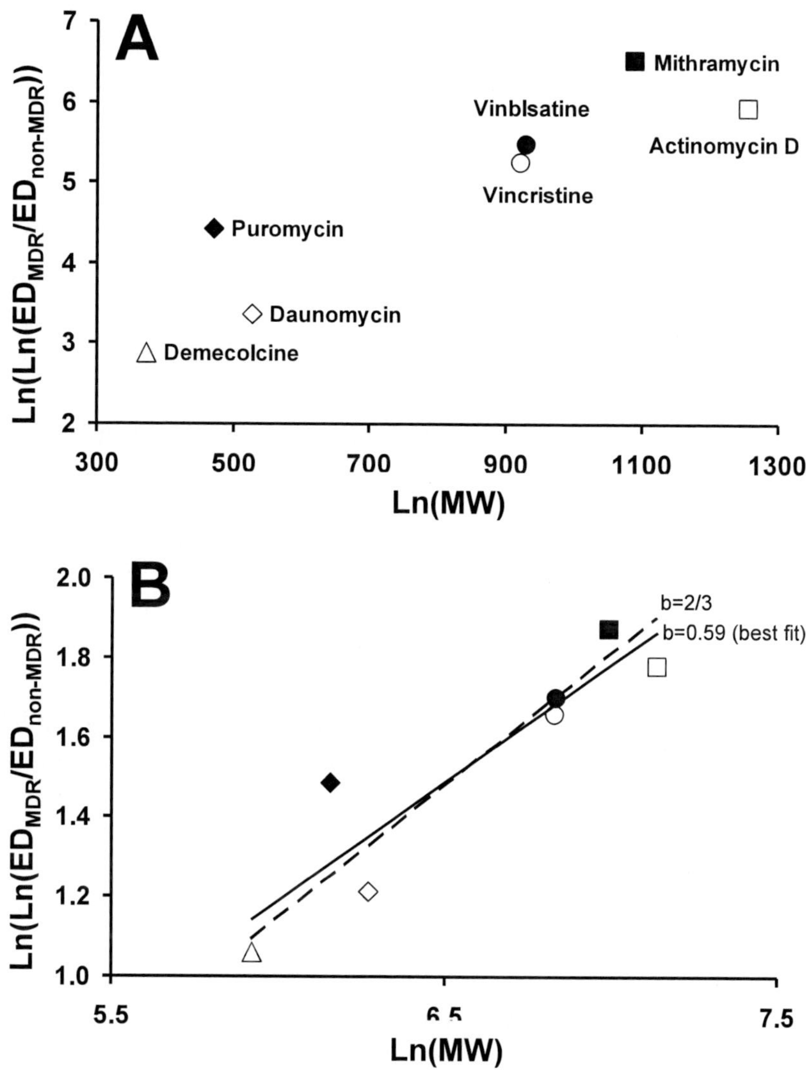

Figure 3: (A) Data from [93]. The Neperian logarithm of relative resistance levels is plotted against the MW of drugs. Drug's name is also given. (B) Same graph as in (A) where the power law predicted by Eq.14 (b=2/3, dashed curve) including the power law deduced from the best fit (b=0.59, plain curve) are plotted together and compared against the experimental data.

Given that there exists an inverse relationship between the ability of drugs to cross the membrane of cells and the dose needed to kill cells, it follows that by noting ED, the effective dose, the ratio between the EDs in drug resistant and sensitive states should be:

$$\ln\left(ED_{MDR} / ED_{non\text{-}MDR}\right) \cong \left(MW / MW_c\right)^{2/3} \cdot \left(k / k_0 - 1\right) \tag{14}$$

The numerical data from Bielder and Riehm's study are plotted in Figure 3A. In order to determine whether a power law exists, a double Neperian logarithm was applied to Bielder and Riehm's data (Figure 3A) and it was found that, indeed, a power law ~0.59±0.11 can be determined, which is similar to the one suggested by the drug/membrane mechanical interaction ~0.66 (2/3~0.66) (Figure 3B).

Thus, we know that the drug/membrane mechanical interaction is fundamental regarding the ability of drugs to cross the membrane and kill cells. A central underpinning, in the general case, is identification of the biological mechanism responsible for the increase in the kinetics of endocytosis in MDR cells. Cytosolic alkalization seems the most likely candidate for this.

III. The Role of pH_i in MDR

A. Why Would the pH_i be an Important Factor in a Cell Membrane's Mechanical Properties?

Given the importance of pH_i in drug resistance, as drug movement across the cell membrane is affected by the differential packing of lipids, it may well be that this differential packing is governed by pH changes. To consider any effect of the pH_i on lipid packing it is central to understand the notion of packing from a physics stand point. At a constant membrane surface area, the lipid packing is given by the optimal area per lipid in the cell membrane. The latter is deduced from the balance between lipid repulsion (including hard core or electrostatic effects) and attraction (aliphatic chain(s)/hydrophobic effects). Any changes in this balance are expected to affect the optimal area per lipid (i.e. their packing). Therefore, as a non negligible fraction (~30%) of the inner leaflet lipids are negatively charged, such as phosphatidylserine, for example [96]; a slight increase in positive ion concentration (e.g. decrease in pH_i) is expected to interact with lipids, "masking" their negative charges and decreasing the electrostatic repulsion between them. Given the size of hydrogen ions (i.e. exchangeable protons) they will have a more pronounced effect on negatively charged lipids than any other cation. As a final result, a low pH_i is more likely to be central in abolishing the physical repulsion between lipids, and thus decreases the surface tension (i.e. the lipid packing of the cytosolic leaflet. Note that both lipid packing and surface tension are proportional to each other). Such a relationship between free electrolytes and the cross section area per lipid in model biomembranes is well known experimentally [97-99]. Conversely, when the cytosolic pH increases (i.e. when cells become resistant to drugs in our case), fewer positive charges will be available to mask the lipids charge, which in turn is expected to increase their repulsions and thus their packing. Thus, this higher lipid packing would increase the surface tension of the leaflet in contact with the milieu of elevated cellular pH in the case of drug resistant cells. So, if the pH affects the packing of lipids, and the packing of lipids affects the intracellular accumulation of drugs, it follows that the cytosolic pH should affect the intracellular accumulation of those drugs.

Finally, the changes in pH_i observed when cells switch their state of resistance may be directly responsible for altering the intracellular accumulation of drugs as a function of their sizes, thus impairing their activity. In due course, this could provide a strong argument for the unification of the fields of drug bioavailability and drug resistance.

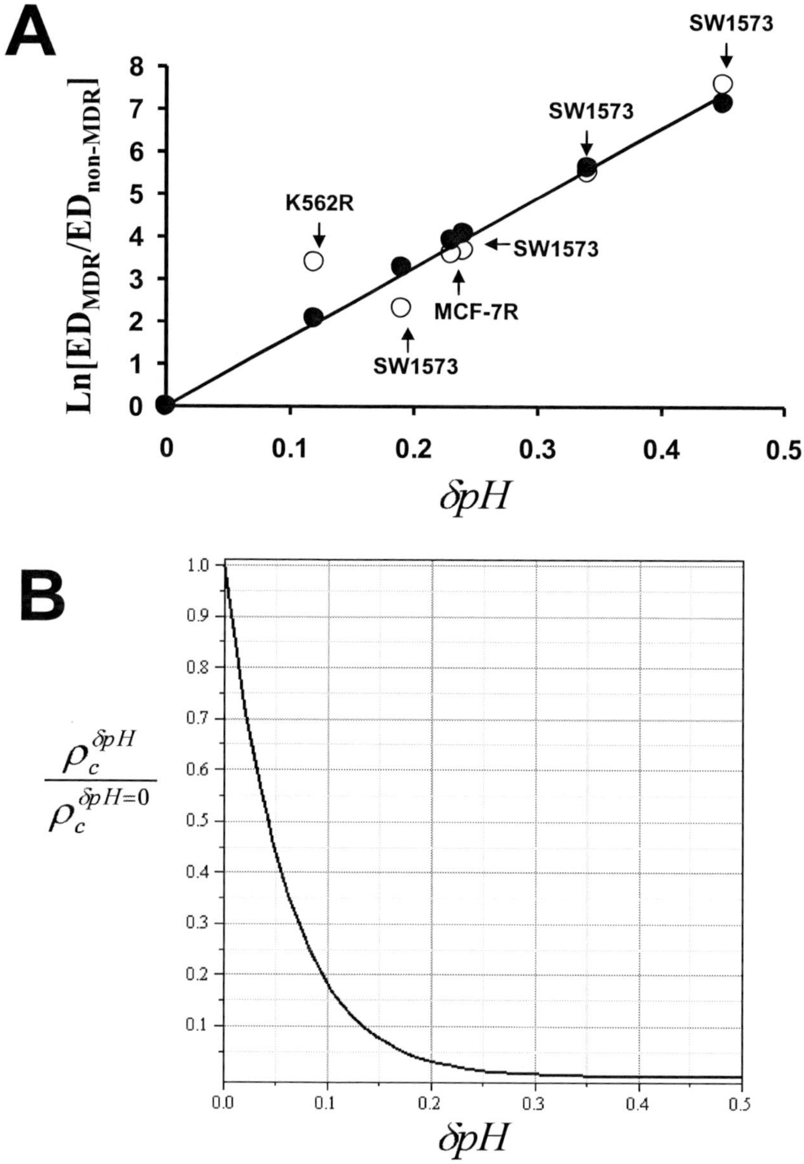

Figure 4. (A) Comparison between experimental (blanked circles) doxorubicin resistance levels obtained in cells and the theory (filled circles- Eq.16) with $\delta N / N_0 = 2.27\%$ (note that this value concerning the lipid asymmetry falls within the error margins defined previously $\delta N / N_0 = 2 \pm 0.5\%$ [84]. The open circles corresponding to SW1573 (lung derived cancer cells), K562R (leukemic cancer cells) and MCF-7R (breast derived cancer cells) are indicated with arrows and labels. Finally the straight line is the linear regression of experimental data which agrees very well with the theory. (B) Effect of pH changes (cytosolic alkalization) on the surface density of Pgp transporters needed to trigger drug resistance. As seen in the figure the number of Pgp can decrease exponentially when the pH increases: the membrane takes over.

B. Fundamental Relationship between pH and MDR Levels

Given Eq.14, it is possible to determine the effect of pH on the EDs ratio. It is possible to demonstrate that if the pH is involved, then the effective doses should be written as follows:

$$\ln\left(\frac{ED_{MDR}}{ED_{non\text{-}MDR}}\right) \cong \left(\frac{MW}{MW_c}\right)^{2/3} \cdot \left[\frac{\left(\frac{1+\left(\frac{1+\gamma}{1+10^{-\delta pH}}\right)^2}{2}\right)^{1/2} - 1}{2\frac{\delta N}{N_0}}\right] - \ln\left(1 - \frac{\rho_{Pgp}}{\rho^c_{Pgp}}\right) \qquad \text{(Eq.15)}$$

In Eq.15, $\delta pH = pH_{MDR} - pH_{non\text{-}MDR}$. is the cytosolic pH difference between the MDR and non MDR states, and $\gamma \cong 1.5$ is a physical constant that describes the probability that a hydrogen ion interacts with a negatively charged lipid in the sensitive state.

From Eq.15, the effect of Pgp mediated drug extrusion is only a Neperian logarithm of the surface density of transporters. This indicates that this term will be dominant only if $\rho_{Pgp} \sim \rho^c_{Pgp}$ (in which case the Neperian logarithm becomes infinite). Note however that when the EDs are determined, the amount of drug added to cells is necessarily higher than the concentration of the same drug in culture condition that maintains the resistant phenotype. Therefore, full drug resistance is never reached when the effective doses are determined. It means therefore that when the effective doses are determined: $\rho_{Pgp} < \rho^c_{Pgp}$ and that in the last term can be omitted. In this condition, it follows that:

$$\ln\left(\frac{ED_{MDR}}{ED_{non\text{-}MDR}}\right) \cong \left(\frac{MW}{MW_c}\right)^{2/3} \cdot \left[\left(\frac{1+\left(\frac{1+\gamma}{1+10^{-\delta pH}}\right)^2}{2}\right)^{1/2} - 1\right] \Big/ 2\frac{\delta N}{N_0} \qquad \text{(Eq.16)}$$

Eq.16 can be plotted against experimental data issued from numerous studies performed in the field of cancer. Accordingly, it is possible to demonstrate the correlation between Eq.16 and the experimental data obtained with doxorubicin (Figure 4A). In turn, this suggests that the effective doses needed to kill cells are not dependent on a drug handling activity by Pgp-like transporters, but on the cytosolic pH changes only.

C. Drug Handling Versus Cytosolic pH: Relative Involvement of Each

At the cellular level, both Pgp expression levels and cytosolic alkalization are correlated with MDR levels. Figure 4A demonstrates that a drug handling activity is not needed to interpret the results. The reason can be traced back to Eq.9. It was then stated that when the kinetic of endocytosis increases, the surface density of Pgp needed to trigger full drug resistance can decrease exponentially. This is because when the kinetic of endocytosis increase, the inner leaflet of the membrane is further packed (Figure 1A & Eq.4) and, as a result, membrane-embedded drugs will remain in the membrane for longer times and diffuse over very long distances. As they diffuse over long distances, there is no need for lots of membrane Pgps. This means that although Pgps can indeed handle drugs, there efficiency and involvement when cytosolic pH changes are taken into consideration, is likely to be low as the interaction between drug size and the membrane's mechanical properties (i.e. the packing of lipids) take over (Figure 4B).

Conclusion

In summary, drug resistance has been attributed to an increase in pH_i. Furthermore, a large variety of MDR modifiers known to be able to revert resistance to chemotherapeutic drugs have been shown to exert their cellular effects through a pH-acidifying mechanism. Conversely, the alkalinizing effect of other pH_i regulatory transporters, like the electrogenic vacuolar H^+-ATPases (V-ATPase), for example, have been shown to be involved not only in the etiology of malignant generation, but also in drug extrusion and resistance to chemotherapy.

No matter what we have learned of the MDR phenomenon in recent years, this is still a complex problem involving multiple and interrelated synergisms. In this chapter, we have summarized how drug transporters, membrane mechanical properties, and cytosolic pH can interact together. A key point that was reached is that even if a drug handling activity is involved, its efficiency is likely to be low. In this line, it is demonstrated that the pumping out of anticancer drugs from the cell, if any, would be relatively inefficient compared to the effect of pH on the membrane. Although other more complex biological mechanisms involved in drug resistance, e.g. anti-apoptotic stimuli linked to cytosolic alkalization [100] might take place, and are certainly not ruled out, the theory presented in this chapter is supported by experimental evidence.

The consistent features reviewed here are of paramount importance in any strategy directed at counteracting and overcoming MDR and, in any attempt to improve the chemotherapeutic approach to anticancer treatment. In summary, the bulk of existent evidence indicates that future attempts to override MDR, no matter what different approaches are considered, should be approached from the perspective afforded by homeostatic alterations of the hydrogen ion. This proposal comes from the fact that MDR reversion can be achieved by lowering pH_i specific to cancer cells and tissues in most, if not in all, kinds of solid tumor cells and leukemias. It is therefore very much worth considering that targeting the cytosolic pH with drugs through a concerted action of different proton transport inhibitors could help to overcome MDR in different clinical situations in oncology.

References

[1] K. Dano, Active outward transport of daunomycin in resistant Ehrlich ascites tumor cells, *Biochem Biophs Acta*, 1973, 323 466-483.

[2] Gajate, C; Mollinedo, F. Biological activities, mechanisms of action and biomedical prospect of the antitumor ether phospholipid ET-18-OCH3 (edelfosine), a proapoptotic agent in tumor cells, *Curr Drug Metab*, 2002, 3, 491-525.

[3] Torigoe, T; Izumi, H; Ise, T; Murakami, T; Uramoto, H; Ishiguchi, H; Yoshida, Y; Tanabe, M; Nomoto, M; Kohno, K. Vacuolar $H(^{+})$-ATPase: functional mechanisms and potential as a target for cancer chemotherapy, *Anticancer Drugs*, 2002, 13, 237-243.

[4] Harguindey, S; Reshkin, SJ; Orive, G; Arranz, JL; Anitua, E. Growth and trophic factors, pH and the Na^{+}/H^{+} exchanger in Alzheimer's disease, other neurodegenerative diseases and cancer: new therapeutic possibilities and potential dangers, *Curr Alzheimer Res.*, 2007, 4, 53-65.

[5] Harguindey, S; Orive, G; Luis Pedraz, J; Paradiso, A; Reshkin, SJ. The role of pH dynamics and the Na^{+}/H^{+} antiporter in the etiopathogenesis and treatment of cancer. Two faces of the same coin--one single nature, *Biochim Biophys Acta*, 2005, 1756, 1-24.

[6] Harguindey, S; Pedraz, JL. Garcia Canero, R; Perez de Diego, J; Cragoe, EJ; Jr., Hydrogen ion-dependent oncogenesis and parallel new avenues to cancer prevention and treatment using a H^{+}-mediated unifying approach: pH-related and pH-unrelated mechanisms, *Crit Rev Oncog*, 1995, 6, 1-33.

[7] Perona, R; Serrano, R. Increased pH and tumorigenicity of fibroblasts expressing a yeast proton pump, *Nature*, 1988, 334, 438-440.

[8] Reshkin, SJ; Bellizzi, A; Caldeira, S; Albarani, V; Malanchi, I; Poignee, M; Alunni-Fabbroni, M; Casavola, V; Tommasino, M. Na^{+}/H^{+} exchanger-dependent intracellular alkalinization is an early event in malignant transformation and plays an essential role in the development of subsequent transformation-associated phenotypes, *FASEB J*, 2000, 14, 2185-2197.

[9] Hanahan, D; Weinberg, RA. The hallmarks of cancer, *Cell*, 2000, 100, 57-70.

[10] Lagarde, AE. Pouyssegur, JM. The Na^{+}:H^{+} antiport in cancer, *Cancer Biochem Biophys*, 1986, 9 1-14.

[11] Rotin, D; Steele-Norwood, D; Grinstein, S; Tannock, I. Requirement of the Na^{+}/H^{+} exchanger for tumor growth, *Cancer Res.*, 1989, 49, 205-211.

[12] Rich, IN; Worthington-White, D; Garden, OA; Musk, P. Apoptosis of leukemic cells accompanies reduction in intracellular pH after targeted inhibition of the $Na(^{+})/H(^{+})$ exchanger, *Blood*, 2000, 95, 1427-1434.

[13] Orive, G; Reshkin, SJ; Harguindey, S; Pedraz, JL. Hydrogen ion dynamics and the Na^{+}/H^{+} exchanger in cancer angiogenesis and antiangiogenesis, *Brit J Cancer*, 2003, 89, 1395-1399.

[14] Cardone, RA; Casavola, V; Reshkin, SJ. The role of disturbed pH dynamics and the Na^{+}/H^{+} exchanger in metastasis, *Nat Rev Cancer*, 2005, 5, 786-795.

[15] Keizer, HG; Joenje, H. Increased cytosolic pH in multidrug-resistant human lung tumor cells: effect of verapamil, *JNCI*, 1989, 81, 706-709.

[16] Simon, S; Roy, D; Schindler, M. Intracellular pH and the control of multidrug resistance, *PNAS*, 1994, 91, 1128-1132.

[17] Oberhaensli, RD; Hilton-Jones, D; Bore, PJ; Hands, LJ; Rampling, RP; Radda, GK. Biochemical investigation of human tumours in vivo with phosphorus-31 magnetic resonance spectroscopy, *Lancet ii*, 1986, 8-11.

[18] Roepe, PD. The role of the MDR protein in altered drug translocation across tumor cell membranes, *Biochim Biophys Acta*, 1995, 1241, 385-405.

[19] Brand, KA; Hermfisse, U. Aerobic glycolysis by proliferating cells: a protective strategy against reactive oxygen species, *FASEB J*, 1997, 11, 388-395.

[20] Fidler, IJ; Ellis, LM. The implications of angiogenesis for the biology and therapy of cancer metastasis, *Cell*, 1994, 79, 185-188.

[21] Murakami, T; Shibuya, I; Ise, T; Chen, ZS; Akiyama, S; Nakagawa, M; Izumi, H; Nakamura, T; Matsuo, K; Yamada, Y; Kohno, K. Elevated expression of vacuolar proton pump genes and cellular pH in cisplatin resistance, *Int J Cancer*, 2001, 93, 869-874.

[22] Thiebaut, F; Currier, SJ; Whitaker, J; Haugland, RP; Gottesman, MM; Pastan, I; Willingham, MC. Activity of the multidrug transporter results in alkalinization of the cytosol: measurement of cytosolic pH by microinjection of a pH-sensitive dye, *J Histochem Cytochem*, 1990, 38, 685-690.

[23] Webb, SD; Sherratt, JA; Fish, RG. Mathematical modeling of tumour acidity: regulation of intracellular pH, *J Theor Biol.*, 1999, 196, 237-250.

[24] Roepe, PD. pH and multidrug resistance, *Novartis Found Symp*, 2001, 240, 232-247.

[25] Raghunand, N; Gillies, RJ. pH and chemotherapy, *Novartis Found Symp*, 2001, 240, 199-211.

[26] Chen, Q; Benson, RS; Whetton, AD; Brant, SR; Donowitz, M; Montrose, MH; Dive, C; Watson, AJ. Role of acid/base homeostasis in the suppression of apoptosis in haemopoietic cells by v-Abl protein tyrosine kinase, *J Cell Sci.*, 1997, 110(Pt 3), 379-387.

[27] Goossens, JF; Henichart, JP; Dassonneville, L; Facompre, M; Bailly, C. Relation between intracellular acidification and camptothecin-induced apoptosis in leukemia cells, *Eur J Pharm Sci.*, 2000, 10, 125-131.

[28] Roepe, PD; Wei, LY; Cruz, J; Carlson, D. Lower electrical membrane potential and altered pH_i homeostasis in multidrug-resistant (MDR) cells: further characterization of a series of MDR cell lines expressing different levels of P-glycoprotein, *Biochemistry*, 1993, 32, 11042-11056.

[29] Simon, S. The multiple mechanisms of multidrug resistance and cellular pH, *Novartis Found Symp*, 2001, 240, 269-281.

[30] El Awad, B; Kreft, B; Wolber, EM; Hellwig-Burgel, T; Metzen, E; Fandrey, J; Jelkmann, W. Hypoxia and interleukin-1beta stimulate vascular endothelial growth factor production in human proximal tubular cells, *Kidney Int.*, 2000, 58, 43-50.

[31] D'Arcangelo, D; Facchiano, F; Barlucchi, LM; Melillo, G; Illi, B; Testolin, L; Gaetano, C; Capogrossi, MC. Acidosis inhibits endothelial cell apoptosis and function and induces basic fibroblast growth factor and vascular endothelial growth factor expression, *Circ Res.*, 2000, 86, 312-318.

[32] Laurencot, CM; Andrews, PA; Kennedy, KA. Inhibitors of intracellular pH regulation induce cisplatin resistance in EMT6 mouse mammary tumor cells, *Oncol Res.*, 1995, 7, 363-369.

[33] Chau, Q; Stewart, DJ. Cisplatin efflux, binding and intracellular pH in the HTB56 human lung adenocarcinoma cell line and the E-8/0.7 cisplatin-resistant variant, *Cancer Chemother Pharmacol*, 1999, 44, 193-202.

[34] Barry, MA; Reynolds, JE; Eastman, A. Etoposide-induced apoptosis in human HL-60 cells is associated with intracellular acidification, *Cancer Res.*, 1993, 53, 2349-2357.

[35] De Milito, A; Fais, S. Tumor acidity, chemoresistance and proton pump inhibitors, *Future Oncol*, 2005, 1, 779-786.

[36] Di Sario, A; Bendia, E; Omenetti, A; De Minicis, S; Marzioni, M; Kleemann, HW; Candelaresi, C; Saccomanno, S; Alpini, G; Benedetti, A. Selective inhibition of ion transport mechanisms regulating intracellular pH reduces proliferation and induces apoptosis in cholangiocarcinoma cells, *Dig Liver Dis.*, 2007, 39, 60-69.

[37] Mellman, I; Fuchs, R; Helenius, A. Acidification of the endocytic and exocytic pathways, *Annu Rev Biochem*, 1986, 55, 663-700.

[38] Ouar, Z; Lacave, R; Bens, M; Vandewalle, A. Mechanisms of altered sequestration and efflux of chemotherapeutic drugs by multidrug-resistant cells, *Cell Biol Toxicol*, 1999, 15, 91-100.

[39] Hoffman, MM; Wei, LY; Roepe, PD. Are altered pH_i and membrane potential in hu MDR 1 transfectants sufficient to cause MDR protein-mediated multidrug resistance?, *J Gen Physiol*, 1996, 108, 295-313.

[40] Yamamoto, C; Takemoto, H; Kuno, K; Yamamoto, D; Nakai, K; Baden, T; Kamata, K; Hirata, H; Watanabe, T; Inoue, K. Cycloprodigiosin hydrochloride, a H^+/Cl^- symporter, induces apoptosis in human colon cancer cell lines in vitro, *Oncol Rep.*, 2001, 8, 821-824.

[41] Cosentini, E; Haberl, I; Pertschy, P; Teleky, B; Mallinger, R; Baumgartner, G; Wenzl, E; Hamilton, G. The differentiation inducers phenylacetate and phenylbutyrate modulate camptothecin sensitivity in colon carcinoma cells in vitro by intracellular acidification, *Int J Oncol*, 2001, 19, 1069-1074.

[42] Marquardt, D; Center, MS. Involvement of vacuolar $H(^+)$-adenosine triphosphatase activity in multidrug resistance in HL60 cells, *J Nat Ca Inst*, 1991, 83, 1098-1102.

[43] Drose, S; Bindseil, KU; Bowman, EJ; Siebers, A; Zeeck, A; Altendorf, K. Inhibitory effect of modified bafilomycins and concanamycins on P- and V-type adenosinetriphosphatases, *Biochemistry*, 1993, 32, 3902-3906.

[44] Ohta, T; Arakawa, H; Futagami, F; Fushida, S; Kitagawa, H; Kayahara, M; Nagakawa, T; Miwa, K; Kurashima, K; Numata, M; Kitamura, Y; Terada, T; Ohkuma, S. Bafilomycin A1 induces apoptosis in the human pancreatic cancer cell line Capan-1, *J Pathol*, 1998, 185, 324-330.

[45] Adams, DJ; Wahl, ML; Flowers, JL; Sen, B; Colvin, M; Dewhirst, MW; Manikumar, G; Wani, MC. Camptothecin analogs with enhanced activity against human breast cancer cells. II. Impact of the tumor pH gradient, *Cancer Chemother Pharmacol*, 2006, 57, 145-154.

[46] Kozin, SV; Shkarin, P; Gerweck, LE. The cell transmembrane pH gradient in tumors enhances cytotoxicity of specific weak acid chemotherapeutics, *Cancer Res.*, 2001, 61, 4740-4743.

[47] Thews, O; Gassner, B; Kelleher, DK; Schwerdt, G; Gekle, M. Impact of extracellular acidity on the activity of P-glycoprotein and the cytotoxicity of chemotherapeutic drugs, *Neoplasia*, 2006, 8, 143-152.

[48] Roepe, PD; Wei, LY; Hoffman, MM; Fritz, F. Altered drug translocation mediated by the MDR protein: direct, indirect, or both?, *J Bioenerg Biomembr*, 1996, 28, 541-555.

[49] Gatenby, RA; Gawlinski, ET. Mathematical models of tumour invasion mediated by transformation-induced alteration of microenvironmental pH, *Novartis Found Symp*, 2001, 240, 85-96.

[50] Sparks, RL; Pool, TB; Smith, NK; Cameron, IL. Effects of amiloride on tumor growth and intracellular element content of tumor cells in vivo, *Cancer Res.*, 1983, 43, 73-77.

[51] Denker, SP; Barber, DL. Ion transport proteins anchor and regulate the cytoskeleton, *Curr Opin Cell Biol.*, 2002, 14, 214-220.

[52] Gottlieb, RA; Nordberg, J; Skowronski, E; Babior, BM. Apoptosis induced in Jurkat cells by several agents is preceded by intracellular acidification, *PNAS*, 1996, 93, 654-658.

[53] Perez-Sala, D; Collado-Escobar, D; Mollinedo, F. Intracellular alkalinization suppresses lovastatin-induced apoptosis in HL-60 cells through the inactivation of a pH-dependent endonuclease, *J Biol Chem.*, 1995, 270, 6235-6242.

[54] Lotem, J; Cragoe, EJ; Jr., L. Sachs, Rescue from programmed cell death in leukemic and normal myeloid cells, *Blood*, 1991, 78, 953-960.

[55] Epand, RF; Epand, RM; Gupta, RS; Cragoe, EJ; Jr., Reversal of intrinsic multidrug resistance in Chinese hamster ovary cells by amiloride analogs, *Brit J Cancer*, 1991, 63 247-251.

[56] Miraglia, E; Viarisio, D; Riganti, C; Costamagna, C; Ghigo, D; Bosia, A. Na^+/H^+exchanger activity is increased in doxorubicin-resistant human colon cancer cells and its modulation modifies the sensitivity of the cells to doxorubicin, *Int J Cancer*, 2005, 115, 924-929.

[57] Radvakova, I; Mirossay, A; Mojzis, J; Mirossay, L. The effect of 5'-(N,N-dimethyl)-amiloride on cytotoxic activity of doxorubicin and vincristine in CEM cell lines, *Physiol Res.*, 2001, 50, 283-287.

[58] Goda, K; Balkay, L; Marian, T; Tron, L; Aszalos, A; Szabo, G; Jr., Intracellular pH does not affect drug extrusion by P-glycoprotein, *J Photochem Photobiol*, 1996, B34, 177-182.

[59] Altenberg, GA; Young, G; Horton, JK; Glass, D; Belli, JA; Reuss, L. Changes in intra- or extracellular pH do not mediate P-glycoprotein-dependent multidrug resistance, *PNAS*, 1993, 90, 9735-9738.

[60] Ambudkar, SV; Dey, S; Hrycyna, CA; Ramachandra, M; Pastan, I; Gottesman, MM. Biochemical, cellular, and pharmacological aspects of the multidrug transporter, *Annu Rev Pharmacol Toxicol*, 1999, 39, 361-398.

[61] Bornmann, WG; Roepe, PD. Analysis of drug transport kinetics in multidrug-resistant cells using a novel coumarin-vinblastine compound, *Biochem*, 1994, 33, 12665-12675.

[62] Eytan, GD. Mechanism of multidrug resistance in relation to passive membrane permeation, *Biomed Pharmacother*, 2005, 59, 90-97.

[63] Germann, UA. P-glycoprotein--a mediator of multidrug resistance in tumour cells, *Eur J Cancer*, 1996, 32A, 927-944.

[64] Nielsen, D; Maare, C; Skovsgaard, T. Influx of daunorubicin in multidrug resistant Ehrlich ascites tumour cells: correlation to expression of P-glycoprotein and efflux. Influence of verapamil, *Biochem Pharmacol*, 1995, 50, 443-450.

[65] Ramu, A; Pollard, HB; Rosario, LM. Doxorubicin resistance in P388 leukemia--evidence for reduced drug influx, *Int J Cancer*, 1989, 44, 539-547.

[66] Raviv, Y; Pollard, HB; Bruggemann, EP; Pastan, I; Gottesman, MM. Photosensitized labeling of a functional multidrug transporter in living drug-resistant tumor cells, *J Biol Chem.*, 1990, 265, 3975-3980.

[67] Sharom, FJ. The P-glycoprotein efflux pump: how does it transport drugs?, *J Membr Biol.*, 1997, 160, 161-175.

[68] Sirotnak, FM; Yang, CH; Mines, LS; Oribe, E; Biedler, JL. Markedly altered membrane transport and intracellular binding of vincristine in multidrug-resistant Chinese hamster cells selected for resistance to vinca alkaloids, *J Cell Physiol*, 1986, 126, 266-274.

[69] Spoelstra, EC; Westerhoff, HV; Dekker, H; Lankelma, J. Kinetics of daunorubicin trasport by P-glycoprotein of intact cancer cells, *Eur J Biochem*, 1992, 207, 567-579.

[70] Stein, WD; Cardarelli, C; Pastan, I; Gottesman, MM. Kinetic evidence suggesting that the multidrug transporter differentially handles influx and efflux of its substrates, *Mol Pharmacol*, 1994, 45, 763-772.

[71] Wang, S; Wan, NC; Harrison, J; Miller, W; Chuckowree, I; Sohal, S; Hancox, TC; Baker, S; Folkes, A; Wilson, F; Thompson, D; Cocks, S; Farmer, H; Boyce, A; Freathy, C; Broadbridge, J; Scott, J; Depledge, P; Faint, R; Mistry, P; Charlton, P. Design and synthesis of new templates derived from pyrrolopyrimidine as selective multidrug-resistance-associated protein inhibitors in multidrug resistance, *J Med Chem.*, 2004, 47, 1339-1350.

[72] Rao, VV; Herman, LW; Kronauge, JF; Piwnica-Worms, D. A novel areneisonitrile Tc complex inhibits the transport activity of MDR P-glycoprotein, *Nucl Med Biol.*, 1998, 25, 225-232.

[73] Drori, S; Eytan, GD; Assaraf, YG. Potentiation of anticancer-drug cytotoxicity by multidrug-resistance chemosensitizers involves alterations in membrane fluidity leading to increased membrane permeability, *Eur J Biochem*, 1995, 228, 1020-1029.

[74] Dudeja, PK; Anderson, KM; Harris, JS; Buckingham, L; Coon, JS. Reversal of multidrug resistance phenotype by surfactants: relationship to membrane lipid fluidity, *Arch Biochem Biophys*, 1995, 319, 309-315.

[75] Frezard, F; Garnier-Suillerot, A. Permeability of lipid bilayer to anthracycline derivatives. Role of the bilayer composition and of the temperature, *Biochim Biophys Acta*, 1998, 1389 13-22.

[76] Liang, X; Huang, Y. Physical state changes of membrane lipids in human lung adenocarcinoma A(549) cells and their resistance to cisplatin, *Int J Biochem Cell Biol.*, 2002, 34, 1248-1255.

[77] Ramu, A; Glaubiger, D; Magrath, IT; Joshi, A. Plasma membrane lipid structural order in doxorubicin-sensitive and -resistant P388 cells, *Cancer Res.*, 1983, 43, 5533-5537.

[78] Regev, R; Assaraf, YG; Eytan, GD. Membrane fluidization by ether, other anesthetics, and certain agents abolishes P-glycoprotein ATPase activity and modulates efflux from multidrug-resistant cells, *Eur J Biochem*, 1999, 259, 18-24.

[79] Altan, N; Chen, Y; Schindler, M; Simon, SM. Tamoxifen inhibits acidification in cells independent of the estrogen receptor, *PNAS*, 1999, 96, 4432-4437.

[80] Sehested, M; Skovsgaard, T; van Deurs, B; Winther-Nielsen, H. Increased plasma membrane traffic in daunorubicin resistant P388 leukaemic cells. Effect of daunorubicin and verapamil, *Brit J Cancer*, 1987, 56, 747-751.

[81] Devaux, PF; Zachowski, A; Favre, E; Fellmann, P; Cribier, S; Geldwerth, D; Herve, P; Seigneuret, M. Energy-dependent translocation of amino-phospholipids in the erythrocyte membrane, *Biochimie*, 1986, 68, 383-393.

[82] Farge, E. Increased vesicle endocytosis due to an increase in the plasma membrane phosphatidylserine concentration, *Biophys J*, 1995, 69, 2501-2506.

[83] Farge, E; Ojcius, DM; Subtil, A; Dautry-Varsat, A. Enhancement of endocytosis due to aminophospholipid transport across the plasma membrane of living cells, *Am J Physiol*, 1999, 276, C725-733.

[84] Rauch, C; Farge, E. Endocytosis switch controlled by transmembrane osmotic pressure and phospholipid number asymmetry, *Biophys*, 2000, J 78, 3036-3047.

[85] Regev, R; Yeheskely-Hayon, D; Katzir, H; Eytan, GD. Transport of anthracyclines and mitoxantrone across membranes by a flip-flop mechanism, *Biochem Pharmacol*, 2005, 70, 161-169.

[86] Cirilli, M; Bachechi, F; Ughetto, G; Colonna, FP; Capobianco, ML. Interactions between morpholinyl anthracyclines and DNA. The crystal structure of a morpholino doxorubicin bound to d(CGTACG), *J Mol Biol.*, 1993, 230, 878-889.

[87] Heijn, M; Roberge, S; Jain, RK. Cellular membrane permeability of anthracyclines does not correlate with their delivery in a tissue-isolated tumor, *Cancer Res.*, 1999, 59, 4458-4463.

[88] Ulander, J; Haymet, AD. Permeation across hydrated DPPC lipid bilayers: simulation of the titrable amphiphilic drug valproic acid, *Biophys J*, 2003, 85, 3475-3484.

[89] Bloom, M; Evans, E; Mouritsen, OG. Physical properties of the fluid lipid-bilayer component of cell membranes: a perspective, *Q Rev Biophys*, 1991, 24, 293-397.

[90] Rudnick, J; Gaspari, G. *Elements of the Random Walk*, Cambridge University Press, Cambridge, 2004.

[91] Ferte, J. Analysis of the tangled relationships between P-glycoprotein-mediated multidrug resistance and the lipid phase of the cell membrane, *Europ J. Biochemistry / FEBS*, 2000, 267, 277-294.

[92] Colin, M; Madoulet, C; Warren, L; Jardillier, JC. Alterations of vinblastine influx in multidrug-resistant lymphoblastic leukaemic CEM cells, *Anticancer Res.*, 1996, 16, 407-412.

[93] Biedler, JL; Riehm, H. Cellular resistance to actinomycin D in Chinese hamster cells in vitro: cross-resistance, radioautographic, and cytogenetic studies, *Cancer Res.*, 1970, 30, 1174-1184.

[94] Selassie, CD; Hansch, C; Khwaja, TA. Structure-activity relationships of antineoplastic agents in multidrug resistance, *J Med Chem.*, 1990, 33, 1914-1919.

[95] Safa, AR; Glover, CJ; Meyers, MB; Biedler, JL; Felsted, RL. Vinblastine photoaffinity labeling of a high molecular weight surface membrane glycoprotein specific for multidrug-resistant cells, *J Biol Chem.*, 1986, 261, 6137-6140.

[96] Alberts, B; Bray, D; Lewis, J; Raff, M; Roberts, K; Watson, JD. Biologie Moleculaire de La Cellule, New York, 1994.

[97] Petelska, AD; Figaszewski, ZA. Effect of pH on the interfacial tension of bilayer lipid membrane formed from phosphatidylcholine or phosphatidylserine, *Biochim Biophs Acta*, 2002, 1561, 135-146.

[98] Petrache, HI; Zemb, T; Belloni, L; Parsegian, VA. Salt screening and specific ion adsorption determine neutral-lipid membrane interactions, *PNAS*, 2006, 103, 7982-7987.

[99] Victorov, AV; Janes, N; Taraschi, TF; Hoek, JB. Packing constraints and electrostatic surface potentials determine transmembrane asymmetry of phosphatidylethanol, *Biophs J*, 1997, 72, 2588-2598.

[100] Lagadic-Gossmann, D; Huc, L; Lecureur, V. Alterations of intracellular pH homeostasis in apoptosis: origins and roles, *Cell Death Differ*, 2004, 11, 953-961.

In: Multiple Drug Resistance
Editors: A. Meszaros, G. Balogh, pp. 153-166
ISBN: 978-1-60741-595-4

Chapter VI

Genetic and Clinical Factors of Antibiotic Resistance in Bacteria

Spyros D. Mentzelopoulos [*] ***and Eleni E. Magira***
First Department of Intensive Care Medicine, University of Athens Medical School, Evaggelismos General Hospital, 45-47 Ipsilandou Street, GR-10675, Athens, Greece.

Abstract

Infectious diseases still remain an important cause of mortality. The emergence of pathogenic bacteria resistant to many antibiotics (multidrug-resistant strains) has created the need for exploring resistance to antimicrobial therapy along with the development of novel therapeutic agents. This need has become urgent, because during the last three decades, only two new classes of antibiotics with novel mechanisms of action (i.e., linezolid and daptomycin) have been introduced. Also, the overall antibiotic consumption has increased. The development of drug resistance over time limits the efficacy of antimicrobial agents and exerts a negative effect on patient outcomes.

Interaction between several genetic host factors, distinct anatomical and other features of the bacteria, and hygiene measures play a paramount role in the treatment of infections caused by multidrug-resistant organisms. The recent progress in molecular biology and bacterial genome analysis has revolutionized our understanding of the infectious diseases mechanisms. The evolution of antibiotic resistance is primarily the result of natural selection acting on variant bacterial phenotypes. Both the rigid base sequence of DNA and the more plastic expression patterns of the genes contribute to the bacterial phenotype. Several categories of antibiotic resistance genes have been identified. Examples include silent genes such as the *E. coli* AmpC gene, which when activated confers potent antibiotic resistance, the glutamate decarboxylase genes, which enable the passage through the acidic environment of the stomach, genes regulating the expression of other genes related to antibiotic resistance, genes encoding beta lactamases, etc.

* Coresponding author: E-mail: sdmentzelopoulos@yahoo.com; sdm@hol.gr; FAX: +30-210-6218493; Phone: +30-6977465832; Home Address: 7 Ydras Street, GR-11257, Athens, Greece.

Crosstransmission is frequent in pathogens causing nosocomial outbreaks. Contact precautions, compliance with universal hand hygiene measures, and maximum barrier precautions should be implemented in hospitals, and particularly, in intensive care units. Multiple drug resistance is a very complicated issue perplexed by various mechanisms that have several implications on the pathogenesis, the epidemiology, and the clinical outcome of the infections. In this article, we attempt to clarify the multiple and different genetic paths involved in the pathogenesis of antibiotic resistance. Furthermore, we describe clinical factors related to multiple drug resistance.

Introduction

Infections are still among the most important and potentially life-threatening human diseases. Although the induction of antimicrobial drugs was broadly implemented, the problem with the infection control is not resolved. One of the reasons was the use and misuse of antibiotics that resulted in antibiotic-resistant bacteria. Infections caused by multidrug-resistant (MDR) Gram-negative bacteria are an increasing problem worldwide. For instance, the prevalence of nosocomial infections in hospital intensive care units (ICUs) due to *Acinetobacter baumannii* currently ranges from 2% to 10% of all Gram-negative bacterial infections in Europe and account for about 2.5% of them in the United States [1,2]. *A. baumannii* exhibits a remarkable ability to rapidly develop antibiotic resistance that led to the emergence of MDR strains i.e. strains susceptible only to carbapenems, minocycline, sulbactam, and colistin within a few decades. Besides *A. baumannii, Stenotrophomonas maltophilia* is increasingly prevalent in many ICUs. *S. maltophilia* is often susceptible only to trimethoprim-sulfamethoxazole [2,3].

Multidrug resistance has also been demonstrated in *Escherichia coli, Salmonella enterica serovar typhimurium*, *Shigella dysenteriae*, *Enterococcus faecium*, *Staphylococcus aureus*, *Mycobacterium tuberculosis*, *Haemophilus influenzae*, *Pseudomonas aeruginosa*, *Klebsiella pneumoniae*, and *Xanthomonas* and *Burkholderia strains* [4].

The interaction among several genetic host factors, distinctive anatomical and other features of the bacteria, and hygiene measures plays a paramount role in the treatment of infections caused by MDR organisms. Antibiotic resistance is the result of natural selection acting on variant bacterial phenotypes. The evolution of antibiotic resistance and its clinical consequences is a topic of major medical importance.

The Modes of Antibiotic Action

The use, overuse, and misuse (erroneous antibiotic prescription for nonbacterial infections, multiple combinations of antibiotics) in medicine and agriculture is the leading cause of antibiotic resistance [5]. According to the reservoir hypothesis, MDR bacteria emerge through the selective pressures exerted by antibiotics, with each antibiotic exhibiting a threshold level for induction and maintainance of resistance. After a decline in the populations of susceptible bacteria from antibiotic treatment, naturally resistant bacteria begin to thrive, thus creating an MDR reservoir.

To understand how resistance genes enable bacteria to survive an attack by an antibiotic, it helps to know exactly what antibiotics are and how they harm bacteria. The antibiotic attacks a group of bacterial cells, which die promptly, if highly susceptible. However, cells with some "intrinsic" resistance from the start, or cells with later-on-acquired resistance through mutation or gene exchange, may survive, especially if the antibiotic dose is not sufficiently high. Surviving cells will then proliferate, in the absence of competition from susceptible bacteria.

The modes of antibiotic action can be divided into five major classes:

1. Interference with cell wall synthesis (6,7)

a. β-lactams (penicillin, cephalosporins)

b. Glycopeptides (vancomycin, teicoplanin, oritavancin)

2. Inhibition of protein synthesis (6,8)

a. Macrolides

b. Aminoglycosides

c. Tetracyclines

3. Interference with nucleic acid synthesis (6)

a. Rifampicin

b. Quinolones

4. Inhibition of a metabolic pathway (6)

a. Sulfonamides (*e.g.* sulfamethoxazole) and trimethoprim

5. Disorganization of the cell membrane (9,10)

a. Polymyxin B, Granicidin, and Daptomycin.

What is Antibiotic Resistance?

Antibiotics have historically been considered as "miracle drugs." Antibiotic resistance is the ability of a bacterial strain to survive exposure to a specific antibiotic. This ability is due to genes confering drug resistance. Antibiotic-resistant bacteria are like other pathogens: to establish themselves in a population, they must be able to colonize new hosts faster than they are cleared. The ongoing development of antibiotic-resistant bacteria increases the risk of treatment failure. Also, diseases thought to have been eradicated have re-emerged. A characteristic example is drug-resistant tuberculosis.

Natural and Acquired Antibiotic Resistance

Antibiotic resistance can be intrinstic-natural, or aquired. Examples of itrinsic resistance to particular antibiotics include that of anaerobes for aminoglycosides; mutations in chromosomal genes encoding drug targets, such as the *gyrAB/parCE* and *rpoB* mutations conferring resistance to fluoroquinolones and rifampicin respectively; and activation of intrinsic low-level resistance loci, such as the broad-spectrum *mar* locus16 and the β-lactamase *ampC* gene. An example of natural resistance is Streptomyces, which has genes encoding resistance to streptomycin.

Acquired bacterial antibiotic resistance can result from a mutation of cellular genes, the acquisition of foreign resistance genes, or a combination of these two mechanisms. Transduction tansfer is mediated by bacteriophages, while transformation involves the uptake of naked DNA. The latter has proven to be important in the evolution of *Streptococcus pneumoniae* β-lactam resistance via a mosaic of penicillin-binding-protein gene structures. Conjugation involves direct cell-to-cell contact for transfer of extra-chromosomal or chromosomal DNA and is believed to be the most important transfer mechanism in the acquisition and spread of antibiotic resistance [11].

Mechanisms of Antibiotic Resistance

Genetic aspects of resistance are related to chromosomal mutations or acquisition of antibiotic resistance genes, or plasmids, or transponsons. Bacteria acquiring resistance genes through mutations spontaneously produce a new resistance trait or strengthen an existing one. These mutations can occur randomly as replication errors or an incorrect repair of a damaged DNA in actively dividing cells. Indeed, nucleic acid-base substitutions can randomly occur as DNA is replicated at a frequency of approximately 10^{-9} to 10^{-10} per gene [12]. Copying errors may lead to the partial or complete deletion of individual genes. Spontaneous mutations constitute an important mode of generating antibiotic resistance not related to selective pressure. For example, the quinolone resistance phenotype in *E. coli* is a result of changes in at least seven positions in the *gyrA* gene, but in only three positions in the *arC* gene [13-15]. Also, mutations can spontaneously occur in the sequences of genes encoding the targets of certain antibiotics. For instance, resistance to rifampicin and fluoroquinolones is caused by mutations in the genes encoding the targets of these two molecules, RpoB and DNA - topoisomerases, respectively.

Bacteria will gain a defense against an antibiotic by taking up resistance genes from other bacterial cells in the vicinity. A variety of genes can be involved in antibiotic resistance either because there are several different targets, and access or protection pathways for the antibiotic in the bacterial cell, or because each pathway requires the expression of several genes. Bacteria also acquire resistance genes through DNA transfer by plasmids, i.e., tiny loops of DNA that can help bacteria survive various hazards in the environment (Figure 1). Often one bacterium will pass resistance traits to others by giving them a useful plasmid. Resistance genes can also be transferred by viruses that occasionally extract a gene from one bacterial cell and inject it into another. Furthermore, when a bacterium dies and releases its contents into the environment, another bacterium will occasionally take up a liberated gene [16].

The resistance phenotype may include alteration of targets of antibacterials, up- or down-regulation of drug-inactivation or efflux systems, and inactivation of uptake pathways (i.e., porins and active transporters) (Table 1, Figure1). Target modification may range from a single mutation, to major alterations achieved by the incorporation of foreign DNA (17-19). Modification of penicillin-binding proteins is the mechanism of resistance in penicillin-resistant *S. pneumoniae*, *Neisseria meningitidis*, and *E. faecium*, and methicillin-resistant *S. aureus*. In Gram negative bacteria, β-lactam antibiotics gain access to the cell through a water-filled, hollow membrane protein known as a porin. In the case of imipenem resistant *P. aeruginosa*, the lack of the specific D2 porin confers resistance, as imipenem cannot penetrate the cell. This mechanism is also seen with low-level resistance to fluoroquinolones and aminoglycosides (20). Alteration of the porin protein of the outer membrane of *P. aeruginosa* results in decreased permeability of the drug, with decreased intracellular concentration. The reduced expression or absence of the OprD porin of *P. aeruginosa* reduces the permeability of the cell wall to carbapenems. Increased efflux via an energy-requiring transport pump is a well-recognised mechanism for resistance to tetracyclines and is encoded by a wide range of related genes, such as tet(A), that have become distributed in the *Enterobacteriaceae*. The mutations leading to increased expression of the efflux systems, in general, confer resistance to multiple antibiotics. Intracellular drug concentration can be reduced by the efflux systems of bacteria (e.g., tetracycline efflux system of *E. coli* and fluoroquinolone efflux system of *Staphylococcus*). Modification of the genes for DNA gyrase confers fluoroquinolone resistance, and various ribosomal alterations contribute to macrolide, tetracycline, rifampin, and mupirocin resistance. Resistance genes can also be activated or inactivated by the migration of insertion sequences. Some of the aminoglycoside resistant *Staphylococci* show decreased uptake of the antibiotic by the bacterial cytoplasmic membrane. B-lactamase production is a classical example of drug inactivation. Target bypass is by means of development of alternate metabolic pathways. Examples of this mechanism include the enterococcal and staphylococcal resistance to vancomycin and the resistance of various bacterial pathogens to the folate antagonists (16).

Many bacteria possessed resistance genes even before commercial antibiotics came into use. How has this happened? It is possible that natural antibiotics were initially elaborated as the result of random genetic mutations. Then the compounds, which turned out to eliminate competitors, enabled the manufacturers to survive and proliferate to possess genes that protected them from their own chemical weapons. Later, these protective genes found their way into other species, some of which were pathogenic.

Regardless of how bacteria acquire resistance genes today, commercial antibiotics can select the survival and propagation of antibiotic-resistant strains. In other words, by encouraging the growth of resistant pathogens, an antibiotic can actually contribute to its own undoing.

Antibiotic Resistance and Food

Another important issue is the acquired antibiotic resistance in lactic acid bacteria (LAB) of food origin. When LAB live in a biotope regularly challenged by antibiotics, acquired antibiotic is found in *Enterococci* and *Lactococci*. The resistant bacteria may transfer resistance by horizontal gene transfer. Probiotic bacteria that are consumed to maintain the microbial balance in the intenstines have the potential to transfer antibiotic resistances to pathogenic bacteria. On the other hand the harmless bacteria that normally reside in the human colon can transfer resistance among themselves and transform into pathogens. Evidence is accumulating to support the hypothesis that antibiotic-resistant bacteria from poultry, pigs and cattle enter the food supply, colonize the human digestive tract, and transfer resistance genes to human commensals [21,22].

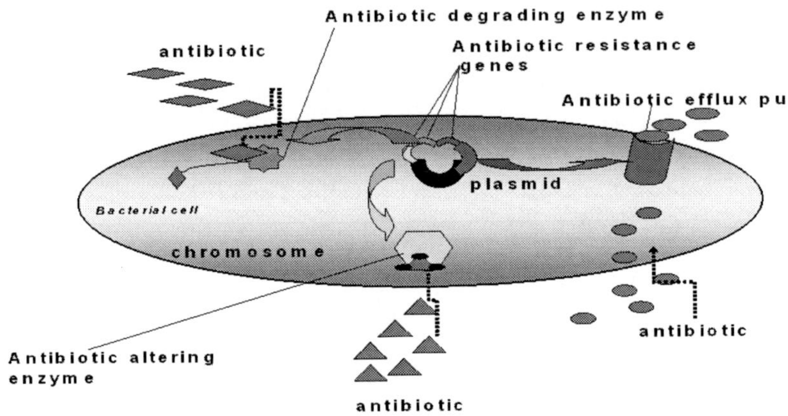

Figure 1. Several different mechanisms of antibiotic resistance. The most common mode is enzymatic inactivation of the antibiotic. An existing enzyme is modified to process the antibiotic and modifies it so that it no longer affects the microorganism. An alternative strategy utilized by bacteria is the alteration of the antibiotic target site. Resistance genes commonly are carried by plasmids, i.e., tiny loops of DNA that can help bacteria survive various hazards in the enviroment (16).

Virulence and Antibiotic Resistance of the Genome of Four of the Most Threatening Microorganisms

a. Staphylococcus aureus

S. aureus continues to be one of the most important human pathogens throughout the community and hospital settings. Lately, there is a growing concern regarding the increasing level of antibiotic resistance in *S. aureus* causing hospital-acquired and community-acquired infections. The accessory genome of *S. aureus* encodes a diverse range of nonessential functions ranging from virulence, drug and metal resistance, to substrate utilization and miscellaneous metabolism. They usually consist of mobile genetic elements (MGEs) that transfer horizontally between strains. These elements include bacteriophages, pathogenicity islands, chromosomal cassettes, genomic islands, and transposons. The identification and characterization of these elements has provided valuable information into how *S. aureus* causes disease and its relative diversity. The multiple insertions of transposons and insertion sequences on the SCC*mec* in the hospital-acquired methicillin-resistant *S. aureus* genomes, the unique feature of the Panton-Valentine leukocidin gene, and the size of the SCC*mec* in two community-acquired *S. aureus* chromosomes (MW2 and FPR3757) have revealed the outstanding ability of this pathogen to evolve and adapt in order to survive in both the hospital and community settings [23,24].

b. Acinetobacter baumannii

Table 1. Main mechanisms of antibiotic resistance in bacteria.

Biochemical aspects	Mechanism	Responsible enzyme	Drug resistance
1) Antibiotic inactivation	Hydrolysis	β-lactamase	Penicillin,cephalosporins
		ESBL	Penicillin, 3rd gen ceph
			Aztreonam
		Esterases	Macrolides
			Fosfomycin
	Group transfer	Transferases	Aminoglycosides
			Chloramphenicol
			Macrolides
			Rifampicin
	Oxidation	TetX enzyme	Tetracycline
2) Target modification	Peptidoglycan structure		Vancomycin
	alteration		
	Protein synthesis interference		Aminoglycosides
			Tetracyclines
			Macrolides
			Chloramphenicol
			Fusidic acid,
			Mupirocin
3) DNA synthesis interference		DNA gyrase	Fluoroquinolones
		Topoisomerase IV	
4) Efflux pumps			Macrolides
			Tetracyclines
			Fluoroquinolones
5) OM permeability changes	Porin proteins		Aminoglycosidesz

Multidraug-resistant *A. baumannii* has increasingly been recognized as being responsible for large and sustained hospital outbreaks, particularly in the ICU [25]. Medical facilities treating patients injured in Iraq and Afghanistan have identified a large number of MDR *A. baumannii* isolates. *A. baumannii* exhibits a remarkable ability to rapidly develop antibiotic resistance. Some strains of *A. baumannii* have become resistant to almost all currently available antibacterial agents, mostly through the acquisition of plasmids, transposons, or integrons carrying clusters of genes encoding resistance to several classes of antibiotics. Phylogenetic analyses confirm that most of the resistance genes found in the *A. baumannii* strain AYE have been recently acquired from bacteria of the genera *Pseudomonas*, *Salmonella*, or *Escherichia* [26,27].

Molecular typing of *A. baumannii* isolates in the medical surgivcal ICU of a university hospital in Rome, Italy during two sequential outbreaks were caused by the spread of two different epidemic clones, which coexisted with unrelated sporadic different strains. The first epidemic clone showed an unstable pulsed-field gel electrophoresis (PFGE) pattern with the presence of several subtypes. The second outbreak episode was caused by the spread of a single different epidemic clone. This is in agreement with other data showing that sequential *A. baumannii* epidemics in the same ICU were caused by different clones, one replacing the other in a well-defined, temporal order [28,29]. Contaminated environmental sources, including humidifiers and monitors, and hand carriage by health-care personnel were identified during the second *A. baumannii* outbreak, suggesting the horizontal transmission of the epidemic strains from one patient to another through the hospital staff. Multivariate analysis has previously identified mechanical ventilation as a major risk factor for *A. baumannii* acquisition in the same ICU ward [28]. Longo et al [30], reported that the range of the minimum inhibitory concentrations in an *A. baumannii* outbreak indicated diminished susceptibility or low resistance. This range appears to be characteristic of *A. baumannii* isolates carrying the OXA-58 carbapenemase. Such isolates, were identified in recent outbreaks occurring in other hospitals in Rome [30-32].

c. Pseudomonas aeruginosa

P. aeruginosa strains are responsible for several recent outbreaks occuring in the intensive care unit environment. In 2005, Pagani et al [34], reported an outbreak of lower respiratory tract infection caused by *P. aeruginosa* producing an IMP-type, metallo-β-lactamase enzyme. Molecular analysis of the metallo-β-lactamase determinant showed the presence of a $bla_{\mathrm{IMP\text{-}13}}$ gene carried on a gene cassette inserted in a class 1 integron which also contained an *aacA4* aminoglycoside resistance cassette encoding an AAC(6_)-Ib enzyme. The $bla_{\mathrm{IMP\text{-}13}}$ gene was not transferable by conjugation and was carried on the chromosome. The *P. aeruginosa* isolates were resistant to carbapenems (imipenem and meropenem), extended-spectrum cephalosporins (ceftazidime and cefepime), and gentamicin, tobramycin, and fluoroquinolones (ciprofloxacin and levofloxacin). In a contemporary outbreak, Deplano et al [35], described an MDR *P. aeruginosa* clone, which exhibited resistance to penicillins, cephalosporins, carbapenems, aminoglycosides, and fluoroquinolones, and remained susceptible only to colistin. The epidemic clone showed an overexpression of the chromosomal cephalosporinase AmpC combined with decreased expression of porin OprD, and absence of metallo-β-lactamase or extended-spectrum β-lactamase. An upregulation of the MexXY efflux system due to an *agrZ* mutation in the *mexZ* regulator was detected. There was also an additional base deletion at aspartic acid position 164 (GAC3 G-C), introducing a frameshift outside the DNA binding region of *mexZ*. In 2007, the proportion of carbapenem-resistant *P. aeruginosa* isolates exceeded 10% in most countries participating in the European Antimicrobial Resistance Surveillance System (Figure 2).

In a more recent outbreak [35], we reported the isolation of a $bla_{\text{VIM-1}}$-like gene positive *P. aeruginosa* strain that was resistant to every available antibiotic, including colistin. The exact mechanism of colistin resistance was not determined. Afflicted patients were effectively treated with a meropenem-amikacin combination, which exhibited additive activity against the pandrug-resistant *P. aeruginosa*.

d. Klebsiella pneumoniae

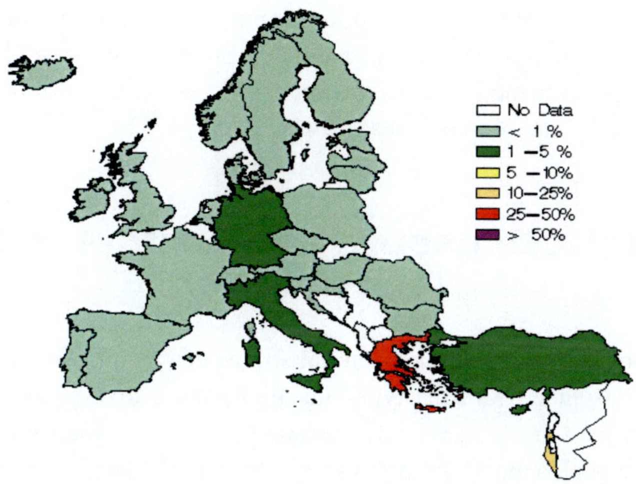

Figure 2. Proportion of carbapenem-resistant *Klebsiella pneumoniae* in participating countries in 2007. The European Antimicrobial Resistance Surveillance System (EARSS). Data are from the EARSS, http://www.rivm.nl/earss/database/.

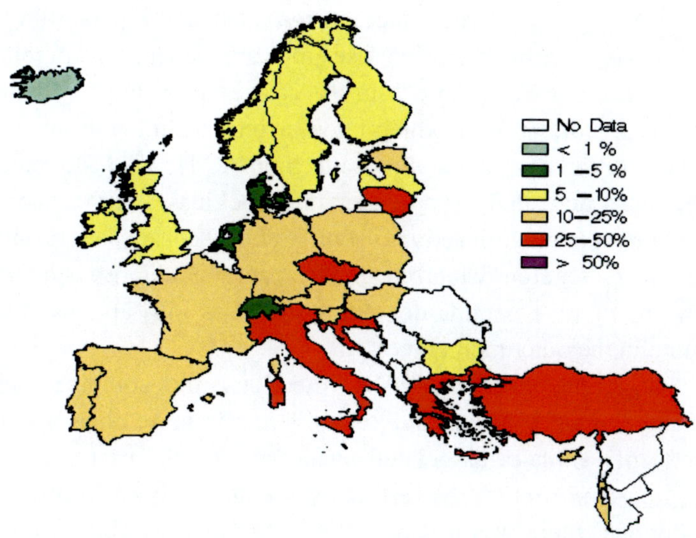

Figure 3. Proportion of carbapenem-resistant *Pseudomonas aeruginosa* in participating countries in 2007. The European Antimicrobial Resistance Surveillance System (EARSS). Data are from the EARSS, http://www.rivm.nl/earss/database/.

In Europe, and especially in Greece, there is an increasing incidence of infections due to carbapenem-resistant *K. Pneumoniae* [36] (Figure 3). This situation seems to be due to the spread of the bla_{VIM-1} cassette among the rapidly evolving multiresistant plasmids and multiresistant or even panresistant strains of mainly *K. pneumoniae*, and also other enterobacterial species [36].

e. Providenzia stuartii

MDR *P. stuartii* infections constitute an emerging problem (37). Antibiotic resistance is due to the production of extended spectrum β-lactamases, the majority of which are derivates of TEM-1 and TEM-2 (common plasmid-mediated β-lactamases of *E. coli*) or SHV-1 (the chromosomal encoded enzyme of *K. pneumoniae*) (38). Bloodtream infections by *P. stuartii* exhibit a high mortality rate of approximately 40% (37).

Antibiotic Exposure and Factors of Cross-Transmission

Antibiotic exposure of susceptible bacterial strains is a major stimulus for the acquisition or emergence of resistance. Both the type and the duration of exposure are important. In a recent study, Martinez et al [39], demostrated that the emergence af resistance to antipseudomonal cephalosporins in previously susceptible strains of *P. aeruginosa* was independently associated with the prior use of pipracillin-tazobactam. Conversely, the exposure to antipseudomonal cephalosporins or quinolones did not promote the acquisition of resistance to these agents. Also, the acquisition of resistance to amikacin was facilitated by prior exposure to amikacin (with exposure defined as the use of amikacin for at least 24 hours), whereas the emergence of resistance to carbapenems, piperacillin-tazobactam, and amikacin was associated with the prior use of carbapenems (for relevant molecular mechanisms of resistance see Table 1). As in the case of β-lactams, colistin, a polypeptide antibiotic, may induce synthesis of enzyme(s) conferring colistin resistance [40]. Polymyxin exposure causes the addition of aminoarabinose to lipid A [41, 42]. The mechanism involves a mutated PmrAB locus activated by a sensor phosphokinase, with concomitant selective suppression of the corresponding, deactivator PmrB phosphatase. This results in constitutive activation of the PmrA regulon which stimulates aminoarabinose synthesis [41]. Other resistance mechanisms involve peptide-degrading elastases [43] and substitution of protein OprH for magnesium in the outer membrane [40].

We showed that in patients with MDR infections, the combined administration of carbapenems for more than 20 days and of colistin for more than 13 days is the sole indpendent predictor of ventilator-associated pneumonia by the first ever isolated, pandrug resistant strain of *P. aeruginosa* [35]. Nevertheless, the outbreak was probably also facilitated by 1) personnel shortage (there was just one physiotherapist per shift, who performed open suctioning procedures in the entire intensive care unit, and the need for frequent suctioning was also associated with the development of the pandrug-resistant infection); and 2) a relatively poor personnel compliance to standard contact precautions. The two prior, large intensive care unit outbreaks of MDR *P. aeruginosa*] were also partly attributed to personnel shortage [33] or contaminated healthcare worker hands [34]. Personnel reinstatement [33] and improved contact precautions and patient isolation [34] facilitated outbreak resolution. In another report [44], patients with MDR *P. aeruginosa* infection received potent antipseudomonal agents for prolonged periods for infections by less resistant Gram-negative bacteria. Also a prior, large outbreak of *A. baumanii* pneumonia was attributed partly to ceftazidime selection pressure; healthcare worker compliance with standard hand washing recommendations was deemed poor and subject to improvement [45]. Poor hand hygiene in conjunction with open suctioning procedures resulting in aerosolization and contamination of healthcare worker hands have recently been suggested as a factor in *A. baumannii* cross-transmission [46].

Conclusion

The use, overuse, and misuse of antibiotics has lead to the development of multiple resistance mechanisms by Gram negative and Gram positive bacteria. In the hospital setting, the spread of MDR infections is facilitated by the poor implementation of standard infection control measures. The potential for synthesis of new antibiotic compounds is clearly overwhelmed by the diversity of the rapidly developing bacterial antibiotic resistance mechanisms. Measures such as standard hand hygiene, environmental and medical device decontamination, prompt isolation of patients with MDR infections, and antibiotic cycling and mixing seem to be the best currently available defense against MDR or pandrug-resistant bacteria.

References

[1] Hanberger, H; Garcia Rodriguez, JA; Gobernado, M; et al. Antibiotic susceptibility among aerobic gram-negative bacilli in intensive care units in European countries. French and Portuguese ICU Study Groups. *JAMA*, 2004, 281, 67-71.

[2] Jones, ME; Draghi, DC; Thornsberry, C; et al. Emerging resistance among bacterial pathogens in the intensive care unit— A European and North American Surveillance study (2000-2002). *Ann Clin Microbiol Antimicrob*, 2004, 3, 14.

[3] Gomez, J; Simarro, E; Banos, V; et al. Six-year prospective study of risk and prognostic factors in patients with nosocomial sepsis caused by *Acinetobacter baumannii*. *Eur J Clin Microbiol Infect Dis*., 1999, 18, 358-361.

[4] Mechanisms of Action of Antibiotics and Mycotoxins. In: Bioactive Secondary Metabolites of Microorganisms, V. Betina (Ed.), Elsevier Science, Amsterdam, *The Netherlands*, 1994, 297-375.

[5] Levy, SB. Balancing the resistance equation. *Trends in Microbiology*, 1994, 2, 341-342.

[6] Strohl, WR. Biotechnology of Antibiotics, *Marcel Dekker Inc*., New York, USA, 1997.

[7] Benton, B; Breukink, E; Visscher, I; et al. Telavancin inhibits peptidoglycan biosynthesis through preferential targeting of transglycosylation: Evidence for a

multivalent interaction between telavancin and lipid II. *Int J Antimicrob Agents (Suppl.)*, 2007, 29, 51-52.

[8] Leach, KL; Swaney, SM; Colca, JR; et al. The site of action of oxazolidinone antibiotics in living bacteria and in human mitochondria. *Mol Cell*, 2007, 26, 393-402.

[9] Tenover, FC. Mechanisms of antimicrobial resistance in bacteria. *Am J Med*, 2006, 119 (Suppl.), 3-10.

[10] Straus, SK; Hancock, REW. Mode of action of the new antibiotic for Gram-positive pathogens daptomycin: comparison with cationic antimicrobial peptides and lipopeptides. *Acta Biochem Biophys.*, 2006, 1758, 1215-1223.

[11] Aminov, RI; Mackie, RI. Evolution and ecology of antibiotic resistance genes, *FEMS Microbiol Lett*, 2007, 271, 147- 161.

[12] Bridges, BA. Hypermutation in bacteria and other cellular systems. *Philos Trans R Soc Lond B Biol Sci.*, 2001, 356, 29-39.

[13] Wang, H; Dzink-Fox, JL; Chen, M; Levy, SB. Genetic characterization of highly fluoroquinolone-resistant clinical *Escherichia coli* strains from China: role of acrR mutations. *Antimicrob Agents Chemother*, 2001, 45, 1515-1521.

[14] Everett, MJ; Jin, YF; Ricci, V; Piddock, LJ. Contributions of individual mechanisms to fluoroquinolone resistance in 36 *Escherichia coli* strains isolated from humans and animals. *Antimicrob Agents Chemother*, 1996, 40, 2380-2386.

[15] Hooper, DC. Emerging mechanisms of fluoroquinolone resistance. *Emerg Infect Dis.*, 2001, 7, 337-341.

[16] Stuart, LB. "The Challenge of Antibiotic Resistance." *Scientific American*, 1998, 278, 46-53.

[17] Wright, GD. Bacterial resistance to antibiotics: Enzymatic degradation and odification. *Adv Drug Deliv Rev.*, 2005, 57, 1451-1470.

[18] Lambert, PA. Bacterial resistance to antibiotics: Modified target sites. *Adv Drug Deliv Rev.*, 2005, 57, 1471-1485.

[19] Kumar, A; Schweizer, HP. Bacterial resistance to antibiotics: Active efflux and reduced uptake. *Adv Drug Deliv Rev.*, 2005, 57, 1486-1513.

[20] Barbosa, TM ; Levy, SB. The impact of antibiotic use on resistance development and persistence. *Drug Resistance Updates*, 2000, 3, 303-311.

[21] The medical impact of the use of antimicrobials in food animals. *Report of a WHO Meeting*, WHO, Berlin, Germany, 1997.

[22] Wegener, HC. Antibiotics in animal feed and their role in resistance development. *Curr Opin Microbiol* 2003, 6, 439-445.

[23] Dumitrescu, O; Boisset, S; Badiou, C; et al. Effect of antibiotics on *Staphylococcus aureus* producing Panton-Valentine Leukocidin. *Antimicrob Agents Chemother*, 2007, 51, 1515-1519.

[24] Baba, T; Takeuchi, F; Kuroda, M; et al. Genome and virulence determinants of high virulence community-acquired MRSA. *Lancet*, 2002, 359, 1819-1827.

[25] Rello, J; Diaz, E. Acinetobacter baumannii: a threat for the ICU? *Intensive Care Med*, 2003, 29, 350-351.

[26] Corbella, X; Montero, A; Pujol, M; et al. Emergence and rapid spread of carbapenem resistance during a large and sustained hospital outbreak of multiresistant *Acinetobacter baumannii*. *J Clin Microbiol*, 2000, 38, 4086- 4095.

[27] Bergogne Berezin, E; Towner, KJ. Acinetobacter spp. as nosocomial pathogens: Microbiological, clinical, and epidemiological features. *Clin Microbiol Rev.*, 1996, 9, 148-165.

[28] Villari, P; Iacuzio, L; Vozzella, EA; Bosco, U. Unusual genetic heterogeneity of *Acinetobacter baumanni* isolates in a university hospital in Italy. *Am J Infect Control*, 1999, 27, 247-253.

[29] Zarrilli, R; Crispino, M; Bagattini, M; et al. Molecular epidemiology of sequential outbreaks of *Acinetobacter baumannii* in an intensive care unit shows the emergence of carbapenem resistance. *J Clin Microbiol*, 2004, 42, 946-953.

[30] Longo, B; Pantosti, A; Luzzi, I; et al. Molecular findings and antibiotic-resistance in an outbreak of *Acinetobacter baumannii* in an intensive care unit. *Ann Ist Super Sanità*, 2007, 43, 83-88.

[31] Coelho, J; Woodford, N; Afzal-Shah, M; Livermore, D. Occurrence of OXA-58-like carbapenemases in *Acinetobacter* spp. Collected over 10 years in three continents. *Antimicrob Agents Chemother*, 2006, 50, 756-758.

[32] Bertini, A; Giordano, A; Varesi, P; et al. First report of the carbapenem-hydrolyzing oxacillinase OXA-58 in *Acinetobacter baumannii* isolates in Italy. *Antimicrob Agents Chemother*, 2006, 50, 2268-2269.

[33] Pagani, L; Colinon, C; Migliavacca, R; et al. Nosocomial outbreak caused by multidrug-resistant Pseudomonas aeruginosa producing IMP-13 metallo-β-lactamase. *J Clin Microbiol*, 2005, 43, 3824-3828.

[34] Deplano, A; Denis, O; Poirel, L; et al. Molecular characterization of an endemic clone of panantibiotic-resistant Pseudomonas aeruginosa. *J Clin Microbiol*, 2005, 43, 1198-1204.

[35] Mentzelopoulos, SD; Pratikaki, M; Platsouka, E; et al. Prolonged use of carbapenems and colistin predisposes to ventilator-associated pneumonia by pandrug-resistant Pseudomonas aeruginosa. *Intensive Care Med*, 2007, 33, 1524-1532.

[36] Vatopoulos, A. High rates of metallo-beta-lactamase-producing Klebsiella pneumoniae in Greece - a review of the current evidence. *Eurosurveillance*, 2008, 1-3, 1-6.

[37] Tumbarello, M; Citton, R; Spanu, T; et al. ESBL-producing multidrug-resistant *Providencia stuartii* infections in a university hospital. *J Antimicrob Chemother*, 2004, 53, 277-282.

[38] Wei, ZQ; Chen, YG; Yu, YS; et al. Nosocomial spread of multi-resistant Klebsiella pneumoniae containing a plasmid encoding multiple *β*-lactamases. *J Med Microbiol*, 2005, 54, 885-888.

[39] Martinez, JA; Delgado, E; Marti, S; et al. Influence of antipseudomonal agents on Pseudomonas aeruginosa colonization and acquisition of resistance in critically ill medical patients. *Intensive Care Med*, 2008, DOI 10.1007/s00134-008-1326-y.

[40] Li, J; Nation, RL; Milne, RW; et al. Evaluation of colistin as an agent against multiresistant Gram negative bacteria. *Int J Antimicrob Agents*, 2005, 25, 11-25.

[41] Moskowitz, SM; Ernst, RK; Miller, SI. Pmr, AB. a two-component regulatory system of Pseudomonas aeruginosa that modulates resistance to cationic antimicrobial peptides and addition of aminoarabinose to lipid A. *J Bacteriol*, 2004, 186, 575-579.

[42] Conrad, RS; Galanos, C. Fatty acid alterations and polymyxin B binding by lipopolysaccharides from Pseudomonas aeruginosa adapted to polymyxin B resistance. *Antimicrob Agents Chemother*, 1989, 33, 1724-1728.

[43] Schmidtchen, A; Frick, IM; Andersson, E; Tapper, H; Bjork, L. Proteinases of common pathogenic bacteria degrade and inactivate the antibacterial peptide LL-37. *Mol Microbiol*, 2002, 46, 157-168.

[44] Wang, CY; Jerng, JS; Cheng, KY; et al. Pandrug-resistant Pseudomonas aeruginosa among hospitalised patients: clinical features, risk-factors and outcomes. *Clin Microbiol Infect*, 2006, 12, 63-68.

[45] Husni, RN; Goldstein, LS; Arroliga, C; et al. Risk factors for an outbreak of multi-drug-resistant Acinetobacter pneumonia among intubated patients. *Chest*, 1999, 115, 1378-1382.

[46] El Shafie, SS; Alishaq, M; Leni Garcia, M. Investigation of an outbreak of multidrug-resistant Acinetobacter baumannii in trauma intensive care unit. *J Hosp Infect*, 2004, 56, 101-105.

In: Multiple Drug Resistance
Editors: A. Meszaros, G. Balogh, pp. 167-194

ISBN: 978-1-60741-595-4

Chapter VII

Bacteriophage Therapies and Enzybiotics: Novel Solutions to Antibiotic Resistance

Noémie Manuelle Dorval Courchesne, Albert Parisien and Christopher Q. Lan*
Department of Chemical and Biological Engineering, University of Ottawa.

Abstract

Bacteriophages (phages) and bacterial cell wall hydrolases (BCWHs) have been recognized as promising alternative antibacterials. Phages are bacterial virsuses that kill bacteria by causing bacteriolysis. It is estimated that there are about 10^{31} phages on earth and approximately 5,100 have been identified and reported towards the end of last century, providing a vast pool of candidates for applications such as phage therapy. Phages are highly effective and specific to target bacteria. They have been generally accepted as effective antibacterials that could potentially provide safe and cost effective means for the treatment and prephylaxis of bacterial infections. BCWHs are lytic enzymes that cause bacteriolysis by hydrolyzing the peptidoglycan of bacterial cell wall. BCWHs are also called enzybiotics because they are enzymes that have antibiotic-like antibacterial activities. They are produced by amost all cellular organisms including microorganisms, plants, and animals. Virolysins (also called lysins, endolysins) are a special group of BCWHs encoded by phages but produced naturally by bacteria infected by lytic phages. They are probably the most promising enzybiotics.

Keywords: Bacteriophage, virolysin, lysin, antibiotic resistance, enzybiotic.

* Corresponding author: E-mail: Christopher.Lan@uottawa.ca.

1. Introduction

For more than half a century, the human society has been relying primarily on antibiotics to treat infectious diseases caused by pathogenic bacteria. However, the emergence of bacterial resistance to antibiotics following widespread clinical, veterinary, and animal agricultural usage [1-3] has made antibiotics less effective. As a result, Gram-positive bacteria have clearly re-emerged as important pathogens world-wide in the past two decades. The hallmark of these Gram-positive pathogens is increasing resistance to available antimicrobial agents. Of particular note is resistance to glycopeptides (Vancomycin), amino glycosides (high-level), and penicillins among the enterococci (especially *E. faecium*), resistance to penicillinase-resistant penicillins (oxacillin and methicillin) and fluoroquinolones (ciprofloxacin and ofloxacin) among staphylococci, and resistance to penicillin, other beta-lactams and macrolides among the pneumococci. The recent detection of decreased susceptibility to vancomycin among S. *aureus* is also quite disturbing. New antibacterials are clearly needed.

The enormous demand has triggered worldwide efforts in developing novel alternative antibacterials. Bacteriophages (phages), bacterial cell wall hydrolases (especially phage encoded virolysins) are among the most promising candidates. In this chapter, we strive on providing a comprehensive picture outlining current developments regarding these alternative antimicrobials.

2. Bacteriophages and Bacteriophage Therapies

Discovered independently by Frederick Twort and Félix d'Hérelle in 1915 and 1917, respectively, bacteriophages (phages) are bacterial viruses that kill bacteria by causing bacteriolysis. Antibacterial properties of phages were assessed in the pre-biotic era and a few Western companies, including French companies Le Laboratoire du Bactériophage and L'Oréal, German company Antipiol and the German Bacteriophage Society, and American companies Eli-Lilly, Swan-Myers of Abbot Laboratories, Squibb and Sons (now belonging to Brystol-Myers, Squibb Company) and the Parke & Davis Company (now a part of Pfizer) manufactured and/or marketed a variety of different phage preparations to treat various infections including abscesses, suppurating wounds, vaginitis, and infections of the upper respiratory tract [4]. Bacteriophages were later abandoned in the western countries in favour of the antibiotics because the mechanism was not well defined. Moreover, the exquisite specificity of this treatment limited their use in the ealy days. Consequently, antibiotics whose mechanisms were understood and had a large spectrum of action became popular in Western countries. Phage therapy was however extensively used in Eastern European countries mainly in the Former Soviet Union and in Georgia. Nevertheless, a revitalization of interests on phage therapy has been observed in the last two decade in Western countries due to the rise of antibiotic resistant bacterial strains, which is marked by a few excellent recent review works [5-13]. In the USA, although no clinic tests have been reported except the pre-antibiotic era practices, some phages were, however, used for medical studies. For instance, phage ϕX174 was used to monitor humoral immune function in treated ADA-deficient patients [14] and analyze the importance of cell surface-associated molecules in modulating the immune response [15]. In both studies, purified phages were administrated intravenously with consent from volunteers. Moreover, in the last two decades, due to the rise of antibiotic resistance in bacteria, the interest in phage therapy has grown in Western countries [16, 17].

2.1. Classification of Phages

It is estimated that there are about 10^{31} phages on earth and approximately 5,100 have been identified and reported towards the end of last century [18]. These phages are classified into 13 families according to their morphological characteristics, type of nucleic acid, and presence or absence of envelope or lipid. It was noticed that 4950 out of the 5,100 phages are "tailed phages", which are composed of an icosahedral head and a tail. All those tailed phages have double-stranded DNA as genome and are lytic phages that encode endolysins (endolysin will be referred to as virolysins from here on) [19, 20]. They are classified into three families according to the morphological features of the tail: *Myoviridae* (contractile tail), *Siphoviridae* (long noncontractile tail and *Podoviridae* (extremely short tail). The rest of the phages, constituting only 4% of the total, are classified into ten families. They are cubic, filamentous, or pleomorphic phages containing double-stranded DNA (dsDNA), single-stranded DNA (ssDNA), double-stranded RNA (dsRNA) or single-stranded RNA (ssRNA) as the genome [18].

Phages can also be conventionally classified into two categories according to the strategies they use to escape their hosts [19, 20]: filamentous phages and lytic phages. Filementous phages continuously extrude from their hosts without causing host lysis, whereas all other phages are lytic phages that encode gene products to compromise or destroy the bacterial cell wall. Lytic phages can be further divided into two classes according to their bacteriolytic mechanisms: those encode a virolysin-holin system to hydrolyse host cell wall and those encode a single lytic factor to compromise the strength of cell wall and cause bacteriolysis. About 96% of known phages are lytic phages encoding virolysin-holin system. They are large phages containing dsDNA genome. Only the simplest phages encode single lytic factors for bacteriolysis and they usually contain ssDNA or ssRNA genome. Single lytic factors encoded by small phages causes host lysis by inhibiting cell wall biosynthesis, inducing host autolytic system, or other mechanisms. In the virolysin-holin lysis system, virolysin is a muralytic enzyme that hydrolyses the peptidoglycan in bacterial cell wall and holin is a small peptide that oligomerizes in the membrane to form disruptive membrane lesions, allowing access of virolysin to the cell wall at a programmed timing of the phage's life cycle [21].

2.2. Mode of Action

The most common mode of action of the bactericidal activitity of phages is that of lytic phages, i.e., sensitive bacteria are killed by means of bacteriolysis. The lytic life of phages involves several stages including adsorption, injection of nucleic acid, commandeering of host machinery, production of phage components (expression of early and late phage genes), assembly of phage particles, and release of phage particles by cell lysis. Bacteriolysis occurs naturally in the latest phase of the life cycle, in which the peptidoglycan network of bacterial cell wall is disrupted by the action of virolysins. This event is initiated by the formation of holin oligomore pores in cytoplasmic membrane, which allows virolysins to access their substrate [22]. Bacteriolysis could also happen in the adsorption stage if a high multiplication of infection (MOI) is used, in which a substantially large number of phage particles attach to each host cell [23, 24].

Another mode of action involves genetically modified phages, especially filamentous ones, which do not cause cell lysis and cannot be used directly for phage therapy. It has been shown that these phages can be genetically modified in such as way that they lose the ability to extrude from host cells but have the ability to digest the nucleic acid of host (the transportation protein gene is replaced by a restriction enzyme gene) [25, 26]. It has been demonstrated that this type of genetically modified filamentous phages can be used as effective anti-infection agents. Besides, they were shown to have the benefit of reduced release of membrane associated endotoxins, leading to significantly higher survival rates of experimental animals in comparison with therapies using lytic phages [25, 26].

Furthermore, as will be discussed later, phage gene products such as endolysins are also promising alternative antimicriobials that may be ultilized in medical and other applications. These gene products have their unique modes of action.

2.3. Antibacterial Efficacy of Phages

The revival of research in phage therapy in Western countries is marked by a series of works on the treatment of *Escherichia coli* infections using experimental mice and calves conducted by Smith and Huggins in late 70s and 80s [27-29]. It was observed that phages multiplied rapidly and profusely after gaining entry to the *E. coli*-infected small intestine of calves, quickly reducing the *E. coli* to numbers that were virtually harmless. It was also demonstrated that a single intramuscular dose of one anti-K1 phage is more effective for treating mice challenged with *E. coli* intramuscularly or intracerebrally than multiple intramuscular doses of tetracycline, ampicillin, chloramphenicol, or trimethoprim plus sulfafurazole.

Since Smith's work, there have been many published reports examining the efficacy of phages against experimental infections by Gram-negative bacteria such as *E. coli*, *Pseudomonas aeruginosa*; *Acinetobacter baumanii*, *Klebsiella pneumoniae*, *Vibrio vulnificus*, *Salmonella* Spp. and Gram-positive bacteria such as *Enterococcus faecium* (vancomycin-resistant strain, VRE) and *Staphylococcus aureus*, mostly in animal models. Nakai *et al.* succeeded in saving the lives of cultured fish challenged by *Lactococcus garvieae* and *Pseudomonas plecoglossicida*. Phages were also shown to be effective for the elimination of food poisoning pathogens such as *Listeria monocytogenes*, *Campylobacter jejuni* and *Salmonella* Spp. On August 18, 2006, FDA approved the use of phages for the treatment of ready-to-eat meat. A combination of six viruses was designed to be sprayed on ready-to-eat meat to eradicate strains of *Listeria monocytogenes*.

Numerous patents have been filed disclosing methods relating the use of phages for treatment and prophylaxis of bacterial infections [30-37]. There are now evidences that phages can be employed to treat infectious diseases caused by both gram-positive and gram-negative bacteria [38, 39]. For instance, the treatment of *E. coli* infections in experimental mice an calves [40] and recent work in animal models have demonstrated the efficacy of phages against experimental infections by gram-negative and gram-positive bacterial pathogens.

Many of these patents also provide innovative technologies to enhance the efficacy and/or safety of phage therapy. For example, an invention [36] provides *Bacillus* phages to prevent and treat the infection of *Bacillus* bacteria, including *Bacillus anthracis*. Methods and materials to decontaminate a surface or an organism that is contaminated with *Bacillus* bacteria or spores is also provided [36]. Treating acne, which is caused by increased colonization of *Propionibacterium acnes* on human skin, using *P. acnes* phages has also been described [37]. It involves the use of a phage that cannot enter a lysogenic cycle, representing an advantage because the phage cannot lie dormant in the bacterial chromosomal DNA. This way, some of the aforementioned safety concerns such as the lysogenic immunity of pathogenic bacteria and the alternation of bacterial virulence can be avoided. Another innovative approach of phage therapy is the use of lysin-deficient phages [41], which can be generated via targeted mutation or selected by screening through phages that have reduced lysis rates. Without a functional lytic enzyme, phages can infect and kill bacterial cells without causing bacteriolysis, resulting in dead but intact bacterial cells. Therefore, the phage therapies have a reduced immunogenicity and toxicity because cell materials of killed bacteria (e.g. endotoxins) are not released [41, 42]. However, the trade-off of this technology is that phages cannot be propagated if there is no bacteriolysis and a larger dosage of phage would have to be used to eliminate all the bacteria in comparison to therapies involving self-propagating phages.

The extreme specificity of phages renders them ideal candidates for applications designed to increase food safety during the production process as phages can be used for biocontrol of bacteria without interfering with the natural microflora or the cultures in fermented products. They have been shown to be effective against poisoning pathogens such as *Listeria monocytogenes*, *Campylobacter jejuni* and *Salmonella spp.* [43]. Another advantage of phage decontamination is that phage compositions are non-toxic and do not alter color, texture or taste of the food to be decontaminated [43, 44]. In fact, application of phages for food decontamination has been considered to be one of the low-handing fruits since the FDA of the USA and other western authorities have much less rigorous regulations towards food decontamination agents in comparison to human therapeutic agents. As an encouraging notion, FDA approved the use of phages for the treatment of ready-to-eat meat, which is a cocktail of six bacteriophages to be sprayed on ready-to-eat meat to eradicate strains of *L. monocytogenes*, in 2006 [45]. *E. coli* 0157:H7 is a leading cause of hemolytic-uremic syndrome (HUS) in the United States and a leading cause of acute renal failure in children. Estimates based on a 1994 outbreak in the Seattle area suggest that more than 20,000 cases occur in the USA each year, and that 250 of them are fatal. This strain of *E. coli* is very dangerous because it can cause disease at very low doses - ingestion of less than 1,000 organisms compared to the more than 10,000,000 needed for *Vibrio cholerae* to cause cholera. Based on continued works, Averback and Gemmell [46] patented *E. coli* phages B1 and B3, which were isolated from raw sewage, and phages 146A and 119U, from a urinary tract infection (UTI) isolate, for the treatment of *E. coli* infections, particularly the enteric diseases caused by the toxin-producing *E. coli 0157:H7* strain [46]. Pasternack and Sulakvelidze [47] patented six *Listeria monocytogenes* phage strains (ATCC Deposit Accession Nos. PTA-5372, PTA-5373, PTA-5374, PTA- 5375, PTA-5376 and PTA-5377), which are capable of controlling the contamination of food products by *L. monocytogenes*. The invention also contemplates the use of these phages, and polynucleotides and polypeptides derived therefrom, for the treatment of host infections or environmental contamination by *L. monocytogenes*.

2.4. Specificity of Phage Therapy

The first essential step of phage infection is the attachment of phage tail to specific receptor on the surface of a bacterial cell. This feature makes phage infection a very specific process. There seem to be some controversies with regard of how specific phage infection really is. While some authors tend to think that phages are generally species-specific [48], it seems to be more accurate to say that phages typically attack bacteria on a strain-specific basis [49]. Nevertheless, there is no doubt that phages are much more specific than antibiotics in therapeutical application. While the high specificity of phages made them less appealing in comparison with broad-spectrum antibiotics in the early days, it is now highly appreciated as a major merit of phage therapy. Because of the high specificity, phage therapies would not affect the microbism of the hosts as antibiotics would normally do.

2.5. Bacterial Resistance to Phages

Bacteria may acquire resistance to phages via at least the following fours mechanisms [11]: 1) integrating a phage into its genome (the lysogenic cycle); 2) losing phage receptor from cell surface; 3) acquiring horizontally a restriction-modification system that degrades the injected phage nucleic acid; and 4) mutating to lose a gene essential for phage replication or assembly. Nevertheless, induced resistance of bacteria to phages is so far not considered a significant obstacle to the clinic applicability of phage therapy. After all, phages mutate at frequences significantly higher than that of bacteria and there are abudant experimental evidences showing that the co-mutation of phages would be enough to maintain the efficacy of phage therapies (Schuch *et al.* 2002). However, the dependence on the co-mutation of phages implies that we would have to deal with a constantly mutating phage population for effective phage therapies. This may, even though not necessarily, present a concern in long term application of phage therapy.

2.6. Advantages and Disadvantages of Phage Therapy

Matsuzaki *et al.* [50] summarized the advantages of phage therapy over chemotherapy as follows: 1) it is effective against multidrug-resistant pathogenic bacteria as the bacterium-killing mechanism of phage is completely different from that of antibiotics; 2) substituted microbism does not occur because the phages have high specificity to target bacteria; 3) it can respond quickly to the appearance of phage-resistant bacterial mutants because the frequency of phage mutation is significantly higher than that of bacteria; 4) the cost of developing a phage system is cheaper than that of a new antibiotics; 5) the side effects are rare. Nevertheless, there are still some concerns need to be addressed such as: 1) lack of pharmacokinetic data; 2) neutralization of phages by the host immune system may lead to failure of phage therapy; 3) some phages may encode toxins [48]; 4) conversion of lytic phages to lysogenic prophages renders immunity (lysogenic immunity) to the bacteria [51] and may also change the virulence of the bacteria [52, 53]; 5) rapid cell lysis of bacteria may result in the release of large amount of membrane-bound endotoxins of the hosts [54].

Some of the aforementioned concerns have been successfully addressed by different approaches. For instance, the rapid release of endotoxin (e.g. lipopolysaccharide, a component of the outer membrane of Gram-negative bacteria) by phage infection was considered to be a potential problem in phage therapy [25, 54]. Recently, a unique method to minimize the release of endotoxin in phage therapy against *P. aeruginosa* was reported [25, 26, 55, 56]. Hagens *et al.* [25, 26, 56] constructed a recombinant phage derived from the *P. aeruginosa* filamentous phage. In this phage, the export protein gene was replaced with a restriction endonuclease gene. The mutant phage therefore could not multiply in *P. aeruginosa* cells but the restriction endonuclease encoded by the injected phage DNA digested the host genomic DNA and consequentially killed the bacteria with minimal release of endotoxin in vitro. This modified phage reduced mortality rate to a greater extent than the wildtype in mice challenged with *P. aeruginosa*. However, large dosage than that of wildtype lytic phages would be essential for therapy involving this type of modified phages because they cannot propagate after administration.

In both Gram-positive and Gram-negative bacteria, temperate bacteriophage may encode toxins and virulence factors in addition to their essential viral proteins [53, 57, 58]. Examples of phage-associated toxins include the CTX cholera toxin [59-61], botulinum toxin, shiga toxin [62, 63], and diphtheria toxin [57]. Phage-associated conversion of Tox^- *Streptococcus pyogenes* into Tox^+ bacteria was also confirmed *in vitro* and *in vivo* [52, 53]. We therefore should have rather thorough studies before selecting a canaditate phage for therapeutical applications.

Despite of concerns over phage therapy due to the lack of pharmacological and pharmacokinetic data, possible toxicity of certain phages, and other uncertainties associated with phage therapies, accumulating evidences have shown that phages are effective antibacterial agents that can be employed for clinic treatment or prevention of infectious diseases caused by Gram-positive and Gram-negative bacteria. Facing the threat presented by the rapid emerging of antibiotic resistant pathogenic bacteria, phage therapy is no doubt one of the most promising alternative antibacterial agents. Furthermore, as will be discussed later, phage-encoded gene products such as virolysins, and lytic factors are also promising alternative antibacterials.

3. Enzybiotics: Bacterial Cell Wall Hydrolases (BCWHs) as Novel Alternatives to Antibiotics

The term “enzybiotics” was first coined for virolysisns, i.e., phage-encoded lytic enzymes, and is now used to describe all bacterial cell wall hydrolases (BCWHs), enzymes that degrade the peptidoglycan, the major component of bacterial cell wall and cause bacteriolysis. The sources of BCWHs include animals, insects, plants, and microbes. Enzymes from different sources, even though may have similar structure and functionalities, do have important differences that may have significant impact on their potential clinic applications. It was proposed to classify BCWHs according to their sources into the following categories [64, 65]: 1) lysozymes, BCWHs of eukaryotic origin; 2) microlysins, BCWHs produced by bacteria and other microorganisms; and 3) virolysins, phage-encoded BCWHs responsible for the lysis of host cells and the release of phage particles at the end of a phage life cycle. The three groups of BCWHs are discussed briefly as follows.

3.1. BCWHs from Different Sources

3.1.1. Lysozymes

Lysozyme is sometimes used as a genric name for BCWHs from different sources. To avoid confusion, it was proposed to explicitly define lysozymes as the BCWHs of eukaryotic origins, e.g., those BCWHs produced by animals and plants. Lysozymes are an important component of the innate defense systems of their hosts and are known to exert antimicrobial activities against a broad spectrum of bacterial, fungal, and viral pathogens [66]. These enzymes, alone or in combinations with other antimicrobials, have found wide applications as food preservatives and pharmaceuticals. A few excellent review works are available on this topic [67-71] , which provide insights regarding the antibacterial properties and mode of action of lysozyme against Gram-positive and Gram-negative bacteria, and the underlying causes of bacterial resistance or sensitivity to lysozyme. The distribution, activity and particularly the number of genes that encode lysozyme vary considerably among species. For instance, it has been reported that in mammals, humans and pigs contain a single lysozyme gene, whereas camels and mice contain 2, cows, sheep, and deer each contain 10 lysozyme genes [72]. In humans, lysozyme presents in various tissues including skin, and secretions such as saliva, tears, urine, milk, respiratory and cervical secretions [70].

3.1.2. Microlysins

Microlysins can be further classified into two subgroups, autolysins and other microlysins. Most bacterial species contain one or more autolysins, which are usually membrane-bound proteins that have BCWH activities [73-75]. A number of autolysins have been identified and have been shown to be involved in a number of physiological cell functions such as cell wall biosynthesis, cell separation, cell adhesion, and virulence. They may also, as the name suggests, cause cell lysis and lead directly to cell death when provoked by various mechanisms [76]. A number of autolysins have been expressed in *E. coli* [77-81]. The concept of activating the autolytic systems of pathogenic bacteria using cationic peptides and other compounds have been investigated with encouraging results [82-87]. Exogenous autolysins such as LytA, an *N*-acetylmuramoyl-L-alanine amidase [88, 89] and the major autolysin of *S. pneumoniae*, which play important roles in the pathogenesis of *S. pneumoniae* [90-92], might be used as vaccines due to its ability to provoke protective responses against streptococci inoculated in the lungs [93, 94].

3.1.3. Virolysins

As aforementioned, virolysins are BCWHs encoded by lytic dsDNA phages and produced in phage-infected bacterial cells toward the end of the lytic cycle. They are capable of degrading peptidoglycan when applied externally (as purified proteins) to the bacterial cell wall, resulting in a rapid lysis of the bacterial cell. The name "virolysin" was first adopted by Rolston et al. in 1950s [95] and was recently suggested to replace the more commonly used but more generic names such as lysozymes, lysins, and lytic enzymes to avoid confusion [64, 65].

The first virolysins was identified as early as in the 1950s [95], however, was reported to be active against dead but not live cells [95]. Then, a second virolysin, PAL (phage-associated virolysin), which lysed dead and live *S. aureus* cells, was identified in the early 1970s [96]. In addition, virolysins from staphylococcal phages Twort [97], 87 [98], phi11 [99], and 80 [100] as well as *Bacillus anthracis* prophage [101], *Listeria monocytogenes* phage and *Clostridium tyrobutyricum* phage, were identified in 1990s. Stimulated by the great potential of virolysins as powerful alternatives to antibiotics, a number of virolysins have been identified and demonstrated to be efficient and safe antimicrobials since 2000 [6, 102-104]. These virolysins have been tested for the control of a variety of pathogens such as *E. faecalis* and *E. faecium*, staphylococci, *B. anthracis*, group A streptococci, *S. pneumoniae*, and Clostridium bacteria [105].

Virolysins possess several important features including a narrow antibacterial spectrum and activity against bacteria regardless of their antibiotic sensitivity. It is also important to notice that there are evidences showing that it is unlikely for sensitive bacteria to develop resstance to virolysins. The results of preclinical studies indicate that the most apparent potential problems associated with phage therapy (e.g., their immunogenicity, the potential toxicity, or the development of resistance) may not be a serious problem to the use of virolysins [10].

3.2. Mode of Action

The primary bactericidal mechanism of BCWHs is the lytic enzymatic activities of these enzymes, which leads to peptidoglycan degradation and consequently bacteriolysis [70].

Bacterial cell wall is a unique structure comprised primary of a peptidoglycan network embedded with other compounds and, in the case of Gram-negative bacteria, surrounded by a lipid-rich outer membrane. The backbone of peptidoglycan is the polymer of the repeat units of two amino sugars, [*N*-acetylglucosamine-*N*-acetylmuramic acid]$_n$. The two amino sugars are linked by a β-1,4 glycoside bond. Tetrapeptides are attached to the D-lactyl moiety of N-acetylmuramic acids. Adjacent tetrapeptide may be cross-linked by an inter-peptide bond (in Gram-positive bacteria) or by an inter-peptide bridge (in Gram-positive bacteria). The tetrapeptides are composed of L-Alanine linked to D-Glutamate, L-lysine and then D-Alanine in the case of gram-positive bacteria. The cross-linked between the two peptide chains connects the L-lysine from one peptide to the D-Alanine of the other. In gram-negative bacteria, such as *E. coli*, L-lysine is replaced by L-diaminopimelic acid (DAP), and this amino acid is cross-linked with the D-Alanine of the other peptide chain. Peptidoglycan forms a closed network around the entire cell that is called the murein sacculus, which defines cellular shape and absorbs cellular turgor pressure [106-110]. Gram-positive bacteria have a thicker peptidoglycan layer (15 to 80nm) than the gram-negative bacteria (10nm) [110]. The peptidolycan is tightly cross-linked on the cytoplamic side and becomes looser for outer layers, and therefore more subject to degradation. Teichoic acid and lipoteichoic acid are two characteristic molecules found in the peptidoglycan layer of gram-positive bacteria. Teichoid acids are chemically bound to peptidoglycan, while lipoteichoic acids are anchored by a fatty acid in the plasma membrane [107]. In the case of gram-negative bacteria, a periplasmic space separates the plasma membrane from a single peptidoglycan layer adjacent to an outer lipopolysaccharide membrane. This outer membrane consists of proteins and lipopolysaccharides, composed of lipid A, the core, and a long repeating O antigen [107].

BCWHs hydrolyse peptidoglycan by attacking specific sites in the peptidolycan network. They can therefore be classified into different groups accordingly: 1) glycosidases, including β-N-acetylmuramidases, attacking the *N*-acetylmuramic acid→*N*-acetylglucosamine β-1-4 glycosidic bond, and β-N-acetylglucosaminidases, hydrolyzing the *N*-acetylglucosamine → *N*-acetylmuramic acid β-1-4 glycosidic bond; 2) transglycosylases, cleaving the same bond that is attacked by β-N-acetylmuramidases but transfering the glycosyl moiety onto the C-6 hydroxyl group of muramic acid; 3) amidases, cleaving the amide bond between the lactyl group of N-acetylmuramic acid and the α-amino group of L-alanine, the first amino acid of the tetrapeptide of peptidoglycan; 4) endopeptidases that cut within the peptide moiety of the peptidoglycan; and 5) other enzymes such as phosphocholine esterase that releases phosphocholine residues from the cell wall teichoic acid (TA) .

The hydrolysis of bacterial cell wall requires two distinct functions of BCWHs: 1) binding to the cell wall leading to the correct positioning of BCWHs as the essential first step; and 2) cleaving specific peptidoglycan bond. These two functions are achieved by two separate domains of BCWHs. It is now clear that most BCWHs have a two-domain modular structure, in which the binding domain is separated from the catalytic domain. For instance, LytA amidase, the major autolysin of pneumococci, has a molecular mass of ~36 kDa and a two-domain modular organization [111]. The C-terminal domain is responsible for the attachment to teichoic or lipoteichoic acid residues on the surface of pneumococci. The N-domain, on the other hand, is responsible for the lytic activity against pneumococcal cell wall. This modular structure is shared by almost all known BCWHs including lysozymes [71, 112-114], autolysins [115-117], and virolysins [101, 118, 119].

A second bactericidal mechanism, the non-lytic mechanism, of BCWHs has also attracted the attention of the research community in recent years [120-122]. The non-lytic mechanism is based on the cationic and amphiphilic properties of BCWH or its peptide derivatives to cause membrane perturbation of its targets through the binding of a certain domains of BCWHs with the bacterial surface or to provoke the autolytic system of bacteria.

As will be discussed later, this non-lytic bactericidal mechanism is shared by other antimicrobial peptides.

3.3. Antimicrobial Efficacy of BCWHs

Extensive studies on the antimicrobial efficacy of different groups of BCWHs, mostly of lysozymes [68-71, 123, 124] and virolysins [105, 125, 126], have been carried out in the last two decades.

Lysosomes are a group of broad-spectrum lytic enzymes that exhibit bactericidal activity toward most Gram-positive bacteria [125]. In addition to their bactericidal activities, lysozymes have also been demonstrated to have anti-fungal (e.g. *Fusarium oxysporum, Fusarium solani, Pythium aphanidermatum, Sclerotium rolfsii, and Botrytis cinerea*) [127] and anti-virus (e.g. HIV) [128] activities. Nevertheless, many virulent Gram-positive bacterial pathogens have acquired resistance to lysolyzymes to survive the innate defense of their hosts [66, 129, 130]. It is therefore not surprising to find that the most significant commercial applications of lysozyme are so far in food preservation and processing [131-133]. Lysozyme also found applications in human medicine and veterinary in different ways. For instance, transgenic mice expressing rat lysozyme cDNA in distal respiratory epithelial cells was generated with a significantly enhanced survival rate in comparison with that of wildtype mice when both were challenged with *Pseudomonas aeruginosa* [134]. Lysozymes also have important roles in surveillance of membranes of mammalian cells, enhancement of phagocytic activity of polymorphonuclear leukocytes and macrophages, and stimulation of proliferation and anti-tumor functions of monocytes [121]. It was suggested that lysozymes might be useful as a food additive in the complex treatment of oncological patients for enhancing antineoplastic chemotherapy efficacy [135].

On the other hand, there are abundant evidences showing that endolysins have the capacity of rapidly killing pathogenic Gram-positive bacteria on a generally species-specific basis, *in vitro* or *in vivo*, with effective dosages in the order of milligrams or even micrograms per liter. Nelson *et* al. [104] studied the efficacy of an endolysin encoded by the streptococcal phage C_1, which is specific for groups A, C, and E streptococci with little or no activity against a number of oral streptococci or other commensal organisms tested. Using purified endolysin, Nelson et al. demonstrated that 1,000 units (10 ng) of the enzyme were sufficient to sterilize an *in vitro* culture of about 10^7 Group A streptococci within 5 seconds. When a single dose of endolysin (250 units) was first added to the oral cavity of mice, followed by 10^7 live group A streptococci, it provided protection from colonization. Furthermore, when endolysin (500 units) was given orally to 9 heavily colonized mice, no detectable streptococci were observed 2 h after endolysin treatment. Loeffler *et* al. [136] showed that Pal, a purified pneumococcal endolysin, was able to kill 15 common serotypes of pneumococci, including highly penicillin-resistant strains within seconds of contact. The addition of 100 U/ml of endolysin reduced the concentration of bacteria by 4-logs in 30 seconds. *In vivo* experiments showed that mice exposed to a 10^8 CFU of *Streptococcus pneumoniae* did not yield a detectable level of bacteria 5 h after administration of 1400 U of endolysin. This experiment was repeated with 500 U of endolysin resulting in 63 % of the mice being free of bacteria and a significant reduction in the bacterial titer in all the animals. It was also shown that *S. pneumoniae* growing on mucous membranes were sensitive to endolysin; and even though some bacteria reappeared after a certain time, the number was not high enough to cause recolonization of the mucous membrane.

A rapid killing of *Streptococcus pneumoniae* in the nasopharynx of mice has also been reported using other two endolysins, Cpl-1 murein hydrolase and the Pal amidase, in a murine sepsis model. Purified Pal amidase and/or Cpl-1 lysozyme were used alone or in combination. It was concluded that those two endolysins, used separatedly or in combinaition, could protect animals from bacteraemia and death. Moreover, a synergic effect *in vivo* was observed with the combined use of 2.5 μg each of Cpl-1 and Pal [137]. The rapid killing of sensitive bacteria by endolysins at relatively low dosage is not only important in the sense of therapy costs, but could be one of the major reasons whereby the enzymes would avoid being neutralized by the immune response or causing severe allergic responses in hosts [105].

3.4. Bacterial Resistance to BCWHs

In general, Gram-negative bacteria are resistant to exogenous BCWHs due to the protection of their outer membrane. As discussed previously, some successful Gram-positive pathogenic bacteria are also resistant to lysozymes. Several resistant mechanisms have been characterized in pathogens such as *S. aureus*. Those include: 1) O-acetylation of the NAM of peptidoglycan as reported in staphylococci [129, 138, 139]; 2) attachment of other polymers (e.g. polysaccharides) to the cell wall, as described for streptococci [139]; 3) D-Asp (D-aspartic acid) incorporation as discovered in the *Lactococcus lactis* peptidoglycan crossbridge [140]; and 4) some microbes may synthesize lysozyme inhibitors to neutralize the enzymatic activity [141-143]. On the other hand, virolysins apparently have a very different mechanism, which allows specific virolysins to be functional to those Gram-positive bacteria that have acquired resistance to lysozymes.

It is worthy mentioning that studies with a number of pathogenic bacteria, including *S. pneumoniae*, *S. pyogenes* and *B. anthracis* [101], have shown that repeated exposure of those bacteria to sub-lethal doses of corresponding virolysins does not lead to the development of enzyme resistant strains. This observation was tentatively explained by the fact that choline, an essential structural component of many Gram-positive cell wall [144], serves as receptor for binding of virolysins to bacterial cell wall [112, 115, 116, 145, 146].

3.5. Prephylaxis using BCWHs

Nearly all infections begin at a mucous membrane site and the human mucous membranes are a reservoir for many pathogenic bacteria (e.g., pneumococci, staphylococci, and streptococci) found in the environment [147-149]. This observation, in combination with the fact that induced resistance to virolysins is rarely developed, led to the proposal of a novel method for the control of pathogens by destroying pathogenic bacteria on mucous membranes [104, 136, 150]. Another potential application is in anti-bioterror warfare. Nelson and Fischetti explore the feasibility of exploiting the specific binding and lytic action of virolysins for the rapid detection and killing of *B. anthracis*. PlyG, an virolysin isolated from the γ phage of *B. anthracis* and specifically kills *B. anthracis* and other members of the *B. anthracis* 'cluster' of bacilli, was found satisfactory as a tool for the treatment and detection of *B. anthracis* [151].

4. Virolysins: Promising Enzybiotics

4.1. General Description of Virolysins

As discussed previously, virolysins are phage-encoded BCWHs. They are naturally expressed by bacteriophages during their lytic cycle, and aid to the phage release from infected cells [105]. Virolysins are regarded as the most promising enzybiotics among the three groups of BCWHs because of 1) their capacity of rapidly killing sensitive bacteria, even for lysozyme-resistant bacteria; 2) general narrow spectra of sensitive bacteria, minimizing the disturbance to normal microflora; 3) the large diversity of different virolysins from differet lytic bacteriophages; and 4) the easily detectable bacteriolytic activity of bacteriophages providing a solid basis for rational selection the sources of virolysins [65].

4.2. Antibacterial Efficacy of Virolysins

Virolysins have several known applications, including food decontamination, treatment of bacterial infections in human and animals, prophylaxis, detection of a specific bacterium and diagnostics. All of these uses are possible because of the capacity of virolysin to rapidly kill bacteria and cause bacteriolysis. Extetensive studies have demonstrated that they could represent a realistic alternative to antibiotics. A few virolysins, their target bacteria, and the corresponding health problems are are summarized in Table 1.

4.2.1. Virolysins against streptococcal bacteria

Some *Streptococcus* species, such as *Streptococcus pneumonia* (a *Streptococcus* Group A species), can cause respiratory illnesses. A recent patent describes an invention to treat these diseases by administrating a virolysin, Pal that reaches the mucosal lining in the oral or nasal cavity [152]. It has also been demonstrated that amidase Pal and endopeptidase Cpl-1 from the pneumococcal phage Cpl-1 can act synergistically to decrease the occurrence or the severity of local and systemic pneumococcal disease or prevent and eliminate pneumococcal colonization [163]. This virolysin can kill 15 common serotypes of pneumococci, including highly penicillin-resistant strains within seconds of contact [136]. A few virolysins that have bacteriolytic activities to Group A, B and C streptococci have been studied intensively. Group A and C streptococci cause illness such as pharyngitis, toxic shock syndrome, rheumatic fever [153], while group B streptococci are often responsible for neonatal bacterial infections [155]. PlyC virolysin from C1 phage has been found to be an effective antimicrobial agent for group A and C streptococci [164]. *Streptococcus pyogenes,* a Group

A *Streptococcus*, can cause diseases such as pharyngitis, rheumatic fever and toxic shock syndrome [153]. The virolysin encoded by the streptococcal phage C1 is also specific for group E streptococci, but has only little or no effect against a number of oral streptococci and other commensal organisms tested [165]. 1,000 units of this enzyme were shown to be sufficient to sterilize *in vitro* culture of about 10^7 Group A streptococci within five seconds, demonstrating the therapeutic efficiency of this virolysin. Its prophylaxis effectiveness has also been verified by administrating first 250 units of virolysin C1 to the oral cavity of mice, followed by 10^7 live Group A streptococci. This prevented colonies to grow [165]. It has also been revealed that *S. pyogenes* is highly sensitive to PlyV12 lysin, a virolysin isolated from the enterococcal bacteriophages Φ1 [166].

In the case of Group B streptococci (GBS), the GBS phage NCTC11261 genomic DNA was sequenced and PlyGBS lysin was discovered to be effective against GBS *in vitro* and *in vivo* [167]. Its gene was over 90% identical to several virolysins from various streptococcal species, including GBS phage B30 lysin, *Streptococcus pyogenes* M1 phage-associated lysin, and *Streptococcus equi* phage-associated protein, both at the nucleotide and amino acid level [164].

Table 1. Recently discovered virolysins that can be used to treat human or animal bacterial infections

Phage / Lysin	Targeted bacteria	Related health disorders	References
Pal phage / Pal lytic enzyme	Oral streptococci	Pneumonia	[152]
C1 phage / PlyC	Group A or C streptococci bacteria	Pharyngitis, toxic shock syndrome, rheumatic fever [153]	[154]
GBS phage/ PlyGBS	Group B streptococci bacteria	Neonatal infections	[155]
Actinomyces naeslundii phage/Av-1 lysin	*Actinomyces naeslundii*	Periodontal disease (gingivitis) and root surface (cementum) caries	[156]
PlyV12 phage	*Staphylococcus aureus*	Acute dermatitis	[157]
Phage K/LysK	*Staphylococcus aureus* and 8 other species *Staphylococcus*	Abscesses, fatal sepsis, endocarditis, pneumonia, mastitis, phlebitis, meningitis and toxinoses	[158]
B. anthracis γ-phage/PlyG	*Bacillus anthracis*	Anthrax	[159]
PlyV12 phage	*Enterococcus faecalis*, *Enterococcus faecium*, *Streptococcus pyogenes*	Nosocomial infections, intraabdominal and pelvic infections	[160]
HL18 phage	*Salmonella typhimurium*	Food-borne illness	[161]
Phage .phi.3626	*Clostridium perfringens*	Necrotic enteritis, gas gangrene, food poisoning	[162]

4.2.2. Virolysins against cariogenic bacteria

A bactericide was prepared with an N-acetylmuraminidase, the auto-mutanolysin (Aml) strongly specific to *Streptococcus sobrinus* and *Streptococcus mutans*, two bacteria found in human oral cavity [168]. This preparation could be used to treat dental caries and periodontal disease and easily incorporated into gum, dentifrice or mouthwash. This concept could also possibly be applicable to virolysins. For instance, the virolysin encoded by *Actinomyces naeslundii* phage Av-1 can prevent gingivitis and root surface caries formation [156]. *A. naeslundii* bacteria are resistant to lysozymes but sensitive to virolysins.

4.2.3. Virolysins against staphylococcus

Phage K, a phage belongs to the Myrovidae phage family, exhibits anti-staphylococcal activity and its virolysin, LysK, has been cloned and expressed in *Lactococcus lactis*. Bioinformatics analysis shows that this enzyme contains two peptidoglycan hydrolase domains at the N- terminus, CHAP and Amidase-2, and a cell wall binding domain at the Cterminus [158]. This virolysin has the advantage of being effective to a wide range of Staphylococci. It was demonstrated that LysK could kill nine species of *Staphylococcus* (*S. aureus, S. epidermidis, S. saprophytics, S. chromogenes, S. captis, S. hominis, S. haemolyticus, S. caprea and S. hyicus*), including some methicillin-resistant *S. aureus* (MRSA) strains that causes serious hospital infections worldwide [169] and the pathogenic *S. aureus* strain associated with bovine mastisis [158]. A patent entitled “Antimicrobial Protein Specific to *Staphylococcus aureus*” also describes a novel virolysin that targets *Staphylococcus aureus* [157]. *S. aureus* is also a bacterial pathogen responsible for nosocomial infections that can be targeted by the PlyV12 virolysin [166]. Methods for controlling the growth and treating the infections of these bacteria using PlyV12 have been patented [160].

4.2.4. Virolysins against bacilli

A promising approach to treat anthrax involves the isolation of virolysins effective to *B. anthracis* from *B. cereus* phages. *B. cereus* is a bacterium closely related to *B. anthracis* but has a different virulent type. It could be theoretically treated as *B. anthracis* cured of its virulent plasmid [151]. *B. cereus* is related to food poisoning while *B. anthracis* has a recognized potential for biological weapons and mass destruction [151, 170]. The phages of both bacterial species can easily be isolated from top soil [171]. Experiments demonstrated that virolysin PlyG can lyse both spores and vegetative cells of diverse *B. anthracis* strains and no resistance from the bacteria has been developed after several expositions to the enzyme. This lytic enzyme is not blocked by the capsule of many *B. anthracis* strains [151]. A patent entitled “Lytic Enzymes and Spore Surface Antigen for Detection and Treatment of *Bacillus anthracis* Bacteria and Spores” describes the methods of PlyG isolation and the application of the virolysin to treat anthrax [159], a disease caused by highly resistant spore forming bacteria that generally infect animals but can be transmitted to humans under three forms: cutaneous anthrax, gastrointestinal anthrax and inhalation anthrax [172].

A recent patent [160] disclosed the methods, compositions and articles of manufacture useful for the treatment of *B. anthracis* and *B. cereus* bacteria and spores and related conditions. This disclosure further relates to methods for the identification of a virolysin to rapidly and specifically detect and kill *B. anthracis* and other bacteria. Related articles of manufacture, methods of degrading spores and methods of treatment of infections of *B. anthracis* are also provided [173].

4.2.5. Virolysins against enterococcus species

Nosocomial infections are caused by *Enterococcus faecalis* and *Enterococcus faecium*, two gram-positive bacteria that normally colonize the lower intestinal track. A PlyV12 phage virolysin has been discovered to have lytic effect on those *enterococcus* species as well as on two vancomycin-resistant *E. faecalis* strains (VRE) and three vancomycin-resistant *E. faecium* strains. Vancomycin is an antibiotic that is considered as the last line of defense against a bacterial pathogen that is already resistant to the other antibiotics [160]. Another patent disclosed a virolysin that is active to various bacteria including both *E. faecalis* and *E. faecium* (including vancomycin resistant strains), as well as other human pathogens [160].

4.2.6. Virolysins against salmonella

Salmonella is a Gram-negative bacterium. Its cell envelope includes a lipopolysaccharide (LPS) layer (the outer membrane), which can protect it from the lysis caused by lytic enzymes. A novel approach was disclosed pertaining the use of lyases, polysaccharide-degrading enzymes that are normally found on tail spikes of phages and create openings through the outer membrane, to allow the lytic enzymes to access the peptideglycan network of bacterial cell wall [161]. A patent provides HL18 phage virolysins and lyases, enzymatic compositions, and methods of producing and using virolysins and lyases from HL18 phage [161]. It was demonstrated that administration of the purified HL18 phage reduces at least 10-fold the *Salmonella* population in animals. Similarly, by isolating this virolysin gene and producing lyase from *Salmonella* infected cells, a lytic system against several *Salmonella* strains, including multi-drug resistant strains, can be obtained [161]. This bacterium is principally found in contaminated food [174] and in consequence, it was suggested that HL18 lytic enzyme could be preventively added to food products to inactivate *Salmonella*.

4.2.7. Virolysins against clostridium

Clostridium perfringens, which colonizes intestinal track, can cause diseases such as necrotic enteritis, food poisoning and growth retardation [162]. A virolysin specific to this bacterium was isolated from Clostridium phage phi3626, which was proposed for the treatment of a disorder, disease or condition associated with a Clostridium patho-genic species, in particular, *C. perfringens*.

4.3. Production of Virolysins

Virolysin production cost is one major obstacle associated with this enzybiotic, which can however be resolved by the fast technology development [65]. Two distinct common methods are employed nowadays for virolysin production. The first approach consists in employing high cell density bacterial culture infected with the corresponding phages to allow bacteriolysis to occur. For example, at the end of each phage lytic cycle, using Group C streptococci and C1 phage, the produced virolysins were liberated into the culture medium [175]. Using a similar technique in combination with an alkylating agent, it is possible to obtain a phage-free virolysin preparation at a large scale. *Vibrio harveyi* cultures, isolated from shrimp farms, hatcheries and seawater, were propagated and sodium thiosulphate was added to the cell lysate as alkylating agent. This compound reacts with the phage nucleic acids and deactivates the phage [176]. A more sophisticated and potentially more cost-effective approach involve the cloing and expression of virolysins as recombinant proteins. In the 1970s and 1980s, molecular cloning of DNA fragments via host cells such as *E. coli* was developed and became a popular technique [102]. At this point of time, virolysins from different phages have started to be expressed and produced in different recombinant bacteria. This consists of the second and more sophisticated approach to produce virolysins, which is more popular and potentially more cost-effective than the infected bacteria strategy. A method was patented in 1985 [103] regarding expression of the lysin gene sequence of phage T7 in *E. coli* [103]. This was one of the experiments that marked the beginning of high level nontoxic expression of cell wall disrupting proteins and numerous patents have been filed thereafter. In a recent patent [84], a plasmid, pSOFLysK, which contains the gene sequence of virolysin LysK, was constructed and transferred to bacterial strain *Lactococcus lactis* NZ9800. The recombinant bacterial strain, which was referred to as *Lactococcus lactis* NZ9800-pSOFLysK and subsequently designated as *Lactococcus lactis* DPC6132, was claimed to be useful for amplifying large quantities of genetic material providing anti-staphylococcal activity [84]. This technique requires the identification of the potential virolysin using bioinformatics tools and by comparing the homology of the new sequences with those of known virolysins in order to find similar functional domains in the genes. Open reading frame (ORF) analysis can also be carried out, such as in the case of the Clostridium phage phi3626 genome, in which a holing gene was found and permitted to discover a lysin gene encoded downstream of the holin one [162].

5. Conclusion Remarks

A vast number of studies have been carried out on phages and phage-encoded virolysins as promising solutions to antibiotic resistance. Phages, when properly selected, offers the most cost-effective alternative antibacterials. They are also highly specific, effective, and safe for the treatment and prevention of infectious diseases. Virolysins have also been estabolished as promising anternative antibacterials, which are effective to antibiotic resistant strains. In a broader scope, virolysins belong to bacterial cell wall hydrolysases, lytic enzymes produced by animals, plants, and microbes for a diversity of different physiological functionalities. Despite of the well-based optimism, however, extensive studies are needed to develop these alternative antimicrobials to practical substitutes for antibiotics in term of efficacy, safety, and affordability.

Acknowledgment

Fincial support from the Natural Science and Engineering Research Council of Canada (NSERC) is gratefully acknowledged.

References

[1] Heuer, O. E., et al., (2006.). Human health hazard from antimicrobial-resistant enterococci in animals and food. *Clinical Infectious Diseases, 43(7)*, 911-916.

[2] Witte, W. (2000). Selective pressure by antibiotic use in livestock. *International Journal of Antimicrobial Agents,* 16(SUPPL. 1).

[3] Teuber, M. (2001). Veterinary use and antibiotic resistance. *Current Opinion in Microbiology, 4(5)*, 493-499.

[4] Kutateladze, M. & Adamia, R. (2008). Phage therapy experience at the Eliava Institute. *Medecine et Maladies Infectieuses, 38(8)*, 426-430.

[5] Brussow, H. (2005). Phage therapy: The E. coli experience. *Microbiology, 151(7)*, 2133-2140.

[6] Godany, A., et al., (2003). Phage therapy: Alternative approach to antibiotics. *Biologia - Section Cellular and Molecular Biology, 58(3)*, 313-320.

[7] Inal, J. M. (2003). Phage therapy: A reappraisal of bacteriophages as antibiotics. *Archivum Immunologiae et Therapiae Experimentalis, 51(4)*, 237-244.

[8] Krylov, V. N. (2001). Phage therapy in terms of bacteriophage genetics: Hopes, perspectives, safety, limitations. *Genetika, 37(7)*, 869-887.

[9] Levin, B. R. & Bull, J. J. (1996). Phage therapy revisited: The population biology of a bacterial infection and its treatment with bacteriophage and antibiotics. *American Naturalist, 147(6)*, 881-898.

[10] Borysowski, J., et al., (2006). Current status and perspectives of phage therapy. *Advances in Clinical and Experimental Medicine, 15(4)*, 575-580.

[11] Skurnik, M. & Strauch, E. (2006). Phage therapy: Facts and fiction. *International Journal of Medical Microbiology, 296(1)*, 5-14.

[12] Murthy, K, A. B., Roman. J. L., Durand, S., Fairbrother, J., Quessy, S. & Mandeville, R. (2002). Phage therapy: an innovative approach to treat antibiotic-resistant bacterial strains. Amer. *Ass. Swine Vet.*, 217 -220.

[13] Mandeville, R., et al., (2003). Diagnostic and Therapeutic Applications of Lytic Phages. *Analytical Letters*, *6(15)*, 3241-3259.

[14] Ochs, H. D., et al., (1992). Antibody responses to bacteriophage ϕX174 in patients with adenosine deaminase deficiency. *Blood*, *80(5)*, 1163-1171.

[15] Ochs, H. D., et al., (1993). Regulation of antibody responses: The role of complement and adhesion molecules. *Clinical Immunology and Immunopathology*, *67(3 II)*.

[16] Brussow, H. (2005). Phage therapy: The E. coli experience. *Microbiology*, *151(7)*, 2133-2140.

[17] Damasko, C., et al., (2005). Studies of the efficacy of enterocoliticin, a phage-tail like bacteriocin, as antimicrobial agent against Yersinia enterocolitica serotype O3 in a cell

culture system and in mice. Journal of Veterinary Medicine Series B: *Infectious Diseases and Veterinary Public Health*, *52(4)*, 171-179.

[18] Ackermann, H. W., (2001). Frequency of morphological phage descriptions in the year 2000. Archives of Virology, *146(5)*, 843-857.

[19] Young, R., Wang, I. N. & Roof, W. D. (2000). Phages will out: Strategies of host cell lysis. *Trends in Microbiology*, *8(3)*, 120-128.

[20] Bernhardt, T. G., et al., (2002). Breaking free: "Protein antibiotics" and phage lysis. *Research in Microbiology*, *153(8)*, 493-501.

[21] Ugorcakova, J. & Bukovska, G. (2003). Lysins and holins: Tools of phage-induced lysis. *Biologia - Section Cellular and Molecular Biology*, *58(3)*, 327-334.

[22] Wang, I. N., Smith, D. L. & Young, R. (2000). Holins: The protein clocks of bacteriophage infections. *Annual Review of Microbiology*, *54*, 799-825.

[23] Loeb, M. R. (1974). Bacteriophage T4 mediated release of envelope components from E. coli. *Journal of Virology*, *13(3)*, 631-641.

[24] Tarahovsky, Y. S., Ivanitsky, G. R. & Khusainov, A. A. (1994). Lysis of E. coli cells induced by bacteriophage T4. *FEMS Microbiology Letters*, *122(1-2)*, 195-199.

[25] Hagens, S. & Blasi, U. (2003). Genetically modified filamentous phage as bactericidal agents: A pilot study. *Letters in Applied Microbiology*, *37(4)*, 318-323.

[26] Hagens, S., et al., (2004). Therapy of experimental Pseudomonas infections with a nonreplicating genetically modified phage. *Antimicrobial Agents and Chemotherapy*, *48(10)*, 3817-3822.

[27] Smith, H. W. & Huggins, M. B.(1977). Treatment of experimental E. coli infection in mice with colicine V. *Journal of Medical Microbiology*, *10(4)*, 479-482.

[28] Williams Smith, H. & Huggins, M. B. (1983). Effectiveness of phages in treating experimental E. coli diarhoea in calves, piglets and lambs. *Journal of General Microbiology*, *129(8)*, 2659-2675.

[29] Williams Smith, H., Huggins, M. B. & Shaw, K. M. (1987). Factors influencing the survival and multiplication of bacteriophages in calves and in their environment. *Journal of General Microbiology*, *133(5)*, 1127-1135.

[30] Fischetti, V. A. & Loeffler, J. (2004). Use of synergistic bacteriophage lytic enzymes for prevention and treatment of bacterial infections,WO/2004/058182.

[31] Rapson, M. E., et al., (2005). bact bacteriophages useful for therapy and prophylaxis of bacterial infections, in european patent.

[32] Jayasheela, M., Sriram, B. & Padmanabhan, S. (2005). *bact defined dose therapeutic phage*, in patent cooperation treaty application.

[33] Piddock, L. J. V. & Woodward, M. J. (2006). *bact use of bacteriophage in medicaments*, in patent cooperation treaty application.

[34] Holland, M. A. & Lenihan, N. (2006). bact bacteriophage for lysis of methylobacterium and compositions and uses thereof, in european patent application.

[35] Pasternack, G. R., Sulakvelidze, A. & Brown, T. (2006). *bact method for vaccination of poultry by bacteriophage lysate*, in european patent application.

[36] Walter, M. H. (2008). *bacteriophages that infect bacillus bacteria (anthrax)*, in united states patent and trademark office pre-grant publication.

[37] West, D., Holland, K. & Bojar, K. (2007). *bact bacteriophage and their uses*, in patent cooperation treaty application.

[38] Bull, J. J., et al., (2002). Dynamics of success and failure in phage and antibiotic therapy in experimental infections. *BMC microbiology [electronic resource]*, *2(1)*, 35.

[39] Stone, R. (2002). Bacteriophage therapy. Stalin's forgotten cure. *Science*, *298(5594)*, 728-731.

[40] Smith, W. H., Huggins, M. B. & Shaw, K. M. (1987). The control of experimental E. coli diarrhoea in calves by means of bacteriophages. *Journal of General Microbiology*, *133(5)*, 1111-1126.

[41] Ramachandran, J., Padmanabhan, S. & Sriram, B. (2003). *lysin-deficient bacteriophages having reduced immunogenicity*, in patent cooperation treaty application.

[42] Ramachandran, J., Padmanabhan, S. & Sriram, B. (2004). *bact incapacitated whole-cell immunogenic bacterial compositions*, in european patent.

[43] Greer, G. G., (2005). Bacteriophage control of foodborne bacteria. *Journal of Food Protection*, *68(5)*, 1102-1111.

[44] Hagens, S. & Loessner, M. J. (2007). Application of bacteriophages for detection and control of foodborne pathogens. *Applied Microbiology and Biotechnology*, *76(3)*, 513-519.

[45] Macgregor, H. E. (2006). *Latest food additive: Viruses*, in Los Angeles Times. Los Angeles. F-1.

[46] Averback, P. & Gemmell, J. (2008). BACT Bacteriophage composition useful in treating food products to prevent bacterial contamination, in european patent application.

[47] Pasternack, G. R. & Sulakvelidze, A. (2008). *novel listeria monocytogenes bacteriophage and uses thereof*, in patent cooperation treaty application.

[48] Merril, C. R., Scholl, D. & Adhya, S. L. (2003). The prospect for bacteriophage therapy in Western medicine. *Nature Reviews Drug Discovery*, *2(6)*, 489-497.

[49] Bradbury, J. (2004). "My enemy's enemy is my friend": Using phages to fight bacteria. *Lancet*, *363(9409)*, 624-625.

[50] Matsuzaki, S., et al., (2005). Bacteriophage therapy: A revitalized therapy against bacterial infectious diseases. *Journal of Infection and Chemotherapy*, *11(5)*, 211-219.

[51] Cheng, C. M., et al., (1999). The primary immunity determinant in modulating the lysogenic immunity of the filamentous bacteriophage cf. *Journal of Molecular Biology*, *287(5)*, 867-876.

[52] Broudy, T. B. & Fischetti, V. A. (2003). In vivo lysogenic conversion of Tox- Streptococcus pyogenes to Tox+ with lysogenic streptococci or free phage. *Infection and Immunity*, *71(7)*, 3782-3786.

[53] Dobrindt, U. & Reidl, J. (2000). Pathogenicity islands and phage conversion: Evolutionary aspects of bacterial pathogenesis. *International Journal of Medical Microbiology*, *290(6)*, 519-527.

[54] Chatterjee, S. N. & Chaudhuri, K. (2006). Lipopolysaccharides of Vibrio cholerae: III. Biological functions. *Biochimica et Biophysica Acta - Molecular Basis of Disease*, *1762(1)*, 1-16.

[55] Matsuda, T., et al., (2005). Lysis-deficient bacteriophage therapy decreases endotoxin and inflammatory mediator release and improves survival in a murine peritonitis model. *Surgery*, *137(6)*, 639-646.

[56] Hagens, S., Habel, A. & Blasi, U. (2006). Augmentation of the antimicrobial efficacy of antibiotics by filamentous phage. *Microbial Drug Resistance*, *12(3)*, 164-168.

[57] Brussow, H., Canchaya, C. & Hardt, W. D. (2004). Phages and the evolution of bacterial pathogens: From genomic rearrangements to lysogenic conversion. *Microbiology and Molecular Biology Reviews*, *68(3)*, 560-602.

[58] McGrath, S., Fitzgerald, G. F. & Van Sinderen, D. (2004). The impact of bacteriophage genomics. Current Opinion in Biotechnology, 15(2), 94-99.

[59] Biswas, B., et al., (2002). Bacteriophage therapy rescues mice bacteremic from a clinical isolate of vancomycin-resistant Enterococcus faecium. *Infection and Immunity*, *70(1)*, 204-210.

[60] Davis, B. M., et al., (2000). CTX prophages in classical biotype Vibrio cholerae: Functional phage genes but dysfunctional phage genomes. *Journal of Bacteriology*, *182(24)*, 6992-6998.

[61] Davis, B. M. & Waldor, M. K. (2003). Filamentous phages linked to virulence of Vibrio cholerae. *Current Opinion in Microbiology*, *6(1)*, 35-42.

[62] Strauch, E., Lurz, R. & Beutin, L. (2001). Characterization of a Shiga toxin-encoding temperate bacteriophage of Shigella sonnei. *Infection and Immunity*, *69(12)*, 7588-7595.

[63] Strauch, E., Schaudinn, C. & Beutin, L. (2004). First-time isolation and characterization of a bacteriophage encoding the Shiga toxin 2c variant, which is globally spread in strains of E. coli O157. *Infection and Immunity*, *72(12)*, 7030-7039.

[64] Parisien, A., et al., (2008). Novel alternatives to antibiotics: Bacteriophages, bacterial cell wall hydrolases, and antimicrobial peptides. *Journal of Applied Microbiology*, *104(1)*, 1-13.

[65] Parisien, A. & Lan, C. Q. (2009). Classification of Bacterial Cell Wall Hydrolysases and Their Potentials as Novel Alternatives to Antibiotics - a response to the letter of Biziulevicius and Kazlauskaite *Journal of Applied Microbiology*, in press.

[66] Abdou, A. M., et al., (2007). Antimicrobial peptides derived from hen egg lysozyme with inhibitory effect against Bacillus species. *Food Control*, *18(2)*, 173-178.

[67] Tenovuo, J., Lumikari, M. & Soukka, T. (1991). Salivary lysozyme, lactoferrin and peroxidases: antibacterial effects on cariogenic bacteria and clinical applications in preventive dentistry. Proceedings of the Finnish Dental Society. *Suomen Hammaslaakariseuran toimituksia*, *87(2)*, 197-208.

[68] Tenovuo, J. (2002). Clinical applications of antimicrobial host proteins lactoperoxidase, lysozyme and lactoferrin in xerostomia: Efficacy and safety. *Oral Diseases*, *8(1)*, 23-29.

[69] Ibrahim, H. R., Aoki, T. & Pellegrini, A. (2002). Strategies for new antimicrobial proteins and peptides: Lysozyme and aprotinin as model molecules. *Current Pharmaceutical Design*, *8(9)*, 671-693.

[70] Masschalck, B. & Michiels, C. W. (2003). Antimicrobial properties of lysozyme in relation to foodborne vegetative bacteria. *Critical Reviews in Microbiology*, *29(3)*, 191-214.

[71] Niyonsaba, F. & Ogawa, H. (2005). Protective roles of the skin against infection: Implication of naturally occurring human antimicrobial agents -defensins, cathelicidin LL-37 and lysozyme. *Journal of Dermatological Science*, *40(3)*, 157-168.

[72] Irwin, D. M., Prager, E. M. & Wilson, A. C. (1992). Evolutionary genetics of ruminant lysozymes. *Animal Genetics*, *23(3)*, 193-202.

[73] Adu-Bobie, J., et al., (2004). GNA33 of Neisseria meningitidis Is A Lipoprotein Required for Cell Separation, Membrane Architecture, and Virulence. *Infection and Immunity*, *72(4)*, 1914-1919.

[74] Blackman, S. A., Smith, T. J. & Foster, S. J. (1998). The role of autolysins during vegetative growth of Bacillus subtilis 168. *Microbiology*, *144(1)*, 73-82.

[75] Garcia, D. L. & Dillard, J. P. (2006). AmiC functions as an N-acetylmuramyl-L-alanine amidase necessary for cell separation and can promote autolysis in Neisseria gonorrhoeae. *Journal of Bacteriology*, *188(20)*, 7211-7221.

[76] Tomasz, A., Albino, A. & Zanati, E. (1970). Multiple antibiotic resistance in a bacterium with suppressed autolytic system. *Nature*, *227(254)*, 138-140.

[77] Beliveau, C., et al., (1991). Cloning, sequencing, and expression in E. coli of a Streptococcus faecalis autolysin. *Journal of Bacteriology*, *173(18)*, 5619-5623.

[78] Vian, A., et al., (1998). Structure of the β-galactosidase gene from Thermus sp. Strain T2: Expression in E. coli and purification in a single step of an active fusion protein. *Applied and Environmental Microbiology*, *64(6)*, 2187-2191.

[79] Croux, C. & Garcia, J. L. (1992). Reconstruction and expression of the autolytic gene from Clostridium acetobutylicum ATCC 824 in E. coli. *FEMS Microbiology Letters*, *95(1)*, 13-20.

[80] Romero, A., Lopez, R. & Garcia, P. (1990). Characterization of the pneumococcal bacteriophage HB-3 amidase: Cloning and expression in E. coli. *Journal of Virology*, *64(1)*, 137-142.

[81] Garcia, E., Garcia, J. L. & Ronda, C. (1985). Cloning and expression of the pneumococcal autolysin gene in E. coli. *Molecular and General Genetics*, *201(2)*,. 225-230.

[82] Diaz, E., et al., (1996). The two-step lysis system of pneumococcal bacteriophage EJ-1 is functional in gram-negative bacteria: Triggering of the major pneumococcal autolysin in E. coli. *Molecular Microbiology*, *19(4)*, 667-681.

[83] Biziulevicius, G. A., et al., (2002). Stimulation of microbial autolytic system by tryptic casein hydrolysate. *International Journal of Antimicrobial Agents*, *20(5)*, 361-365.

[84] Wootton, M., et al., (2005). Reduced expression of the atl autolysin gene and susceptibility to autolysis in clinical heterogeneous glycopeptide-intermediate Staphylococcus aureus (hGISA) and GISA strains. *Journal of Antimicrobial Chemotherapy*, *56(5)*, 944-947.

[85] Isturiz, R., Metcalf, J. A. & Root, R. K. (1985). Enhanced killing of penicillin-treated gram-positive cocci by human granulocytes: Role of bacterial autolysins, catalase, and

granulocyte oxidative pathways. *Yale Journal of Biology and Medicine*, *58(2)*, 133-143.

[86] Ginsburg, I. (2002). Cationic polyelectrolytes from leukocytes might kill bacteria by activating their autolytic systems: Enigmatically, the relevance of this phenomenon to post-infectious sequelae is disregarded [6]. Intensive Care Medicine, *28(8)*, 1188.

[87] Ginsburg, I. (2001). Cationic peptides from leukocytes might kill bacteria by activating their autolytic enzymes causing bacteriolysis: Why are publications proposing this concept never acknowledged? *Blood*, *97(8)*, 2530-2531.

[88] Ronda, C., Garcia, J. L. & Garcia, E. (1987). Biological role of the pneumococcal amidase. Cloning of the lytA gene in Streptococcus pneumoniae. *European Journal of Biochemistry*, *164(3)*, 621-624.

[89] Lopez, R., et al., (1992). Structural analysis and biological significance of the cell wall lytic enzymes of Streptococcus pneumoniae and its bacteriophage. *FEMS Microbiology Letters*, *100(1-3)*, 439-447.

[90] Romero, P., Lopez, R. & Garcia, E. (2004). Characterization of LytA-like N-acetylmuramoyl-L-alanine amidases from two new Streptococcus mitis bacteriophages provides insights into the properties of the major pneumococcal autolysin. *Journal of Bacteriology*, *186(24)*, 8229-8239.

[91] Berry, A. M., et al., (1989). Contribution of autolysin to virulence of Streptococcus pneumoniae. *Infection and Immunity*, *57(8)*, 2324-2330.

[92] Sato, K., et al., (1996). Roles of autolysin and pneumolysin in middle ear inflammation caused by a type 3 Streptococcus pneumoniae strain in the chinchilla otitis media model. *Infection and Immunity*, *64(4)*, 1140-1145.

[93] Canvin, J. R., et al., (1995). The role of pneumolysin and autolysin in the pathology of pneumonia and septicemia in mice infected with a type 2 pneumococcus. *Journal of Infectious Diseases*, *172(1)*, 119-123.

[94] Lock, R. A., Hansman, D. & Paton, J. C. (1992). Comparative efficacy of autolysin and pneumolysin as immunogens protecting mice against infection by Streptococcus pneumoniae. *Microbial Pathogenesis*, *12(2)*, 137-143.

[95] Ralston, D. J., et al., (1955). Virolysin: a virus-induced lysin from staphylococcal phage lysates. *Proc. Soc. Exp. Biol. and Med.*, *89*, 502.

[96] Sonstein, S. A., Hammel, J. M. & Bondi, A. (1971). Staphylococcal bacteriophage-associated lysin: a lytic agent active against Staphylococcus aureus. *Journal of Bacteriology*, *107(2)*, 499-504.

[97] Loessner, M. J., et al., (1998). The two-component lysis system of Staphylococcus aureus bacteriophage Twort: A large TTG-start holin and an associated amidase endolysin. *FEMS Microbiology Letters*, *162(2)*, 265-274.

[98] Loessner, M. J., Gaeng, S. & Scherer, S. (1999). Evidence for a holin-like protein gene fully embedded out of frame in the endolysin gene of Staphylococcus aureus bacteriophage 187. *Journal of Bacteriology*, *181(15)*, 4452-4460.

[99] Navarre, W. W., et al., (1999). Multiple enzymatic activities of the murein hydrolase from staphylococcal phage 11: Identification of a D-alanyl-glycine endopeptidase activity. *Journal of Biological Chemistry*, *274(22)*, 15847-15856.

[100] Bon, J., Mani, N. & Jayaswal, R. K. (1997). Molecular analysis of lytic genes of bacteriophage 80 of Staphylococcus aureus. *Canadian Journal of Microbiology*, *43(7)*, 612-616.

[101] Low, L. Y., et al., (2005). Structure and lytic activity of a Bacillus anthracis prophage endolysin. *Journal of Biological Chemistry*, *280(42)*, 35433-35439.

[102] Hermoso, J. A., et al., (2003). Structural basis for selective recognition of pneumococcal cell wall by modular endolysin from phage Cp-1. *Structure*, *11(10)*,. 1239-1249.

[103] Monterroso, B., et al., (2005). Unravelling the structure of the pneumococcal autolytic lysozyme. *Biochemical Journal*, *391(1)*, 41-49.

[104] Fischetti, V. A., Nelson, D. & Schuch, R. (2006). Reinventing phage therapy: Are the parts greater than the sum? *Nature Biotechnology*, *24(12)*, 1508-1511.

[105] Fischetti, V. A. (2005). Bacteriophage lytic enzymes: Novel anti-infectives. *Trends in Microbiology*, *13(10)*, 491-496.

[106] Strominger, J. L. & Ghuysen, J. M. (1967). Mechanisms of enzymatic bacteriolysis. *Science*, *156(3772)*, 213-221.

[107] Bower, S. & Rosenthal, K. S. (2006). The bacterial cell wall: The armor, artillery, and Achilles heel. *Infectious Diseases in Clinical Practice*, *14(5)*, 309-317.

[108] Meroueh, S. O., et al., (2006). Three-dimensional structure of the bacterial cell wall peptidoglycan. *Proceedings of the National Academy of Sciences of the United States of America*, *103(12)*, 4404-4409.

[109] Dmitriev, B., Toukach, F. & Ehlers, S. (2005). Towards a comprehensive view of the bacterial cell wall. *Trends in Microbiology*, *13(12)*, 569-574.

[110] Borysowski, J., Weber-Dabrowska, B. & Gorski, A. (2006). Bacteriophage endolysins as a novel class of antibacterial agents. *Experimental Biology and Medicine*, *231(4)*, 366-377.

[111] Garcia, P., et al., (1986). Nucleotide sequence and expression of the pneumococcal autolysin gene from its own promoter in E. coli. *Gene*, *43(3)*, 265-272.

[112] Lopez, R. & Garcia, E. (2004). Recent trends on the molecular biology of pneumococcal capsules, lytic enzymes, and bacteriophage. *FEMS Microbiology Reviews*, *28(5)*, 553-580.

[113] Imoto, T. (1996). Engineering of lysozyme. *EXS*, *75*, 163-181.

[114] Qian, S. J., et al., (1995). Studies on the engineering of human lysozyme. *Annals of the New York Academy of Sciences*, *750*, 180-184.

[115] Mesnage, S. & Fouet, A. (2002). Plasmid-encoded autolysin in Bacillus anthracis: Modular structure and catalytic properties. *Journal of Bacteriology*, *184(1)*, 331-334.

[116] Briese, T. & Hakenbeck, R. (1985). Interaction of the pneumococcal amidase with lipoteichoic acid and choline. *European Journal of Biochemistry*, *146(2)*, 417-427.

[117] Lopez, R., et al., (1997). The pneumococcal cell wall degrading enzymes: A modular design to create new lysins? *Microbial Drug Resistance*, *3(2)*, 199-211.

[118] Morita, M., et al., (2001). Functional analysis of antibacterial activity of Bacillus amyloliquefaciens phage endolysin against Gram-negative bacteria. *FEBS Letters*, *500(1-2)*, 56-59.

[119] Cheng, X., et al., (1994). The structure of bacteriophage T7 lysozyme, a zinc amidase and an inhibitor of T7 RNA polymerase. *Proceedings of the National Academy of Sciences of the United States of America*, *91(9)*, 4034-4038.

[120] Masschalck, B., Deckers, D. & Michiels, C. W. (2002). Lytic and nonlytic mechanism of inactivation of gram-positive bacteria by lysozyme under atmospheric and high hydrostatic pressure. *Journal of Food Protection*, *65(12)*, 1916-1923.

[121] Ibrahim, H. R., Matsuzaki, T. & Aoki, T. (2001). Genetic evidence that antibacterial activity of lysozyme is independent of its catalytic function. *FEBS Letters*, *506(1)*, 27-32.

[122] De Vries, J., et al., (1999). The bacteriolytic activity in transgenic potatoes expressing a chimeric T4 lysozyme gene and the effect of T4 lysozyme on soil- and phytopathogenic bacteria. *Systematic and Applied Microbiology*, *22(2)*, 280-286.

[123] Laube, D. M., et al., (2006). Antimicrobial peptides in the airway. *Current topics in microbiology and immunology.*, *306*, 153-182.

[124] Sava, G. (1996). Pharmacological aspects and therapeutic applications of lysozymes. *EXS*, *75*, 433-449.

[125] Loessner, M. J. (2005). Bacteriophage endolysins - Current state of research and applications. *Current Opinion in Microbiology*, *8(4)*, 480-487.

[126] Bull, J. J. & Regoes, R. R. (2006). Pharmacodynamics of non-replicating viruses, bacteriocins and lysins. *Proceedings of the Royal Society - Biological Sciences (Series B)*, *273(1602)*, 2703-2712.

[127] Wang, S., et al., (2005). First report of a novel plant lysozyme with both antifungal and antibacterial activities. *Biochemical and Biophysical Research Communications*, *327(3)*, 820-827.

[128] Lee-Huang, S., et al., (2005). Structural and functional modeling of human lysozyme reveals a unique nonapeptide, HL9, with anti-HIV activity. *Biochemistry*, *44(12)*, 4648-4655.

[129] Bera, A., et al., (2005). Why are pathogenic staphylococci so lysozyme resistant? The peptidoglycan O-acetyltransferase OatA is the major determinant for lysozyme resistance of Staphylococcus aureus. *Molecular Microbiology*, *55(3)*, 778-787.

[130] Solovykh, G. N., et al., (2004). Lysozyme of the mollusk Unio pictorum and the sensitivity of alkanotrophic rhodococci to its effect. *Applied Biochemistry and Microbiology*, *40(5)*, 482-489.

[131] Nattress, F. M., Yost, C. K. & Baker, L. P. (2001). Evaluation of the ability of lysozyme and nisin to control meat spoilage bacteria. *International Journal of Food Microbiology*, *70(1-2)*, 111-119.

[132] Pellegrini, A., Schumacher, S. & Stephan, R. (2003). In-vitro activity of various antimicrobial peptides developed from the bactericidal domains of lysozyme and β-lactoglobulin with respect to Listeria monocytogenes, E. coli O157, Salmonella spp. and Staphylococcus aureus. *Archiv fur Lebensmittelhygiene*, *54(2)*, 34-36.

[133] Cagri, A., Ustunol, Z. & Ryser, E. T. (2004). Antimicrobial edible films and coatings. *Journal of Food Protection*, *67(4)*, 833-848.

[134] Akinbi, H. T., et al., (2000). Bacterial killing is enhanced by expression of lysozyme in the lungs of transgenic mice. *Journal of Immunology*, *165(10)*, 5760-5766.

[135] Shcherbakova, E. G., et al., (2002). Lysozyme effect on the mouse lymphoma growth and antineoplastic activity of cyclophosphamide. *Antibiotiki i Khimioterapiya, 47(11)*, 3-8.

[136] Loeffler, J. M., Nelson, D. & Fischetti, V.A. (2001). Rapid killing of Streptococcus pneumoniae with a bacteriophage cell wall hydrolase. *Science, 294(5549)*, 2170-2172.

[137] Jado, I., et al., (2003). Phage lytic enzymes as therapy for antibiotic-resistant Streptococcus pneumoniae infection in a murine sepsis model. *Journal of Antimicrobial Chemotherapy, 52(6)*, 967-973.

[138] Argueso, P. & Sumiyoshi, M. (2006). Characterization of a carbohydrate epitope defined by the monoclonal antibody H185: Sialic acid O-acetylation on epithelial cell-surface mucins. *Glycobiology, 16(12)*, 1219-1228.

[139] Fedtke, I., Gotz, F. & Peschel, A. (2004). Bacterial evasion of innate host defenses - The Staphylococcus aureus lesson. *International Journal of Medical Microbiology, 294(2-3)*, 189-194.

[140] Veiga, P., et al., (2006). Identification of an essential gene responsible for D-Asp incorporation in the Lactococcus lactis peptidoglycan crossbridge. *Molecular Microbiology, 62(6)*, 1713-1724.

[141] Bukharin, O. V. & Valyshev, A. V. (2006). Microbial inhibitors of lysozyme. *Zhurnal mikrobiologii, epidemiologii, i immunobiologii., (4)*, 8-13.

[142] Nakimbugwe, D., et al., (2006). Inactivation of gram-negative bacteria in milk and banana juice by hen egg white and lambda lysozyme under high hydrostatic pressure. *International Journal of Food Microbiology, 112(1)*, 19-25.

[143] Callewaert, L., et al., (2005). Purification of Ivy, a lysozyme inhibitor from E. coli, and characterisation of its specificity for various lysozymes. *Enzyme and Microbial Technology, 37(2)*, 205-211.

[144] Fischer, W. (2000). Phosphocholine of pneumococcal teichoic acids: Role in bacterial physiology and pneumococcal infection. *Research in Microbiology, 151(6)*, 421-427.

[145] Jedrzejas, M. J. (2001). Pneumococcal Virulence Factors: Structure and Function. Microbiol. *Mol. Biol. Rev., 65(2)*, 187-207.

[146] Tomasz, A., Zanati, E. & Ziegler, R. (1971). DNA uptake during genetic transformation and the growing zone of the cell envelope. *Proceedings of the National Academy of Sciences of the United States of America, 68(8)*, 1848-1852.

[147] Coello, R., et al., (1994). Prospective study of infection, colonization and carriage of methicillin-resistant staphylococcus aureus in an outbreak affecting 990 patients. *European Journal of Clinical Microbiology and Infectious Diseases, 13(1)*, 74-81.

[148] De Lencastre, H., et al., (1999). Carriage of respiratory tract pathogens and molecular epidemiology of Streptococcus pneumoniae colonization in healthy children attending day care centers in Lisbon, Portugal. *Microbial Drug Resistance, 5(1)*, 19-29.

[149] Von Eiff, C., et al., (2001). Nasal carriage as a source of Staphylococcus aureus bacteremia. *New England Journal of Medicine, 344(1)*, 11-16.

[150] Fischetti, V. A., (2003). Novel method to control pathogenic bacteria on human mucous membranes. *Annals of the New York Academy of Sciences, 987*, 207-214.

[151] Schuch, R., Nelson, D. & Fischetti, V. A. (2002). A bacteriolytic agent that detects and kills Bacillus anthracis. *Nature, 418(6900)*, 884-889.

[152] Fischetti, V. & Loomis, L. (2006). Use of bacterial phage associated lysing enzymes for treating upper respiratory illnesses, US Patent 6432444.

[153] Cunningham, M. W. (2000). Pathogenesis of group a streptococcal infections. *Clinical Microbiology Reviews*, *13(3)*, 470-511.

[154] Nelson, D. C. & Fischetti, V. A. (2002). *C1 bacteriophage lytic system*, in united states patent and trademark office pre-grant publication.

[155] Fischetti, V. A. & Cheng, Q. (2007). *ply-gbs mutant lysins*, in patent cooperation treaty application.

[156] Delisle, A. L., Barcak, G. J. & Guo, M. (2004). bacteriophage-encoded antibacterial enzyme for the treatment and prevention of gingivitis and root surface caries, in patent cooperation treaty application.

[157] Yoon, S., Kang S., Kyound S., Choi Y., Son J., (2008). *Antimicrobial protein specific to staphylococcus aureus*, patent: WO/2008/016240.

[158] Ross, P. & Coffey, A. (2008). Recombinant staphylococcal phage lysin as an antibacterial agent, patent: WO/2008/001342 .

[159] Fischetti, V. A. & Schuch, R. (2005). *lytic enzymes and spore surface antigen for detection and treatment of*, in patent cooperation treaty application.

[160] Yoong, P., et al., (2007). *Bactiophage lysins for Enterococcus faecalis, Enterococcus faecium and other bacteria*, in United States patent and trademark office pre-grant publication.

[161] Harris, D. L. & Lee, N. (2003). *Bacteriophage and enzymes lytic to salmonellae*, WO/2003/103578.

[162] Zimmer, M., Loessner, M. & Morgan, A. J. (2005). *Novel protein*, in united states patent and trademark office pre-grant publication.

[163] Fischetti, V. & Loomis, L. (2005). Therapeutic treatment of upper respiratory infections using a nasal spray. United States Patent 6893635 .

[164] Fischetti, V. A., Nelson, D. & Schuch, R. (2004). *Nucleic acids and polypeptides of c1 bacteriophage and uses thereof*, in patent cooperation treaty application.

[165] Nelson, D. C. & Fischetti, V. A. (2003). C1 bacteriophage lytic system.

[166] Yoong, P., et al., (2004). Identification of a broadly active phage lytic enzyme with lethal activity against antibiotic-resistant Enterococcus faecalis and Enterococcus faecium. *Journal of Bacteriology*, *186(14)*, 4808-4812.

[167] Nelson, D., Loomis, L. & Fischetti, V. A. (2001). Prevention and elimination of upper respiratory colonization of mice by group A streptococci by using a bacteriophage lytic enzyme. *Proceedings of the National Academy of Sciences of the United States of America*, *98(7)*, 4107-4112.

[168] Yoshimura, G., et al., (2006). Identification and molecular characterization of an N-acetylmuraminidase, Aml, involved in Streptococcus mutans cell separation. *Microbiology and Immunology*, *50(9)*, 729-742.

[169] Hiramatsu, K., et al., (2001). The emergence and evolution of methicillin-resistant Staphylococcus aureus. *Trends in Microbiology*, *9(10)*, 486-493.

[170] Zhong, W., et al., (2007). Differentiation of Bacillus anthracis, B. cereus, and B. thuringiensis by using pulsed-field gel electrophoresis. *Applied and Environmental Microbiology*, *73(10)*, 3446-3449.

[171] Walter, M. H. & Baker, D. D. (2003). Three Bacillus anthracis bacteriophages from topsoil. *Current Microbiology*, *47(1)*, 55-58.

[172] Yoong, P., Schuch R., Nelson D., and FISCHETTI, (2008). *Bactiophage lysins for bacillus anthracis*, WO/2008/018854.

[173] Fischetti, V. A., Schuch, R. & Nelson, D. (2008). *Phage-associated lytic enzymes for treatment of Bacillus anthracis and related conditions*, in united states patent and trademark office granted patent.

[174] Cetinkaya, F., et al., (2008). Shigella and Salmonella contamination in various foodstuffs in Turkey. *Food Control*, *19(11)*, 1059-1063.

[175] Yang, H. H., Hiu, S. F. & Harris, J. L. (1989). *PROD Production of phage and phage-associated lysin*, in United States patent and trademark office granted patent.

[176] Alday-Sanz, V., Karunasagar, I. & Karunasagar, I. (2007). prod + app compositions comprising lytic enzymes of bacteriophages for treating bacterial infections, in patent cooperation treaty application.

In: Multiple Drug Resistance
Editors: A. Meszaros, G. Balogh, pp. 195-202
ISBN: 978-1-60741-595-4

Chapter VIII

Nutrition and Tuberculosis

***Wing Wai Yew*[1] *and Chi Chiu Leung*[2*]**
[1]Chief of Service, Tuberculosis and Chest Unit, Grantham Hospital, Hong Kong, China.
[2]Consultant Chest Physician, Tuberculosis and Chest Service, Centre for Health Protection, Department of Health, Hong Kong, China.

Abstract

Evidences are accumulating in both human and animal studies that undernutrition is associated with increased risk and severity of tuberculosis. In addition, obesity appears to protect against tuberculosis. Diabetes mellitus increases risk of tuberculosis, but poor diabetic control contributes to the bulk of such risk. In both under-nutrition and poor diabetic control, the increased risk is seen mainly in the pulmonary form of the disease, and the exact reason for relative sparing of the extrapulmonary sites remains unclear. Undernutrition has also been associated with worsened prognosis, poorer response to treatment and increased risk of relapse. Data from randomized controlled trials are scanty, as nutritional supplementation trials are often costly and difficult to implement. Micronutrients have been shown to decrease the risk of reversion of sputum culture to positivity after initial conversion, but there was no significant effect on mortality. With the putative roles of systemic inflammatory responses in tuberculosis manifestations, adjunctive corticosteroid administration treatment has been found to afford earlier and more significant body weight gain, albeit no differences in sputum bacteriological conversion and disease relapse rate. Further studies, with better study designs and serial monitoring of relevant nutritional parameters, are required to clarify the complex situation.

[*] Corresponding author: Email: cc_leung@dh.gov.hk, Tel.: 852-25353864, Fax:852-29775940.

Introduction

Tuberculosis is commonly associated with poverty and under-nutrition in both developed and developing countries [1-4]. However, the presence of multiple potential confounders often poses considerable difficulties in delineating the exact relationship. With the often chronic and insidious nature of the disease, and its multiple nutritional / metabolic effects, the exact direction of causality is generally obscure in most cross-sectional or case-control studies.

Nutrition and Risk of Tuberculosis

In recent years, a number of systematic reviews [5-6] have helped to summarize the previous human and animal studies on the subject. Two previous prospective studies showed higher risk of tuberculosis among underweight subjects, but the authors attributed such effect to body build [7-8]. A prospective cohort study not only reconfirmed the previous observations, but also demonstrated a substantially decreased risk of tuberculosis among those subjects who were obese at the baseline, as compared to their normal-weight counterparts [9]. The linear relationship between body mass index and tuberculosis risk suggested a close link between the nutritional status and the immune defense mechanism against the tubercle bacillus. Improving socioeconomic conditions have been associated with the decline of tuberculosis well before the advent of effective treatment in the last century [10]. Increased availability of cheaper food associated with improving socioeconomic conditions could have played a pivotal role [10]. While severe malnutrition is uncommon at peace time in developed areas nowadays, milder degree of undernutrition is probably fairly common, even among these areas, and overall nutrition status is likely to continue to have a major impact of the epidemiology of tuberculosis.

Various defects in cellular immune mechanism have also been demonstrated in animal studies, especially those on protein deprivation in the guinea pig model [11-12]. However, the interaction is likely to go beyond those related to simple nutrient deficiencies. A cholesterol-rich diet has also been shown to accelerate bacteriologic sterilization in pulmonary tuberculosis [13]. Adipose tissue is now recognized to have major endocrine functions [14]. Increasing evidence suggests that leptin differentially regulates metabolic, neuroendocrine and immune functions in human [15]. The administration of leptin in human congenital leptin deficiency has demonstrated beneficial effects on obesity, T-cell hyporesponsiveness and neuroendocrine / metabolic dysfunction [16]. Leptin-deficient ob/ob mice have been shown to be highly susceptible to pulmonary infection by *Mycobacterium tuberculosis* [17]. A better understanding of the complex interplay between the tubercle bacillus and our body is likely an important step for the discovery of new intervention targets in our battle against this long-standing enemy of humanity.

Diabetes Mellitus

Diabetes mellitus has been well reported to be associated with increased risk of tuberculosis [18-19]. In a recent prospective cohort study in Hong Kong [20], diabetes mellitus (mainly type 2) was associated with a modest increase in risk of active, culture-confirmed and pulmonary but not extrapulmonary tuberculosis, with adjusted hazard ratios of 1.77, 1.91, 1.89 and 1.00 respectively [20]. The increased risk was observed only among diabetic patients with baseline glycosylated hemoglobin HbA1c ≥ 7%. They had a three-fold increase in risk in comparison with those diabetic subjects with baseline HbA1c <7%, who were not at increased risk. Substantial heterogeneity in tuberculosis risk is observed among diabetic subjects in different localities [18-21]. Apart from possible constitutional differences, including the relative proportion of type 1 and 2 diabetes, barriers of access to care and differences in diabetic control might have contributed to the ethnic differences as observed. In-vitro immune studies and skin testing among diabetic subjects have shown possible impairment of adaptive immune responses [22-25]. Similar to the effect of body mass index [8, 9], the increased risk of diabetes mellitus was relatively specific for pulmonary tuberculosis but not extrapulmonary tuberculosis. Higher prevalence of diabetes mellitus was also observed among patients with pulmonary tuberculosis as compared to those with extrapulmonary tuberculosis in a case-control study [26]. Diabetes mellitus has also been reported to modify the disease manifestation, with more frequent lower lung field involvement and cavity formation [27-28]. A close interplay between the energy metabolism and immune system could well be implicated in the relatively specific pulmonary effect of both body mass index and diabetic control.

Severity of Disease

Nutritional status has been well reported to be associated with the severity of disease [29, 30]. Again, because of the profound metabolic effect of tuberculosis, it might be difficult to be certain of the direction of causality in a cross-sectional or case-control analysis. With the increased risk of tuberculosis among the underweight, immunological effect of protein depletion in animal models, and modified disease manifestations in DM or immunocompromizing conditions, it is biological plausible that malnutrition does increase the severity of disease.

Response to Treatment

Malnutrition has also been associated with poor response to treatment [30-31]. Nutritional deficit has also been found as a negative prognostic factor in patients with miliary tuberculosis [32]. Using a nutritional risk score comprising four factors (low body mass index, hypoalbuminemia, hypocholesterolemia, and severe lymphocytopenia), the independent and major prognostic values of nutritional status on both acute respiratory failure and 90-day mortality among 56 patients with miliary tuberculosis were demonstrated. Again with the retrospective design and observational nature of this study, it might be difficult to pinpoint the exact cause and effect direction between nutrition status and tuberculosis severity / outcome.

Underweight at baseline was shown to be independently associated with relapse risk among HIV-negative tuberculosis patients in a randomized chemotherapy trial [33]. On reanalysis of the data in the same trial, the two-year relapse rates were 4.2%, 11.9, and 20.3% among those not underweight, those underweight but gaining > 5% weight at two months, and those underweight and not gaining weight, respectively, and lack of early weight gain was found to be an independent predictor of relapse in underweight tuberculosis patients (OR 2.4, P = 0.03), after controlling for other risk factors including, among others, cavity and sputum culture positivity at two months [34]. As much as 61% of relapse in that trial occurred among those ≥10% underweight at diagnosis, and 62% of these in turn occurred in those failing to gain > 5% weight in the induction phase of treatment. On the other hand, a previous study in Tanzania concluded that weight gain during tuberculosis therapy was an unreliable indicator of overall treatment response [35]. However, that study, besides including HIV-infected subjects, did not specifically examine the effect of weight change during the initial phase among patients who were underweight at diagnosis. In the absence of randomized intervention targeting at nutritional status, the question still remains regarding whether the weight gain helps to augment host defense against the mycobacterial pathogen, or just reflects successful control of the disease by the chemotherapy [36].

Nutritional Supplementation

Tuberculosis carries a very substantial degree of mortality, especially for the more disseminated forms of the disease in debilitated / immunocompromized host. If poor nutritional status does predispose to major complication(s) and death, specific intervention targeting at improving the nutritional status would be indicated to decrease the associated morbidity and mortality. Anti-tuberculosis drug resistance is an increasing concern globally. With our currently limited armament, it might be difficult to work out an effective regimen for those patients suffering from extensively drug-resistant tuberculosis. As only one in ten infected persons, on average, will ever develop disease in his / her lifetime, host factors appears to be critical in the defense against the tubercle bacillus. Where we are almost back to the pre-chemotherapy era, it might also be worthwhile to re-examine the role of nutritional supplementation, either alone or as adjunct to chemotherapy / surgery, in the humanitarian and active management of these unfortunate patients.

Unfortunately, systematically collected data are notably scarce in this area. In a randomized controlled trial design, micronutrients have also been shown to decrease the risk of reversion of sputum culture to positivity after initial conversion at the first month in both HIV-infected and non-infected patients, but there was no significant effect on mortality [37]. However, micronutrients benefitted HIV-uninfected subjects the most in that trial, whereas the opposite was the case in a previous trial in the same locality [38]. In anti-tuberculosis chemotherapy, bacteriological cure with absence of relapse is probably the most clinically relevant endpoint. While it is generally acceptable to use validated surrogate endpoints, such as two-month culture conversion [39] or time-to-culture conversion [40], to decrease the sample size requirement and shorten the duration of follow-up in explorative trials, caution might have to be exercised in the employment of less well characterized endpoints such as culture reversion after a single negative sputum culture at the first month. Minor variation in sputum collection technique and / or sputum processing could have produced a single negative culture when the bacillary load was lowered after a month of treatment. When multiple endpoints and subgroups were evaluated in a single trial, results should also be interpreted with care.

As tuberculosis is generally more prevalent in developing areas and nutritional supplementation is likely to show the greatest effects among those with malnourishment, an adequately powered trial will probably have to be implemented in a resources-limited area. Micronutrient deficiencies often occur in midst of global nutritional deficits. As both of them might play a role in modulating our body defense against tuberculosis, careful documentation of both overall nutritional status and specific nutrient deficiencies is desirable, so that maximal amount of information can be extracted from these often costly trials. Unfortunately, neither of the above two trials on micronutrient supplementation contained specific information on total protein-calorie intake or serial measurements of body weight or body mass index to allow clear inference.

Other Adjunctive Therapy

Systemic inflammatory responses also appear to play an important role in the development of severe complications in tuberculosis. In a study just alluded to, elevated C-reactive protein level was also shown to be an independent predictor of acute respiratory failure [32]. Poor appetite and decreased food intake may also be associated with advanced tuberculosis disease. Adjunctive corticosteroid administration during tuberculosis treatment has been found to afford earlier and more significant body weight gain, albeit no differences in sputum bacteriological conversion and disease relapse rate [41]. Such form of treatment might also merit reappraisal in clinical situations associated with heightened inflammatory responses, especially when simple dietary manipulation does not appear to result in significant improvement in the nutrition status.

Reference

[1] Barr, RG; Diez-Roux, AV; Knirsch, CA; Pablos-Mendez, A. Neighborhood poverty and the resurgence of tuberculosis in New York City 1984-1992. *Am J Public Health*, 2001, 91, 1487-93.

[2] World Health Organization. Addressing poverty in tuberculosis control. WHO/HTM/ TB/2005.352. *World Health Organization*, 2005, Geneva.

[3] van Lettow, M; Harries, AD; Kumwenda, JJ; et al. Micronutrient malnutrition and wasting in adults with pulmonary tuberculosis with and without HIV co-infection in Malawi. BMC *Infect. Dis,* 2004, 4, 61.

[4] Schwenk, A; Macallan, DC. Tuberculosis, malnutrition and wasting. *Curr Opin Clin Nutr Metab Care.*, 2000, 3, 285-91.

[5] Cegielski, JP; McMurray, DN. The relationship between malnutrition and tuberculosis: evidence from studies in humans and experimental animals. *Int J Tuberc Lung Dis*, Mar, 2004, 8, 286-298.

[6] Africa's Health in 2010 project / Academy for Educational Development. Nutrition and Tuberculosis: A review of the literature and considerations for TB control programs. *United States Agency for International Development*, 2008, Washington.

[7] Palmer, CE; Jablon, S; Edwards, PQ. Tuberculosis morbidity of young men in relation to tuberculin sensitivity and body build. *Am Rev Tuberc*, 1957, 76, 517-39.

[8] Tverdal, A. Body mass index and incidence of tuberculosis. *Eur J Respir Dis.*, 1986, 69, 355-62.

[9] Leung, CC; Lam, TH; Chan, WM; et al. Lower risk of tuberculosis in obesity. *Arch Intern Med*, 2007, 167, 1297-304.

[10] Fairchild, AL; Oppenheimer, GM. Public health nihilism vs pragmatism: history, politics, and the control of tuberculosis. *Am J Public Health*, 1998, 88, 1105-17.

[11] Dai, G; McMurray, DN. Altered cytokine production and impaired antimycobacterial immunity in protein malnourished guinea pigs. *Infect Immun.*, 1998, 66, 3562-3568.

[12] Mainali, ES; McMurray, DN. Adoptive transfer of resistance to pulmonary tuberculosis in guinea pigs is altered by protein deficiency. *Nutr Res.*, 1998, 118, 309-317.

[13] Perez-Guzman, C; Vargas, MH; Quinonez, F; Bazavilvazo, N; Aguilar, AA. cholesterol-rich diet accelerates bacteriologic sterilization in pulmonary tuberculosis. *Chest*, 2005, 127, 643-51.

[14] Rondinone, CM. Adipocyte-derived hormones, cytokines, and mediators. *Endocrine*, 2006, 29, 81-90.

[15] Chan, JL; Matarese, G; Shetty, GK; et al. Differential regulation of metabolic, neuroendocrine, and immune function by leptin in humans. *Proc Natl Acad Sci U S A*, 2006, 103, 8481-6.

[16] Farooqi, IS; Matarese, G; Lord, GM; et al. Beneficial effects of leptin on obesity, T cell hyporesponsiveness, and neuroendocrine/metabolic dysfunction of human congenital leptin deficiency. *J Clin Invest*, 2002, 110, 1093-103.

[17] Wieland, CW; Florquin, S; Chan, ED; et al. Pulmonary Mycobacterium tuberculosis infection in leptin-deficient ob/ob mice. *Int Immunol*, 2005, 17, 1399-408.

[18] Kim, SJ; Hong, YP; Lew, WJ; et al. Incidence of pulmonary tuberculosis among diabetics. *Tuber Lung Dis*, 1995, 76, 529-33.

[19] Coker, R; McKee, M; Atun, R; et al. Risk factors for pulmonary tuberculosis in Russia: case-control study. *BMJ*, 2006, 332, 85-7.

[20] Leung, CC; Lam, TH; Chan, WM; et al. Diabetic Control and Risk of Tuberculosis: A Cohort Study. *Am J Epidemiol*, 2008, 167, 1486-94.

[21] Olmos, P; Donoso, J; Rojas, N; et al. Tuberculosis and diabetes mellitus: a longitudinal-retrospective study in a teaching hospital. *Rev Med Chil*, 1989, 117, 979-83.

[22] Casey, JI; Heeter, BJ; Klyshevich, KA. Impaired response of lymphocytes of diabetic subjects to antigen of Staphylococcus aureus. *J Infect Dis*, 1977, 136, 495-501.

[23] Eibl, N; Spatz, M; Fischer, GF; et al. Impaired primary immune response in type-1 diabetes: results from a controlled vaccination study. *Clin Immunol*, 2002, 103, 249-259.

[24] Pozzilli, P, Pagani, S; Arduini, P; et al. In vivo determination of cell mediated immune response in diabetic patients using a multiple intradermal antigen dispenser. *Diabetes Res.*, 1987, 6, 5-8.

[25] Spatz, M; Eibl, N; Hink, S; et al. Impaired primary immune response in type-1 diabetes. Functional impairment at the level of APCs and T-cells. *Cell Immunol*, 2003, 221, 15-26.

[26] Antony, SJ; Harrell, V; Christie, JD; et al. Clinical differences between pulmonary and extrapulmonary tuberculosis: a 5-year retrospective study. *J Natl Med Assoc*, 1995, 87, 187-92.

[27] Perez-Guzman, C; Torres-Cruz, A; Villarreal-Velarde, H; et al. Atypical radiological images of pulmonary tuberculosis in 192 diabetic patients: a comparative study. *Int J Tuberc Lung Dis*, 2001, 5, 455-61.

[28] Shaikh, MA; Singla, R; Khan, NB; et al. Does diabetes alter the radiological presentation of pulmonary tuberculosis. *Saudi Med J*, 2003, 24, 278-81.

[29] van Lettow, M; Kumwenda, JJ; Harries, AD; et al. Malnutrition and the severity of lung disease in adults with pulmonary tuberculosis in Malawi. *Int J Tuberc Lung Dis*, 2004, 8, 211-7.

[30] Zachariah, R; Spielmann, MP; Harries, AD; Salaniponi, FM. Moderate to severe malnutrition in patients with tuberculosis is a risk factor associated with early death. *Tran R Soc Trop Med Hyg*, 2002, 96, 291-4.

[31] Harries, AD; Nkhoma, WA; Thompson, PJ; Nyangulu, DS; Wirima, JJ. Nutritional status in Malawian patients with pulmonary tuberculosis and response to chemotherapy. *Eur J Clin Nutr.*, 1988, 42, 445-50.

[32] Kim, DK; Kim, HJ; Kwon, SY; et al. Nutritional deficit as a negative prognostic factor in patients with miliary tuberculosis. *Eur Respir J*, 2008, 32, 1031-6.

[33] Benator, D; Bhattacharya, M; Bozeman, L; et al. Tuberculosis Trials Consortium. Rifapentine and isoniazid once a week versus rifampicin and isoniazid twice a week for treatment of drug-susceptible pulmonary tuberculosis in HIV-negative patients: a randomized clinical trial. *Lancet*, 2002, 360, 528-534.

[34] Khan, A; Sterling, TR; Reves, R; Vernon, A; Horsburgh, CR. Tuberculosis Trials Consortium. Lack of weight gain and relapse risk in a large tuberculosis treatment trial. *Am J Respir Crit Care Med*, 2006, 174, 344-8.

[35] Kennedy, N; Ramsay, A; Uiso, L; Gutmann, J; Ngowi, FI; Gillespie, SH. Nutritional status and weight gain in patients with pulmonary tuberculosis in Tanzania. *Trans R Soc Trop Med Hyg*, 1996, 90, 162-166.

[36] Yew, WW; Leung, CC. Prognostic significance of early weight gain in underweight patients with tuberculosis. *Am J Respir Crit Care Med*, 2006, 174, 236-7.

[37] Villamor, E; Mugusi, F; Urassa, W; et al. A Trial of the Effect of Micronutrient Supplementation on Treatment Outcome, T Cell Counts, Morbidity, and Mortality in Adults with Pulmonary Tuberculosis. *J Infect Dis*, 2008, 197, 1499-1505.

[38] Range, N; Changalucha, J; Krarup, H; Magnussen, P; Andersen, AB; Friis, H. The effect of multi-vitamin/mineral supplementation on mortality during treatment of pulmonary tuberculosis: a randomised two-by-two factorial trial in Mwanza, Tanzania. *Br J Nutr.*, 2006, 95, 762-70.

[39] Mitchison, DA. Assessment of new sterilizing drugs for treating pulmonary tuberculosis by culture at 2 months. *Am Rev Respir Dis*, 1993, 147, 1062-1063.

[40] Holtz, TH; Sternberg, M; Kammerer, S; et al. Time to sputum culture conversion in multidrug-resistant tuberculosis: predictors and relationship to treatment outcome. *Ann Intern Med*, 2006, 144, 650-9.

[41] Bilaceroglu, S; Perim, K; Buyuksirin, M; Celikten, E. Prednisolone: a beneficial and safe adjunct to anti-tuberculous treatment? A randomized controlled trial. *Int J Tuberc Lung Dis*, 1999, 3, 47-54.

In: Multiple Drug Resistance
Editors: A. Meszaros, G. Balogh, pp. 203-211
ISBN: 978-1-60741-595-4

Chapter IX

Reversal of Multidrug Resistance (MDR) by the Isoquinoline Alkaloid Glaucine

Yonggang Ma[1] and Michael Wink[2*]
[1]School of Pharmacy, Nankai University, Tianjin, China
[2]University of Heidelberg, Institute of Pharmacy and Molecular Biotechnology, INF 364, 69120 Heidelberg, Germany

Abstract

The most important mechanism for multidrug resistance (MDR) in tumor cells is that mediated by highly expressed ABC transporters, such as P-gp and BCRP. These transporters expel various lipophilic anti-cancer drugs, which can enter cells by free diffusion. In this study, 96-well plate based assays and flow cytometry analysis were employed to screen natural products for P-gp and BCRP inhibition. The isoquinoline alkaloid glaucine inhibits P-gp and BCRP activity. Glaucine (10 μM) can enhance the cytotoxicity of doxorubicin in P-gp expressing Caco-2 and CEM ADR5000 cells 2.5 and 5.4-fold, respectively. In a BCRP overexpressing breast cancer cell line (MDA-MB-231) the cytotoxicity of mitoxantrone was increased 2.5 fold at 1 μM and that of camptothecin 2.9-fold at 5 μM. Glaucine may be a candidate for the development of broad spectrum reversal agents.

Keywords: Glaucine, MDR, BCRP, P-gp, Reversal agent.

1. Introduction

P-glycoprotein (P-gp) and Breast Cancer Resistance Protein (BCRP) are important components of multidrug Resistance (MDR) observed in many tumour cells (You and Morris,

[*] Corresponding author: wink@uni-hd.de

2007). These transporters belong to ATP binding cassette (ABC) superfamily. Both of them export different kinds of cytotoxins and help cells to protect themselves against cytotoxicity (Twentyman and Bleehen, 1991; Steinbach et al., 2002).

P-gp has two ATP binding domains, which bind and hydrolyze ATP and two transmembrane domains, which recognize, bind, and transport substrates. P-gp utilizes the energy of binding and hydrolysis of ATP to change conformation and expel substrates. Although BCRP functions in a similar mode as P-gp, BCRP is a "half transporter", which has one ATP bind domain and one transmembrane domain. Usually BCRP forms dimeric protein complexes, which function as a full transporter (Ambudkar et al., 1999; Krishnamurthy and Schuetz, 2006).

During the course of chemotherapy, tumor cell may up-regulate the expression of one or more types of MDR transporters. BCRP and P-gp can be present simultaneously. Most chemotherapeutics used in cancer treatment are lipophilic and can enter cells by simple diffusion. The transporters can export the diffused anti-cancer drugs out of the cells (Gottesman, 2002). Thus they decrease the accumulation of cytotoxins, and protect tumor cells. P-gp exports anthracenes, anthracyclines, taxanes, Vinca alkaloids, many other alkaloids etc (Wink, 2007). The substrate spectrum of BCRP is similar; it exports anthracyclines, anthracenes, camptothecin, etc. The substrate range of them do not fully overlapped (Schinkel and Jonker, 2003; Krishnamurthy and Schuetz, 2006). If the activity of the drug transporters is inhibited, the resistance can be reversed and the outcome of chemotherapy might be improved. Developing broad-spectrum MDR reversal agents is an important task of pharmaceutical research.

When screening for MDR reversal agents among natural products (Ma and Wink, 2008a; Ma and Wink, 2008b), we discovered the isoquinoline alkaloid glaucine (Figure. 1); it shows high BCRP inhibition and moderate P-gp inhibition. Apparently, glaucine could be a good candidate to develop lead compound for new MDR reversal agents.

2. Materials and Methods

2.1. Chemicals

RPMI 1640 and DMEM medium were purchased from GIBCO. Fetal bovine serum was from Biochrom AG. Fumitremorgin C (FTC) was from Alexis. Glaucine, verapamil, doxorubicin, 3-(4,5-dimethylthiazole-2-yl)-2,5-diphenyl tetrazolium bromide (MTT), rhodamine 123, G418, mitoxantrone, and other chemicals were from Sigma Aldrich.

2.2. Cell Culture

The MDA-MB-231pcDNA3-BCRP-clone23 cell line was derived from breast cancer cell line MDA-MB-231. The parental cell line was transfected with BCRP cDNA to produce BCRP overexpressing subline, which was maintained in RPMI 1640 medium supplemented with 10% fetal bovine serum and 800 ng/mL G418 (Efferth et al., 2003). A human colon adenocarcinoma cell line, Caco-2 cells, was maintained in DMEM medium supplemented with 10% fetal bovine serum and 2mM glutamine and 1% non-essential amino acid. The leukemia cell line, CEM ADR5000, a P-gp overexpressing subline of CCRF-CEM, was maintained in RPMI 1640 medium supplemented with 10% fetal bovine serum and 5 μg/mL doxorubicin (Efferth et al., 2003). Caco-2 was kindly provided by Prof. Dr. G. Fricker (IPMB, University of Heidelberg, Heidelberg, Germany) and CEM ADR5000 and MDA-MB-231pcDNA3-BCRP-clone23 were kindly provided by Apl. Prof. Dr. T. Efferth (DKFZ, Heidelberg, Germany).

2.3. Mitoxantrone Efflux assay

About 1 × 10^4 BCRP expressing cells were seeded into 96-well plates per well and incubated at 37 °C with 5% CO_2 for 4 days. Glaucine was pipetted at different concentration into the wells 10 minutes after 10 μM of the chemotherapeutic mitoxantrone had been added. After 5 hours the plates were washed twice with ice-cold PBS. The plates were scanned with a Fluoroskan Ascent fluorescence reader (Labsystems) at excitation wavelength of 584 nm and emission wavelength of 670 nm. Fluorescence intensity of cells treated with 20 μM FTC (as a positive control for BCRP inhibition) was set 100% (Rabindran et al., 2000). Experiments were conducted in triplicates and repeated at least three times independently. The interference of quenching or auto fluorescence of the alkaloid had been excluded.

2.4. Flow Cytometry Analysis

Tubes containing 2.5 × 10^5 CEM ADR5000 cells each were placed on ice, incubated with 10 μg/mL rhodamine 123 for 120 minutes. Cells were washed and incubated with 20 μM glaucine at 37 °C and 5% CO_2 for 120 minutes. Cells were centrifuged and washed with ice-cold medium. Cells were then re-suspended in ice-cold medium. Samples were analysed by FACSCalibur flow cytometry (Becton-Dickinson).

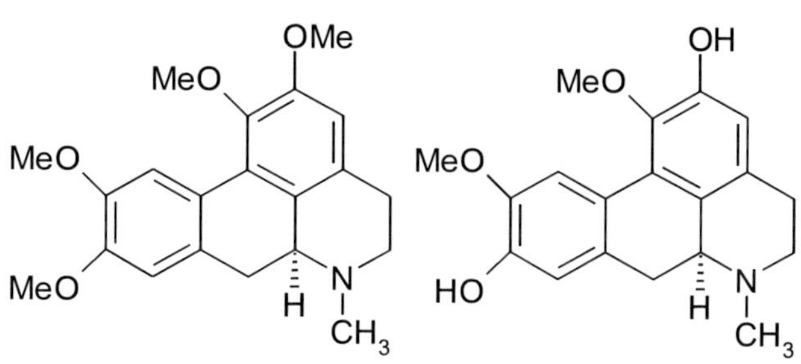

Figure 1. Structures of glaucine and boldine.

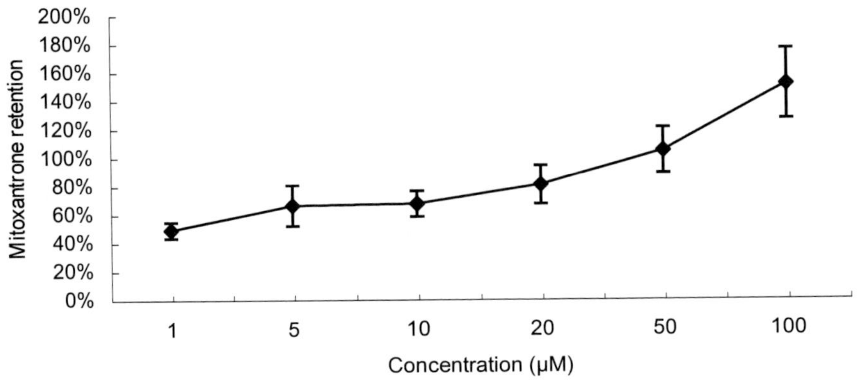

Figure 2. Effects of glaucine on mitoxantrone retention in the cells as measured by an in crease of fluorescence intensity. Values are expressed as mean±SD.

2.5. Rhodamine 123 Efflux Assay

This assay was performed as described before with some modifications (Schwab et al., 2003). 2×10^4 Caco-2 cells per well were seeded into 96-well plates; plates were incubated at 37 °C and 5% CO_2 for 6 days. Glaucine was applied at different concentrations into wells 20 minutes after 1 μg/mL rhodamine 123 had been added. After incubation for 4 hours the plates are washed twice with ice cold PBS. The plates were scanned with a Fluoroskan Ascent fluorescent reader (Labsystems) at excitation wavelength of 485 nm and emission wavelength of 538 nm. Fluorescence intensity of cells treated with 20 μM verapamil (as a positive control for P-gp inhibition) was set 100% (Salmon et al., 1991). Experiments were conducted in triplicates and repeated at least three times independently. The interference of quenching or auto fluorescence of the alkaloid had been excluded.

2.6. Cytotoxicity Assay

About 1.5×10^4 (Caco-2), 2×10^4 (CEM ADR5000) or 1×10^4 (MDA-MB-231pcDNA3-BCRP-clone23) cells per well were seeded into 96-well plates. Different concentration of cytotoxic agents and 10 μM glaucine or different concentration of glaucine were added into three triplicate wells, cells were incubated for 24 hours at 37 °C and 5% CO_2. Then cells were incubated for another 48 hours. MTT at a final concentration of 0.5 μg/mL were added and incubated for 4 hours. The medium was discarded and replaced by formazon crystal dissolved in 100 μl DMSO. The plates were shaken 15 minutes before they were read at 570 nm with a spectrophotometric plate reader (Bio-Rad).

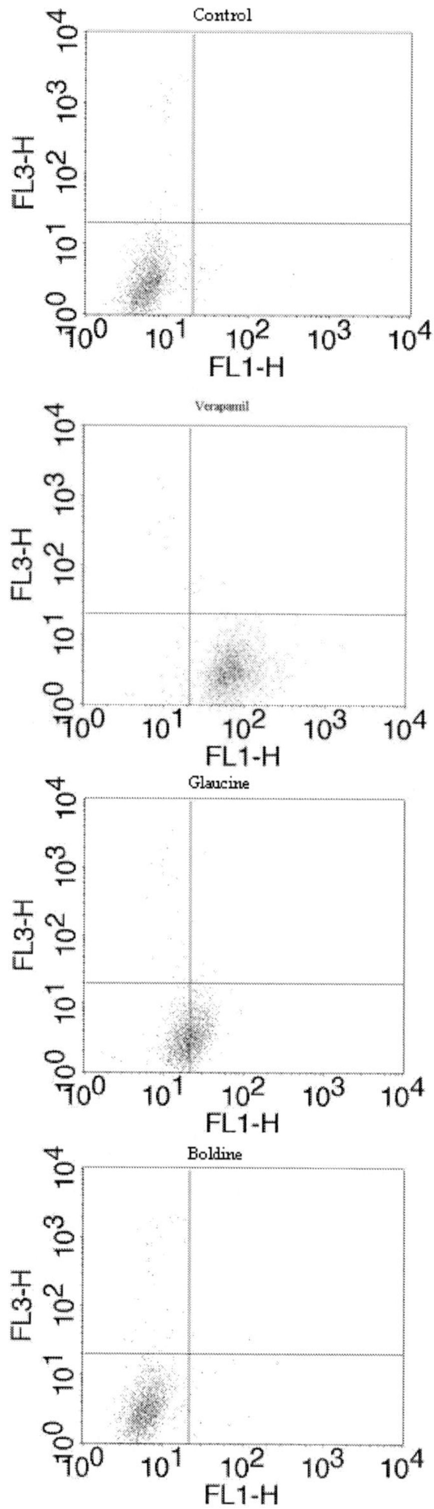

Figure 3. Flow cytometric analysis of CEM ADR5000 cells treated with 20 μM glaucine, 20 μM verapamil and 20 μM boldine. Dot plots of control and treated cells that were stained with rhodamine 123.

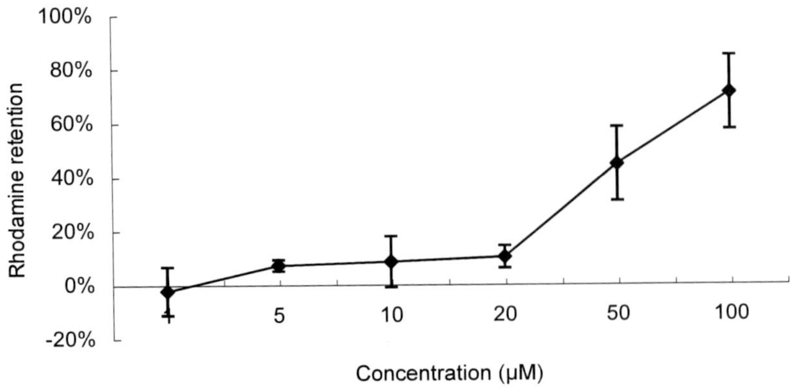

Figure 4. Effects of glaucine on P-gp expressing Caco-2 cells determined from rhodamine 123 retention. Values are expressed as mean ± SD.

2.7. Data Analysis

All experiments were repeated at least three times. Data are presented as mean ± SD. The significance of differences of means was tested using unpaired two-tailed t-test P values < 0.05 were considered significant. Inhibition efficacy was defined as (fluorescence intensity of glaucine treated cells minus fluorescence of untreated control)/(fluorescence intensity of FTC or verapamil treated minus fluorescence of untreated control). IC_{50} was defined as the concentration of drugs required to inhibit cells by 50% as compared to controls. IC_{50} was calculated with GraphPad Prism 4.

3. Results

3.1. Mitoxantrone Efflux Assay in MDA-MB-231pcDNA3-BCRP-Clone23

Mitoxantrone is a fluorescent substrate of BCRP. It was used as the indicator of BCRP activity in BCRP over-expressing cells. If BCRP was inhibited, mitoxantrone would accumulate in the cells and the fluorescence intensity would increase. This system was used to determine the inhibitory activity of glaucine. Significant differences of fluorescence intensity between treated and control groups were obtained with glaucine concentrations higher than 1 μM (Figure. 2). Thus, glaucine apparently inhibits BCRP quite effectively.

3.2. Flow Cytometry Analysis in CEM ADR5000

Activity of P-gp over-expressing cell line, CEM ADR5000, was determined using the rhodamine 123 efflux assay. Rhodamine 123 would accumulate in cells if P-gp was inhibited. Upon inhibition FACS signals of these cells shift to lower right region of the dot plots.

Otherwise signals stayed at lower left region. Figure 3 shows that 20 μM glaucine can significantly inhibit rhodamine 123 efflux.

3.3. Rhodamine 123 Efflux Assay in Caco-2 Cells

Inhibitory activity of glaucine was measured by Caco-2 cells, which express P-gp. Rhodamine 123, a fluorescent substrate of P-gp, would accumulate in cells upon P-gp inhibition and increase fluorescent intensity. Significant differences of fluorescence intensity between treated and control groups were obtained with glaucine concentrations higher than 20 μM (Figure. 4).

3.4. Cytotoxicity Assay

Cytotoxicity of glaucine in Caco-2 was IC50 120.5±19.32 μM, in CEM ADR5000 IC50 91.05±17.07 μM to and MDA-MB-231pcDNA3-BCRP-clone23 cells IC50 132.8 ± 27.49 μM. Cell lines expressing P-gp or BCRP are resistant or less sensitive to cytotoxic agents. In case of co-treatment with an effective P-gp or BCRP substrate, we should expect an enhanced cytotoxicity of the chemotherapeutic agent; i.e. resistance is reversed. Co-treatment of the cells with non-toxic concentrations of glaucine (1 and 10 μM) substantially increased the cytotoxicity of the chemotherapeutic drug: Glaucine (10 μM) can enhance the cytotoxicity of doxorubicin in P-gp expressing Caco-2 and CEM ADR5000 cells 2.5 and 5.4-fold, respectively. In a BCRP overexpressing breast cancer cell line (MDA-MB-231) the cytotoxicity of mitoxantrone was increased 2.5 fold at 1 μM and that of camptothecin 2.9-fold at 5 μM. Thus glaucine can re-sensitize multidrug resistant cells (Table 1 and Table 2).

Table 1. IC50 of doxorubicin in P-gp expressing cells (Caco-2 and CEM ADR5000) in the presence or absence of 10 μM glaucine. Values are expressed as mean±SD.

	IC50 in Caco-2 (μg)	IC50 in CEM ADR5000 (μg)
Doxorubicin	1.11 ± 0.21	51.57 ± 5.36
Doxorubicin + 10 μM glaucine	0.44 ± 0.01	9.53 ± 0.57

Table 2. IC50 values of mitoxantrone and camptothecin in BCRP over-expresing cells(MDA-MB-231pcDNA3-BCRP-clone23 cell) in the presence or absence of glaucine. Values are expressed as mean±SD.

	IC50 (μM)
Mitoxantrone	6.71 ± 0.76
Mitoxantrone + 1 μM glaucine	2.71 ± 0.36
Camptothecin	2.95 ± 0.36
Camptothecin + 5 μM glaucine	1.00 ± 0.22

4. Discussion

BCRP and P-gp are highly expressed at the apical membrane of blood-brain barrier, placenta, liver, and intestine, etc (Schinkel and Jonker, 2003). They can translocate xenobiotics or metabolites to lumen and thus play a protective role in these organs by limiting access of drugs to the vital organs and fetus. Tumor cells often develop MDR to different classes of anti-cancer drugs by over-expressing BCRP and P-gp. They can effectively pump out Vinca alkaloids, anthracyclines, mitoxantrone, camptothecin and other lipophilic drugs, that have entered cells by free diffusion (You and Morris, 2007). In order to achieve a successful chemotherapy, a strategy could be to inhibit the transporters and thus reverse MDR.

In this study it was shown, that the aporphine alkaloid glaucine can inhibit both BCRP and P-gp mediated drug efflux at concentrations that showed no cytotoxicity. Its toxicity (LD50) in mice was about 4.8 mg/kg body weight (equivalent to 13 μM) (Harborne and Baxter, 1993). Glaucine belongs to the class of aporphine alkaloids, a subclass of the isoquinoline alkaloids. It has been isolated from several members of the Papaveraceae (including Fumariaceae) and Lauraceae. Glaucine is biologically active, it inhibits respiration, lowers blood pressure and blood glucose levels in animals (Harborne and Baxter, 1993).

Glaucine increases the concentration of anti-cancer drugs, such as doxorubicin, mitoxantrone, or camptothecin, in cells and thus enhances their cytotoxicity. Although BCRP and P-gp differ in their substrate specificities, glaucine apparently inhibits both. That suggested that BCRP and P-gp share some common features of drug binding, but that the affinity is different. Boldine, a related aporphine alkaloid (Figure. 1), does not inhibit P-gp at 20 μM in Caco-2 cells (data not shown) and CEM ADR5000 (Figure. 4), but it inhibits BCRP at 20 μM (data not shown), though its efficiency is much lower than glaucine. Glaucine has two extra methoxy groups, which makes the alkaloid more lipophilic and provides more hydrophobic interactions between glaucine and the binding site in the transporter.

Because glaucine inhibits both BCRP and P-gp, it is likely a promising lead compound for the development of a broad-spectrum MDR reversal agent. This property is rare (Wink, 2007): We have recently shown, that the beta-carboline alkaloid harmaline is a specific inhibitor of BCRP (Ma and Wink, 2008b) whereas the piperidine alkaloid lobeline is active as a P-gp reversal agent (Ma and Wink, 2008a).

Acknowledgments

This work was supported by the National Natural Science Foundation of China (Grant No. 30950014), Tianjin Natural Science Foundation (Grant No. 08JCYBJC25900), and the Foundation Landesstiftung Baden-Wuerttemberg.

References

Ambudkar, S. V., Dey, S., Hrycyna, C. A., Ramachandra, M., Pastan, I. & Gottesman, M. M. (1999). Biochemical, cellular, and pharmacological aspects of the multidrug transporter. *Annu Rev Pharmacol Toxicol*, *39*, 361-398.

Efferth, T., Sauerbrey, A., Halatsch, M. E., Ross, D. D. & Gebhart, E. (2003). Molecular modes of action of cephalotaxine and homoharringtonine from the coniferous tree Cephalotaxus hainanensis in human tumor cell lines. *Naunyn Schmiedebergs Arch Pharmacol*, *367*, 56-67.

Gottesman, M. M. (2002). Mechanisms of cancer drug resistance. *Annu Rev Med, 53*, 615-627.

Harborne, J. B. & Baxter, H. (1993). Phytochemical dictionary. Raylor and Francis, London.

Krishnamurthy P and Schuetz JD (2006) Role of ABCG2/BCRP in biology and medicine. *Annu Rev Pharmacol Toxicol*, *46*, 381-410.

Ma, Y. & Wink, M. (2008). Lobeline, a piperidine alkaloid from Lobelia can reverse P-gp dependent multidrug resistance in tumor cells. *Phytomedicine, 15,* 754-758.

Ma, Y. & Wink, M. (2008). The beta-carboline alkaloid Harmine inhibits BCRP and can reverse resistance to the anticancer drugs mitoxanthrone and camptothecin. *Phytother Res* (Epub ahead of print).

Rabindran, S. K., Ross, D. D., Doyle, L. A., Yang, W. & Greenberger, L. M. (2000). Fumitremorgin C reverses multidrug resistance in cells transfected with the breast cancer resistance protein. *Cancer Res.*, *60*, 47-50.

Salmon, S. E., Dalton, W. S., Grogan, T. M., Plezia, P., Lehnert, M., Roe, D. J. & Miller, T. P. (1991). Multidrug-resistant myeloma: laboratory and clinical effects of verapamil as a chemosensitizer. *Blood*, *78*, 44-50.

Schinkel, A. H. & Jonker, J. W. (2003). Mammalian drug efflux transporters of the ATP binding cassette (ABC) family: an overview. *Adv Drug Deliv Rev.*, *55*, 3-29.

Schwab, D., Fischer, H., Tabatabaei, A., Poli, S. & Huwyler, J. (2003). Comparison of in vitro P-glycoprotein screening assays: recommendations for their use in drug discovery. *J Med Chem.*, *46*, 1716-1725.

Steinbach, D., Sell, W., Voigt, A., Hermann, J., Zintl, F. & Sauerbrey, A. (2002). BCRP gene expression is associated with a poor response to remission induction therapy in childhood acute myeloid leukemia. *Leukemia*, *16*, 1443-1447.

Twentyman, P. R. & Bleehen, N. M. (1991). Resistance modification by PSC-833, a novel non-immunosuppressive cyclosporin. *Eur J Cancer*, *27*, 1639-1642.

Wink, M. (2007). Molecular modes of action of cytotoxic alkaloids- From DNA intercalation, spindle poisoning, topoisomerase inhibition to apoptosis and multiple drug resistance. In "The Alkaloids, (G. Cordell, ed.), *Elsevier*, Vol. *64*, 1-48.

You, G. & Morris, M. E. (2007). Drug transporters- Molecular characterization and role in drug disposition. Wiley-Interscience, Hoboken, New Jersey.

In: Multiple Drug Resistance
Editors: A. Meszaros, G. Balogh, pp. 213-217

ISBN: 978-1-60741-595-4

Chapter X

Uncommon *Acinetobacter Baumannii* Isolation from Leukemic Patients and Emerging of Tigecycline-Resistance

Vincenzo Savini[1], Chiara Catavitello[1], Marzia Talia[1], Andrea Balbinot[1], Fabio Febbo[1], Assunta Manna[1], Arianna Pompilio[2], Giovanni Di Bonaventura[2], Raffaeele Piccolomini[2] and Domenico D'Antonio[1]*

[1]Department of Transfusion Medicine, 'Spirito Santo' Hospital, Pescara, Italy.
[2]Department of Biomedical Sciences, 'Gabriele d'Annunzio' University School of Medicine of Chieti-Pescara, Italy.

Abstract

Acinetobacter baumannii is associated with nosocomial outbreaks worldwide. Particularly, it has been known to be responsible for significant morbidity and mortality among immunosuppressed patients, mostly those admitted to intensive care units (ICU). We isolated only three *A. baumannii* strains over a 2-year period from leukemic patients. Two of them were found to be commensal of the upper airways, wheras the third one was collected from stool, and played an uncertain role as the cause of an enteritis episode. All of strains were found to be multidrug-resistant. Surprisingly, they also exerted tigecycline-resistance. Authors emphasize the role of multidrug-resistant *A. baumannii* as an emerging bacterium in haematologic hosts. Also, the first enteric isolation of this species is reported, althoug its role as the cause of the patient's diarrhoea remained controversial.

* Coresponding author: Phone number: 320-6265740, E-mail: vincsavi@yahoo.it.

Three *A. baumannii* strains were collected from leukemic patients in May 2008, whereas no organisms of this species had been isolated during the previous 2 years. Strains were named an *ab138*, *ab139*, and *ab140*, according to the storage position assigned. *Ab 138* and *139* were isolated as part of mixed flora from sputum of patients without signs or symptoms of respiratory disease, whereas *ab143* was collected from a stool sample of an enteritis patient with a heavy pure growth (> 200 c.f.u. per plate). No other organisms (bacteria, fungi) of known enteric pathogenicity were detected. Also, *Clostridium difficile* was not cultured, and *C. difficile* A/B toxins were not revealed by the immunoenzimatic test performed (*Clostridium difficile* Panel, Biosite). Further, *Giardia lamblia*, *Cryptosporidium parvum* and *Entamoeba histolytica* antigens were not revealed by the Biosite immunoenzimatic test we carried out (Parasite Panel, Biosite). So, the enteric isolate was considered as the probable cause of the patient's diarrhoea, whereas the ones from sputum appeared as colonizing organisms.

Strain identifications were obtained by using Vitek 2 System (bioMérieux), and confirmed by performing an rRna sequencing. Instead, MICs were provided by the same bioMérieux instrument, except for tigecycline, whose *in vitro* activity was evaluated by an E-test method (tigecycline commercial strips provided by AB BIODISK), according to instructions contained in the product package. All of the three strains study appeared to be multidrug-resistant (MDR). Particularly, they all showed resistance or reduced susceptibility to ampicillin, amoxicillin/clavulanate, piperacillin/tazobactam, cefoxitin, cefepime, ceftazidime, aztreonam, ciprofloxacin, levofloxacin, tetracycline, tobramycin, cotrimoxazole. Further, at least one of the isolates tested exerted resistance or reduced sensitivity to imipenem, meropenem, amikacin and gentamicin, whereas all of them were found to be ampicillin/sulbactam- and colistin-susceptible. Surprisingly, tigecycline-resistance was documented in all of the three cases. MIC values are reported in table 1.

Over the past years, treatment of *A. baumannii* has been limited to ceftazidime, carbapenems, fluoroquinolones, cotrimoxazole, amikacin, tetracycline. Unfortunately, this bacterium commonly expresses several mechanisms of resistance, which are usually able to reduce susceptibility to several or all classes of antimicrobial compounds. Class A extended-spectrum betalactamases (ESBLs) have been recently found in this species (PER-1, VEB-1, SHV-12, TEM 116, CTX-M-2), and make producing strains resistant to all betalactams except for cephamycins, ampicillin/sulbactam, amoxicillin/clavulanate, piperacillin/ tazobactam, and carbapenems. Unfortunaltely, *A. baumannii* ESBL detection has not been standardized, yet, and is complicated by the expression of chromosome-encoded cephalosporinases, so that it is unclear to what extent ESBLs are distributed in this species. Class B metallo-enzymes (IMP and VIM carbapenemases) are able to hydrolyze all betalactams (including carbapenems), except for aztreonam, whereas chromosomally encoded class C beta-lactamases commonly confer resistance to narrow- and extended-spectrum cephalosporins, but not imipenem and meropenem. On the basis of recent phylogenic analysis, these AmpC enzymes appear as more closely related to each other than to AmpC cephalosporinases expressed by other Gram negative species, so that they have been proposed to form a distinct family of beta-lactamases, named ADCs (*Acinetobacter-*derived cephalosporinases). A further group of enzymes are represented by *A.baumannii* naturally occurring class D OXA-type penicillinases, which are robust chromosome- or plasmid-mediated oxacillinases able to confer resistance to all betalactams, including monobactam and carbapenems. Reduced membrane permeability due to loss of OMPs (outer membrane porins) has also been known to contribute to *A. baumannii* drug resistance, although porin changes are difficult to be studied and compared, at present. Also, reduced expression of PBP (penicillin-binding proteins)-2 may be responsible for resistance to betalactams, including carbapenems. Multidrug resistance can be due to contemporary beta-lactamases production and loss of OMPs, to cotransferring of MDR-related genes on ESBL plasmids, and to biofilm formation. Also, efflux pumps represent a unique phenomenon, as a single mechanism is cause for resistance to several class of antimicrobials. These pumps mediate the efflux of toxic molecules, including drugs. The *A. baumannii* AdeABC pump confers resistance to aminoglycosides, cefotaxime, tetracyclines, erythromycin, chloramphenicol, trimetoprim, and fluoroquinolones, whereas the recently described AbeM is able to only pump fluoroquinolones, among drugs. [2-4].

Resistance or reduced sensitivity to carbapenems is emerging all over the world and represents a great clinical concern, given that these compunds commonly play a role as first choice therapy, and represented a viable option for treatment of *A. baumannii* infections until 2000 in Italy, particularly.[3]

Table 1. MICs (S, susceptible - I, intermediate - R, resistant)

	A. baumannii 138	A. baumannii 139	A. baumannii 143
Antimicrobial	MIC (mg/liter)	MIC (mg/liter)	MIC (mg/liter)
Ampicillin	≥32 (R)	≥32 (R)	≥32 (R)
Ampicillin/sulbactam	8 (S)	4 (S)	≥32 (R)
Amoxicillin/clavulanic acid	≥32 (R)	≥32 (R)	≥32 (R)
Piperacillin/tazobactam	≥128 (R)	≥128 (R)	≥128 (R)
Aztreonam	≥64 (R)	≥64 (R)	≥64 (R)
Cefoxitin	≥64 (R)	≥64 (R)	≥64 (R)
Ceftazidime	≥64 (R)	≥64 (R)	≥64 (R)
Cefepime	≥64 (R)	≥64 (R)	≥64 (R)
Imipenem	≤1 (S)	≥16 (R)	≥16 (R)
Meropenem	1 (S)	8 (I)	≥16 (R)
Ciprofloxacin	≥4 (R)	≥4 (R)	≥4 (R)
Levofloxacin	≥8 (R)	≥8 (R)	≥8 (R)
Gentamicin	4 (S)	4 (S)	≥16 (R)
Amikacin	32 (I)	4 (S)	4 (S)
Tobramycin	8(I)	8(I)	≥16 (R)
Cotrimoxazole	≥320 (R)	≥320 (R)	≥320 (R)
Tetracycline	≥16 (R)	≥16 (R)	≥16 (R)
Tigecycline	8 (R)	12 (R)	6 (R)
Colistin	≤0.5 (S)	≤0.5 (S)	≤0.5 (S)

The *Tigecyline Evaluation and Surveillance Trial (T.E.S.T.)* program reported a 1 mg/L MIC for most of the strains studied, and further European studies documented the activity of this bacteriostatic antimicrobial against MDR *A. baumannii* strains, with a MIC of 2 mg/L. Also, tigecycline has been approved for treatment of complicated skin and intra-abdominal infections, whereas the commonly shown activity against *A. baumannii* and the high concentration reached in lung tissue have indicated its use for respiratory tract infections by MDR organisms of this species, too. Further, this compound activity does not seem to be affected by other mechanisms of resistance (such as to carbapenems). Unfortunately, MICs we found do not agree with the mentioned data and this is surely a cause for concern, as tigecyline-resistance (which is thought to be due to a multidrug efflux pump) by *A. baumannii* has been rarely reported, so far.[3] This drug will surely gain importance in the future years, and makes it mandatory to monitor *A. baumannii* isolates in order to assist physicians in deciding on its use, and to further investigate the possible mechanisms underlying resistance and eventual diffusion of the latter by plasmid DNA.[7] Should multidrug-resistance be expressed by *A. baumanni* isolates, colistin may represent the last line of defense.[8] In any case, polymyxin resistant strains have been recently reported, such as colistin dose-dependent nephrotoxicity,[3] but correct intavenous administration of the drug may make it safe of remarkable side-effects.[6,9,10].

Though *A. baumannii* commonly affects all sorts of immunosuppressed hosts, most data in the literature regard ICU patients, except for the findings of Chang et al. [11] who showed as hematological or oncological diseases were the main underlying illnesses in a 52 pediatric patients population harbouring MDR *A. baumannii.* Our findings emphasize the role of this bacterium as a an emerging colonizing and pathogenic organism in haematologic hosts; further, we documented tigecycline-resistance in all of the three cases, and this is also cause for clinical concern. Though it is often difficult to distinguish *A. baumannii* infection from simple colonization, both conditions are believed to behave as indicator of serious illness, with an associated mortality of about 30%.[4] Also, though two of the isolates sudied seemed to simply colonize the upper airways, all of the three strains showed multidrug-resistance, probably to due prior exposure to ceftazidime, piperacillin/tazobactam, fluoroquinolones, and carbapenems.[1] Tigecycline was not administered to none of the three patients, so that we could think of a probable co-transfer of resistance between tigecycline, on the one hand, and other classes of antimicrobials, on the other ones, but this is only speculative, for the moment. Also, *A. baumanni* enteric colonization has been never cited so far. Only isolation from gastric juice has been already reported, [11] so that our finding appears as the first isolation of this commonly respiratory organisms from gut, althoug its role as the causative agent of the mentioned diarrhoea remained unclear.

Funding

The Authors state that no funding of any sort has been received for this work.

Acknowledgments

The Authors thank Mrs Annarita Perfetti for her aid.

Transparency Declarations

None to declare.

References

[1] Mai, MH; Tsai, HC; Lee, SSJ; et al. Multidrug-resistant Acinetobacter baumannii in ventilator associated pneumonia at a medical center in southern Taiwan. *J Microbiol Immunol Infect*, 2007, 40, 401-405.

[2] Robert, E; Siegel, MD. Emerging Gram-negative antibiotic resistance: daunting challenges, declining sensitivities, and dire consequences. *Respiratory Care*, 2008, 53(4), 471-479.

[3] Mezzatesta, ML; Trovato, G; Gona, F; et al. *In vitro* activity of tigecycline and comparators against carbapenem-susceptible and resistant *Acinetobacter baumannii* clinical isolates in Italy. *Ann Clin Microb Antimicrob*, 2008, **7**, 4.

[4] Perez, F; Hujer, AM; Hujer, KM; Decker, BK; Rather, PN; Bonomo, RA. Global challenge of multidrug-resistant *Acinetobacter baumannii*. *Antimicrob Agents Chemother*, 2007, 51(10), 3471-3484.

[5] Hu, WS; Yao, SH; Fung, CP; Hsieh, YP; Liu, CP; Lin, JF. An OXA-66/OXA-51-like carbapenemase and possibly an efflux pump are associated with resistance to imipenem in *Acinetobacter baumannii*. *Antimicrob Agents Chemother*, 2007, 51(11), 3844-3852.

[6] Ho, YH; Wang, LS; Chao, HJ; Chang, KC; Su, CF. Successful treatment of meningitis caused by multidrug-resistant *Acinetobacter baumannii* with intravenous and intrathecal colistin. *J Microbiol Immunol Infect*, 2007, 40, 537-540.

[7] Schafer, JJ; Mangino, JE. Multidrug-resistant *Acinetobacter baumannii* osteomyelitis from *Iraq*. *Em Inf Dis*, 2008, 14(3) , 512-514.

[8] Kroeger, LA; Laurie, BH; Mitropoulos, IF, Schafer, J; Rotschafer, JC. Colistin methanesulfonate against multidrug-resistant Acinetobacter baumannii in an in vitro pharmacodynamic model. *Antimicrobial Agents Chemother*, 2007, 51(9), 3431-3433.

[9] Bassetti, M; Repetto, E; Righi, E; et al. Colistin and rifampicin in the treatment of multidrug-resistant Acinetobacter baumannii infections. *J Antimicrob Chemother*, 2008, 61(2), 417-420.

[10] Pankuch, GA; Lin, G; Seifert, H; Appelbaum, PC. Activity of meropenem with and without ciprofloxacin and colistin against Pseudomonas aeruginosa and Acinetobacter *baumannii*. *Antimicrob Agents Chemother*, 2008, 52(1), 333-336.

[11] Chang, PY; Hsueh, PR; Wu, PS; et al. Multidrug-resistant Acinetobacter baumannii isolates in pediatric patients of a university hospital in Taiwan. *J Microbiol Immunol Infect*, 2007, 40, 406-410.

In: Multiple Drug Resistance
Editors: A. Meszaros, G. Balogh, pp. 219-223

ISBN: 978-1-60741-595-4

Chapter XI

Finding the Genetic Solution for Cancer in the Mechanism of Taxol Cytotoxicity

Frank Un[1*]

[1]Dept. of Clinical & Molecular Pharmacology City of Hope National Medical Center
1500 E. Duarte Rd. Duarte, Calif. 91010, USA.

Abstract

For almost five decades, chemotherapy has played a vital role in managing cancer. With the combination of targeted therapies such as *Cetuximab* targeting EGF receptor, chemotherapy has seen even greater efficacy in clinics. Yet, the advances have been limited to prolonging the survival rather than decreasing mortality. This is largely due to the problem of drug resistance that remains unresolved. Even with the introduction of targeted therapeutics, the inherent ability of the cancer cells to mount resistance through genetic alterations eventually depreciates the therapy. It explains the nearly unchanged percentage of mortality for those with metastatic cancers amongst others. Multi-drug resistance (MDR) phenomenon is associated with the expression of ABC (ATP-binding cassette) transporters, which includes p-glycoprotein, MRP2, ABCG2, and possibly MRP3. By limiting to MDR, i.e. the drug import step, these traditional approaches have largely avoided addressing the drug induced lytic mechanism directly. This is, in part, due to our lack of knowledge concerning the molecular mechanism through which these drugs kill human cancer cells. By limiting to MDR, physicians remain incapable of countering drug resistance occurring as a result of cancer cell's interference with the steps lying further downstream in the lytic path. Instead, we need to develop counter-strategies based on the lytic path. In this commentary, the discovery of 'hyperploid progression-mediated death (HPMD)', a tumor specific lytic path targeting cancers mutated in tumor suppressor genes like RB or p53, is described. HPMD was discovered serendipitously while investigating the mechanism through which Taxol (widely used to treat breast cancer) induces aneuploidy in human cancer cells [*Carcinogenesis* 20, 1161-8 (99)]. The

* Corresponding author: Tel. 626-256-4673; Fax. 626-471-7204, E-mail address: fhong@coh.org

discovery of the lytic path provides a mechanistic basis for understanding how resistance to chemotherapy arise, thus providing a framework to develop counter strategies in a methodical way.

Introduction

Recently, much has been asked about why we cannot cure cancer. The question is a valid one as approximately half a million are expected to die from cancer this year in the U. S. alone despite having spent several hundreds of billions of dollars on research. Back in 1994, sitting across the Pacific Ocean watching the sunset as a post-doctoral fellow at the world renown Salk Institute, F. Hong began to feel that continued research into the biology of RB (retinoblastoma) tumor suppressor gene, one that he helped to clone and characterize during late 1980s through early 1990s at the University of California at San Diego [1-9], may not yield a cure for cancer. Thus, he decided to enter the clinical ward to first learn from physicians why we still cannot cure cancer. To his dismay, he found that there was no real "science" or "field" of cytotoxic cancer therapy. Yet, a glimmer of hope lay in the few patients who survived cancer through chemotherapy though the underlying mechanism was unknown. In other words, the clue to curing cancer lay in deciphering how chemotherapeutics destroyed cancer in these patients.

So, he began the study of Taxol (Paclitaxel). Taxol is considered the top drug for treating a variety of human cancers at the top-ranked University of Texas M. D. Anderson Cancer Center, where he worked as faculty during late 1990s through early 2000s. Specifically, the process through which Taxol induces the genetic abnormality known as aneuploidy in human brain cancer cells was investigated. Aneuploidy refers to abnormality in chromosomes that contain the genetic material of our cells. During the course, the mechanism through which Taxol kills human astrocytoma (a form of brain cancer) cells was discovered by serendipity [10]. It reminded of how Saul Roseman used to explain of his discovery of phosphate transferase system (PTS) at the Johns Hopkins University where he stayed as a graduate student briefly during 1980s. The discovery, which was reported in 1999, came unexpectedly while examining the effect of blocking an intermediated step in the path to aneuploidy induced by antimitotic drugs. Previously it was suggested that continued cell cycling without cytokinesis is necessary to induce aneuploidy. This was inferred from the data obtained using the cell cycle inhibitor $p27^{kip1}$. In mammalian cells, transit through the restriction point from G1 to S phase requires the activation of CDKs (cyclin dependent kinases). CDKs are kinases that require complexing with appropriate cyclins for functional activation. $p27^{kip1}$ is a member of a family of kinase inhibitors with specificity toward cyclin D-CDK4/6 and cyclin E-CDK2 complexes that govern the progression through early and late G1 phase, respectively.

To confirm the above, hydroxyurea was used instead to inhibit cell cycling after first incubating human astrocytoma cells with antimicrotubule drugs. Hydroxyurea is an inhibitor of ribonucleotide reductase that functions by quenching the free radicals necessary for the catalysis. Ribonucleotide reductase is the sole enzyme in human cells that converts ribonucleotides into the deoxy form necessary for DNA synthesis during the S phase. By surprise, it led to a near complete cessation of cell death despite the prolonged incubation. The effect was very pronounced with nocodazole. With Taxol, the study was more complicated as it was known to trigger multiple lytic paths within human cells. At doses higher than that required to interfere with microtubule assembly, it kills cells indiscriminately, i.e. both tumor and normal cells. It is also capable of killing cells at doses lower than that required to disrupt microtubules, which also occurs nonspecifically. Nevertheless, by blocking the cell cycling necessary for aneuploidy induction, greater than half the extent of cell death due to Taxol was blocked. The block in lethality could last as long as 4 days, which was quite a feat to achieve (given that several other independent lytic paths were triggered by Taxol in these cancer cells simultaneously).

The lytic process triggered turned out to be more complicated than previously envisioned. First, the triggering of the lytic process—termed '*hyperploid progression mediated death* (HPMD)'—requires inactivation of tumor suppressor gene RB or p53. In mammalian cells, RB or p53 plays a critical role as part of the checkpoint that oversees the progression from G1 to S. Checkpoints are built-in mechanisms that delays cell cycle progression in the event of a DNA damage to allow time for its repair. We now know that both of these genes also play a role in S/M checkpoint, which inhibits progression into S phase in the event mitosis is not properly completed. Disrupting RB or p53 function through mutation leads to the loss of S/M checkpoint, resulting in the continued cell cycle progression without cytokinesis resulting in cell death. Hence, the HPMD lytic path discovered is tumor-specific at the genetic level.

Second, the cellular consequence of triggering the HPMD lytic path is drastic and probably represents the one-and-only solution for cancer. Further researches in the ensuing periods revealed that it causes 'mitotic catastrophe' with the disintegration of the cancer cells' genetic material. As no cells can survive without the genetic material, it represents "the genetic solution" for the cancer problem. Thus, a tumor specific lytic path (TSLP) exploiting defective S/M checkpoint caused by inactive RB or p53 (the *Achilles* heel for cancer) was elucidated and the science of cytotoxic therapy based on cancer genetics was established. With additional tumor suppressor genes (potentially $p16^{INK4a}$, ATM, $p19^{ARF}$) participating in this checkpoint, the list of human cancers that could be treated with the HPMD-based therapy is likely to grow. This is echoed by the fact that nearly all human cancers are inactivated in the "RB pathway" which governs the above checkpoint.

Finally, a case in point concerns breast cancer. As recognized by many, the genetic mutations that have been identified to date that give rise to the familial form of breast cancer account for only a minor subset of all breast cancers. BRCA-1 and BRCA-2 tumor suppressor genes represent the key genetic determinants for the onset of inherited breast cancers. It follows that BRCA-1 and BRCA-2 as genetic target for developing therapeutics may have a limited application—i.e. as most breast cancer patients do not carry the mutation. Against this backdrop, the frequent occurrence of RB or p53 mutation amongst human breast cancers provides an opportune window to intervene therapeutically. As noted above, the HPMD pathway targets these mutations as its triggering requires RB or p53 gene defect. Depending on the cancer type, RB is mutated 30% to >90% (ex. small cell lung cancer) while p53 is mutated in nearly 50% of all human cancers [11-14]. Hence, the successful development of HPMD-eliciting therapeutics may eradicate breast cancer selectively. Likewise, such drugs may eliminate side effects arising from the disruption of microtubules or inciting of additional nonspecific lytic paths. In a similar vein, the elucidation of the HPMD allows one to comprehend the phenomenon of resistance from the perspective of antimitotic drug-induced lytic path, allowing one to conceive a therapeutic scheme to preempt the resistance based on the mechanism [15,16].

References

[1] Hong, F. & Lee, W. H. (1991). Sequence similarity between part of human retinoblastoma susceptibility gene product and a neurofilament protein subunit. *Biosci. Rep.*, *11*, 159-63.

[2] Hong, F. D., Huang, H. J., To, H., Young, L. J., Oro, A., Bookstein, R., Lee, E. Y. & Lee, W. H. (1989). Structure of the human retinoblastoma gene. *Proc. Natl. Acad. Sci. USA*, *86*, 5502-6.

[3] Hong, F. D. (1992). Retinoblastoma protein has properties similar to the characteristics associated with structural proteins. *University of California at San Diego*, San Diego.

[4] Lee, W. H., Xu, Y., Hong, F., Durfee, T., Mancini, M. A., Ueng, Y. C., Chen, P. L. & Riley, D. J. (1994). The corral hypothesis: a novel regulatory mode for retinoblastoma protein function. *Cold Spr. Harb. Symp. Quant. Biol.*, *59*, 97-107.

[5] Lee, W. H., Hollingsworth, R. E. J., Qian, Y. W., Chen, P. L., Hong, F. & Lee, E. Y. (1991). RB protein as a cellular "corral" for growth-promoting proteins. *Cold Spr. Harb. Symp. Quant. Biol.*, *56*, 211-7.

[6] Lee, W. H., Bookstein, R., Hong, F., Young, L. J., Shew, J. Y. & Lee, E. Y. (1987). Human retinoblastoma susceptibility gene: cloning, idenfication, and sequence. *Science*, *235*, 1394-9.

[7] Lee, W. H., Shew, J. Y., Hong, F. D., Sery, T. W., Donoso, L. A., Young, L. J., Bookstein, R. & Lee, E. Y. (1987). The retinoblastoma susceptibility gene encodes a nuclear phosphoprotein associated with DNA binding activity. *Nature*, *329*, 642-5.

[8] Bookstein, R., Rio, P., Madreperla, S. A., Hong, F., Allred, C., Grizzle, W. E. & Lee, W. H. (1990). Promoter deletion and loss of retinoblastoma gene expression in human prostate carcinoma. *Proc. Natl. Acad. Sci. USA*, *87*, 7762-6.

[9] Hensey, C. E., Hong, F., Durfee, T., Qian, Y. W., Lee, E. Y. & Lee, W. H. (1994). Identification of discrete structural domains in the retinoblastoma protein. Amino-terminal domain is required for its oligomerization. *J. Biol. Chem.*, *269*, 1380-7.

[10] Hong, F. D., Chen, J., Donovan, S., Schneider, N. & Nisen, P. D. (1999). Taxol, vincristine or nocodazole induces lethality in G1 checkpoint-defective human astrocytoma U373MG cells by triggering hyperploid progression. *Carcinogenesis*, *20*, 1161-8.

[11] Lee, E. Y., To, H., Shew, J. Y., Bookstein, R., Scully, P. & Lee, W. H. (1988). Inactivation of the retinoblastoma susceptibility gene in human breast cancers. *Science*, *241*, 218-221.

[12] Knudson, A. (2001). Two genetic hits (more or less) to cancer. *Nat. Rev. Cancer*, *1*, 157-162.

[13] Philips, S. M., Barton, C. M., Lee, S. J., Morton, D. G., Wallace, D. M., Lemoine, N. R. & Neoptolemons, J. P. (1994). Loss of the retinoblastoma susceptibility gene (RB1) is a frequent and early event in prostatic tumorigenesis. *Br. J. Cancer*, *70*, 1252-1257.

[14] Riley, D. J., Lee, E. Y. & Lee, W. H. (1994). The retinoblastoma protein: more than a tumor suppressor. *Ann. Rev. Cell Biol.*, *10*, 1-29.

[15] Un, F., Qi, C., Prosser, M., Wang, N., Zhou, B., Bronner, C. & Yen, Y. (2006). Modulating ICBP90 to suppress human ribonucleotide reductase M2 induction restores sensitivity to hydroxyurea cytotoxicity. *Anticancer Res.*, *26*, 2761-1767.

[16] Un, F. (2007). G1 arrest induction represents a critical determinant for cisplatin cytotoxicity in G1 checkpoint retaining human cancers. *Anticancer Drugs*, *18*, 411-417.

In: Multiple Drug Resistance
Editors: A. Meszaros, G. Balogh, pp. 225-244
ISBN: 978-1-60741-595-4

Chapter XII

Genetic Regulation, Physiology, Assessment and Inhibition of Efflux Pumps Responsible for Multi-Drug Resistant Phenotypes of Bacterial Pathogens

L. Amaral*[*1,2,3], S. Fanning [3,4], M. McCusker [3,4], G. Spengler [1,2], L. Rodrigues [1,2], C. Iversen [4], M. Martins [1,2], A. Martins [1,2], M. Viveiros [1,3] and I. Couto[1,5]

[1]Unit of Mycobacteriology and [2] UPMM, Instituto de Higiene e Medicina Tropical, Universidade Nova de Lisboa (IHMT/UNL),
Rua da Junqueira 96, 1349-008 Lisboa, Portugal
[3]COST ACTION BM0701 (ATENS) of the European Commission/ European Science Foundation
[4]Centres for Food Safety and Food-borne Zoonomics, UCD Veterinary Sciences Centre, University College Dublin, Belfield, Dublin 4, Ireland
[5]Centro de Recursos Microbiológicos (CREM), Faculdade de Ciências e Tecnologia, Universidade Nova de Lisboa, 2829-516 Caparica, Portugal

Abstract

The response of bacteria to a given antibiotic or other toxic agent that does not immediately kill them results in an adaptive response that secures their survival. This response may involve a number of distinct mechanisms, among which is the activation of genes that promote the appearance of transporters that extrude the agent prior to its

* Corresponding author: Leonard Amaral, Unit of Mycobacteriology, Instituto de Higiene e Medicina Tropical, Universidade Nova de Lisboa (IHMT/UNL). Rua da Junqueira, 96, 1349-008 Lisboa, Portugal. Tel: +351 21 365 2600, Fax: +351 21 363 2105. E-mail: lamaral@ihmt.unl.pt.

reaching its target. These transporters extrude a large variety of chemically unrelated compounds and hence they bestow on the bacterium a multi-drug resistant (MDR) phenotype. The appearance of this MDR phenotype during therapy makes therapy problematic. Understanding the genetic and physiological properties of MDR efflux pumps is an absolute requirement if MDR bacterial infections are to be successfully managed. There is much to learn and methods that afford the needed understanding will eventually pave the way for the successful management of an MDR bacterial infection. Therefore, the application of recently developed methods that assess the MDR bacterium at its genetic and physiological levels is the focus of this chapter. The material presented in this chapter is only the beginning for the evaluation and assessment of MDR efflux pumps.

Introduction

Multi-drug resistance of bacterial clinical isolates to representative antibiotics from two or more unrelated classes, is now accepted to be due to over-expressed efflux pumps which extrude the antibiotics prior to their reaching their intended targets [1-5]. Although the manner by which multi-drug resistance develops during infection is still not precisely demonstrated, prolonged *in vitro* exposure of reference bacterial strains to increasing concentrations of given antibiotics results in the appearance of a multi-drug resistant (MDR) phenotype. In this manner, prolonged exposure of *Staphylococcus aureus*, *Escherichia coli*, and *Mycobacterium tuberculosis*, to increasing concentrations of oxacillin [6] tetracycline [7, 8] and isoniazid [9], respectively, renders the respective organism resistant to the antibiotic to which it has been exposed, as well as to other classes of antibiotics. MDR phenotypes can also result from prolonged exposure to increasing concentrations of ethidium bromide (EB) [10], thereby reminding us that as far as the organism is "concerned", the response is due to exposure to a noxious agent, be it an antibiotic or other toxic substances. The response to prolonged exposure to a noxious agent may be considered to be one of "adaptation" inasmuch as when the organism is transferred to drug-free medium, restoration of initial susceptibility to the antibiotic takes place, albeit, over a lengthy number of replications in drug-free medium [8, 9]. Because agents that are known to inhibit efflux pump activity [11, 12] can also render the MDR bacterium susceptible to the antibiotics to which it had been induced to high-level resistance [6-10], the demonstration of reversal of resistance by a given agent constitutes *prima facia* evidence that the agent inhibits the efflux pump system of the MDR bacterium, provided that the resistance has been demonstrated to be due to efflux [1]. To this extent, thousands of compounds have been studied for their effects on over-expressed efflux pumps of MDR bacteria [13, 14] and as of this writing, although many agents have been shown to be effective efflux pump inhibitors (EPIs) [15-19], they have little clinical relevance since they are toxic. Phenothiazines and their derivatives have been shown to have inhibitory activity against many types of over-expressed multi-drug resistance mediating efflux pump systems [6, 8-12, 20-23] and because many have been used for the therapy of non-infectious pathology and produce few serious side effects [24-28], it is this class of compounds which will eventually yield an effective adjuvant for the therapy of MDR bacterial infections. It is therefore the intent of this chapter to discuss these compounds and the mechanism by which they affect efflux pumps of important MDR bacterial pathogens.

Efflux Pumps of MDR Bacteria: The Major Facilitator Superfamily

The Major Facilitator Superfamily (MFS) of transporters is a diverse superfamily that consists of more than a thousand aminoacid sequenced members. They catalyze the exchange of monovalent cations H^+ or Na^+ for unrelated and structurally different antibiotics. Most are of 400-600 aminoacid residues in length and possess either 12, 14 or 24 putative transmembrane α-helical spanning domains although with respect to Gram-negative bacteria, most MFS transporters are of a 12-domain type. The energy that drives the pump and therefore expels the antibiotic from the region immediately medial to the outer component of the cytoplasmic membrane is the proton motive force (PMF). In Gram-positive bacteria, efflux of antibiotics is mainly mediated by MFS-type transporter proteins. About 10% of the total transport proteins of Gram-positive bacteria are putative MFS-type multi-drug efflux pumps which when over-expressed are solely responsible for the MDR phenotype (29 and see also www.membranetransport.org). Examples of this type of pump is the *S. aureus* NorA, which when over-expressed renders the organism resistant to fluoroquinolones [10, 29-31] and the Qac system of efflux, which makes the organism extremely resistant to biocides [32-34]; and, the PmrA efflux pump of *Streptococcus pneumoniae* that when over-expressed results in resistance to fluoroquinolones (FQs) (35). Examples of inhibitors of the MFS-type efflux pump are: an ofloxacin-based EPI that is a potent inhibitor of NorA [36]; phenothiazines [11, 12], reserpine [11, 12, 35], citral derived amides [37], pyrazine derivatives [38] and N-caffeoylphenalkylamide derivatives [39]. Omeprazole derivatives have also been recently shown to inhibit the NorA efflux pump [40].

The NorA Efflux Pump of *Staphylococcus Aureus*

Susceptibility of wild-type *S. aureus* to FQs is dependent upon the permeability of the cell envelop and to the presence of intrinsic efflux pump systems, most commonly NorA, that extrudes the antibiotic, albeit, weakly [41]. Increased resistance to FQs is due to mutations that result in lower affinity of the gyrases GrlA and GyrA for FQs [41, 42]. In *S. aureus* most of these mutations occur in *grlA*. Greater than 97% of all clinical isolates that show resistance to norfloxacin, enoxacin, ciprofloxacin, fleroxacin, sparfloxacin and levofloxacin possess mutations in *grlA* and *gyrA*. Double mutations in both loci result in high-level resistance to these and newer FQs [42]. Examples of single mutations found in the GrlA and which produce intermediate to high-level resistance to ciprofloxacin are: Ser-80-->Phe or Tyr or Glu-84-->Lys or Ala-116-->Glu or Pro or a combination of Ser-80>Phe and Glu-84>Val. When these aminoacid substitutions are combined with alterations in GyrA, namely, Ser-84>Leu or Lys or Glu-88>Lys or Val, high-level resistance results [43].

Although the above mutations account for the vast majority of resistance to FQs, resistance has also been shown to involve the over-expression of the NorA efflux pump [41]. Although mutations of the promoter region of *norA* can lead to the over-expression of NorA [44], over-expression has been shown for some isolates to be independent of changes within the promoter region [45]. Over-expression has been reported in the absence of any mutation within the *norA* promoter region [46, 31].

Efflux mediated resistance to FQs can be induced in *S. aureus* by exposure to substrates recognized by the NorA efflux pump system (47). Among these substrates is EB, which when present in ever-increasing concentration, over-time, promotes the development of extreme resistance of wild-type *S. aureus* to the agent [minimum inhibitory concentration (MIC) increases from 5 to over 150 mg/L] [10]. Accompanying this increased resistance is resistance to FQs which can be reversed upon exposure to reserpine, and a more pronounced effect is seen with phenothiazines chlorpromazine and thioridazine [10]. Evaluation of the activity of *norA* and other efflux pump-encoding genes, active efflux of EB, along with the sequencing of the *norA* gene, yielded a 35-fold increase in the activity of *norA*, no change in the activity of other genes that encode other efflux pumps, a 4-fold increase in the efflux of EB and no mutations within *norA*. However, a 70 bp deletion was noted within the *norA* promoter region [10]. The precise genetic mechanism by which an efflux pump substrate of NorA that has no structural relationship to FQs can initiate the above, remains to be elucidated. These observations are not surprising inasmuch as the mechanism, by which efflux-mediated resistance is normally brought about in FQs resistant clinical isolates, is yet to be defined.

Other Intrinsic Efflux Pumps of Gram-Positive Bacteria

Intrinsic MFS-type efflux pumps of bacteria have not been readily studied due to the lack of sensitivity of the systems employed. However, the main intrinsic MFS-type efflux pump of the Gram-positive *Enterococcus faecalis* is the EmeA pump which has been characterized by Lee et al. [48], and as is the case for all MFS-type pumps, derives the energy needed for its activity from the PMF (48). We have studied the efflux of EB by the *E. faecalis* ATCC29212 reference strain under conditions which are more physiological than those usually employed. These studies were undertaken in the presence of a source of metabolic energy, at different medium pHs [ranging from 5 to 8] and an incubation temperature of 37ºC [49] using a semi-automated method that utilizes the common efflux pump substrate EB [50]. At pH 5, metabolic energy is not required for efflux of EB; in contrast at pH 8 catabolism of glucose is required to energise efflux. These physiological conditions are summarized in Figure 1 showing an increase in EB accumulation at pH 8, with the concomitant increase in slope of the line at this pH, as efflux decreased. In contrast, at pH 5, EPIs such as thioridazine, verapamil and reserpine and the uncoupler of the PMF, carbonyl cyanide m-chlorophenylhydrazone (CCCP) have no effect on the efflux of EB. In the presence of these EPIs, at pH 8 efflux is completely eliminated (as shown for CCCP in Figure 2). These results suggest that at pH 5 the PMF is capable of energizing efflux as a result of the potential difference across the membrane, due to the high concentrations of protons. At pH 8, the PMF is somewhat dissipated and hence the concentration of CCCP that had no affect on efflux at pH 5 completely inhibited efflux at pH 8 by collapsing the proton gradient. If the PMF was to be the only source required to energise this MFS-type efflux, then EPIs which are known to inhibit the hydrolysis of ATP, such as thioridazine, should have no affect on efflux. A similar scenario would be expected to occur in the absence of a source of metabolic energy. Thus, whereas an MFS-type efflux pump readily derives energy from protons at pH 5, when the availability of those protons is reduced as would be the case at pH 8, energy must be provided through the hydrolysis of ATP. Moreover, unlike other Gram-positive bacteria, *E. faecalis* has another efflux system, namely the EfrAB that can extrude antibiotics. This pump is a member of the ATP-Binding Cassette (ABC) superfamily [51] and derives its energy from the hydrolysis of ATP [52], by ATPase enzymes that are inhibited by phenothiazines at pH 8 and not at pH 5 [53].

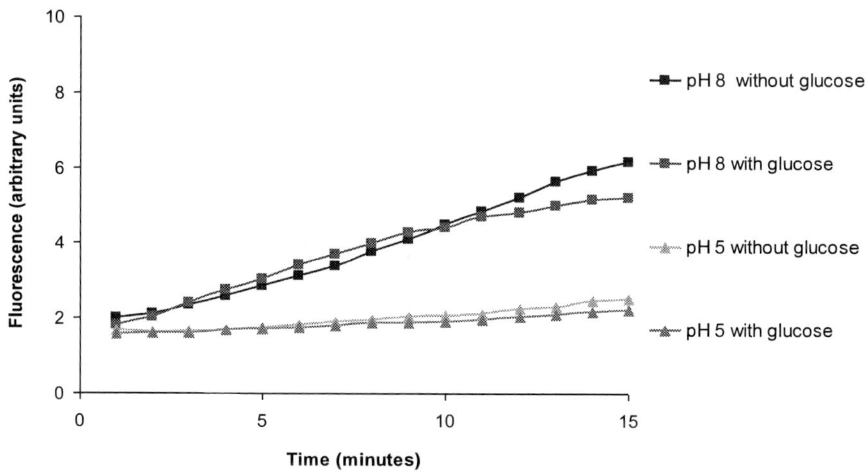

Figure 1. Accumulation of EB at 0.5 mg/L by E. faecalis ATCC29212 at pH 8 and 5 in the presence and absence of glucose 0.6%.

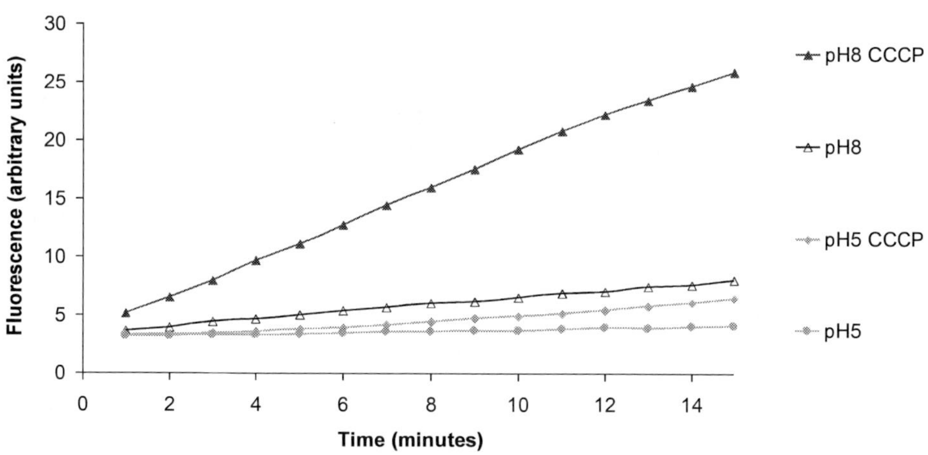

Figure 2. Effect of CCCP 100 μM (½ MIC) on accumulation of EB at 0.5 mg/L by *E. faecalis* ATCC29212 at pH 8 and 5 in the presence of glucose 0.6%.

Efflux Pumps of Gram-Negative Bacteria: The Resistance Nodulation Division (RND) Family

The efflux pumps of Gram-negative bacteria that promote an MDR phenotype when over-expressed, are part of the Resistance Nodulation Division (RND) family of transporters, and consist of tripartite units that span the plasma membrane from the outer membrane to the inner membrane being closely associated with the interstitial periplasm. These tripartite pumps comprise an outer-membrane channel, TolC, which connects to the transporter located in the inner-membrane and which transduces the electrochemical energy of proton gradients. A fusion protein then links the transmembrane component in the periplasm with TolC [54-56]. Although more than two dozen structures of the inner-membrane transporter protein AcrB have been determined for various ligand (substrate) bound states [57, 58], the actual structure as it exists in the cell envelope remains for now as a conjecture. Nevertheless, a variety of models have been presented to represent the relationship of the transporter component to TolC along with its anchorage to the cytoplasmic side of the inner membrane [59-61]. Figure 3 presents such a model (62) which in the opinion of the authors, seems to be supported by the studies of others.

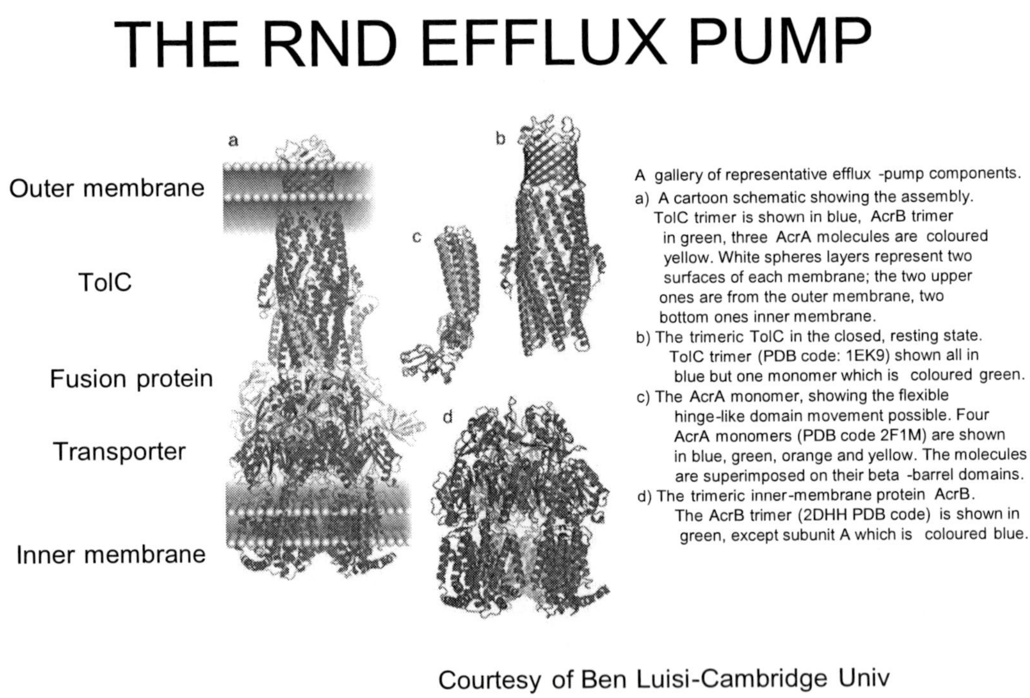

Figure 3. Model representing the assembly of TolC, the transporter protein AcrB and the fusion protein AcrA. Adapted from Pietras Z. et al. (63).

The mechanism by which unrelated antibiotics are extruded by this tripartite efflux pump of Gram-negative MDR bacteria is thought to involve the transport of a proton from the surface of the cell where the proton gradient is strongest through the TolC channel and finally, through the transporter itself. The passage of the proton energises the transporter component to expell the antibiotic from the region of the inner membrane to the TolC where it makes its way to the outside of the cell. The physical chemistry behind this process is beyond the scope of this review and the reader is encouraged to refer to an excellent review by Ben Luisi et al. [62].

Genetic Regulation of Efflux Pumps of Gram-Negative Bacteria (ex. *Escherichia coli*)

E. coli has at least eight tripartite efflux pumps that, when over-expressed, contribute to the MDR phenotype of the organism [7]. Over-expression of these RND efflux pumps results when the organism is exposed to increasing concentrations of an antibiotic, such as tetracycline [7, 8]. The over-expression of these efflux pumps renders the bacterium increasingly resistant to tetracycline along with other antibiotics [7]. At the onset of exposure to tetracycline, the stress regulator genes *soxS* and *rob* are immediately increased. Soon thereafter, the first regulatory gene showing an increased expression is *marB* which is soon followed by *marA*. After the regulatory genes are activated, the expression of the stress genes begins to decrease and the expression of genes that code for the transporters of the main efflux pumps of *E. coli*, namely, *acrB*, *acrF* and *yhiV* are progressively increased with each increase in tetracycline concentration to which the bacterium is exposed.

Figure 4 summarises these findings. Following transfer of the tetracycline induced resistant strain ($AG100_{TET}$) to drug-free media (and hence the removal of the transient selective pressure) initial susceptibility to tetracycline, as well as to the other antibiotics that constituted this MDR phenotype, is restored [7]. Therefore, under these conditions, the genetic response to exposure to increasing concentrations of the antibiotic may be considered as one of adaptation. However, if the tetracycline induced strain is serially passed in medium containing a constant concentration of tetracycline such as 10 mg/L, the organism becomes increasingly resistant, reaching levels of resistance greater than 120 mg/L of tetracycline even though it had never been exposed to a concentration of the agent above 10 mg/L. The expression of genes that encode the global regulators of efflux pumps such as *marA, marB,* stress genes such as *soxR* and *soxS,* and genes that encode the transporters *acrB* and *acrF* of this high-level tetracycline induced resistant strain is now similar to that of the parental wild-type.

To determine whether any broader pleiotrophic effects could be recognized, these strains were investigated using a phenotypic microarray. The complete panel of reactions was analysed and when compared to the isogenic wild-type strain *E. coli* AG100, demonstrated a large number of potential genetic targets whose activities had been altered (data not shown). Moreover, because this strain did not revert to initial susceptibility [to tetracycline (MIC of 2 mg/L)] after greater than 50 serial passages in 500 mL of drug-free medium, the existence of one or more mutations cannot be ruled out. The possibility that such mutations had taken place as a consequence of a master mutator gene, as described by Chopra et al. [63], may represent a reasonable hypothesis.

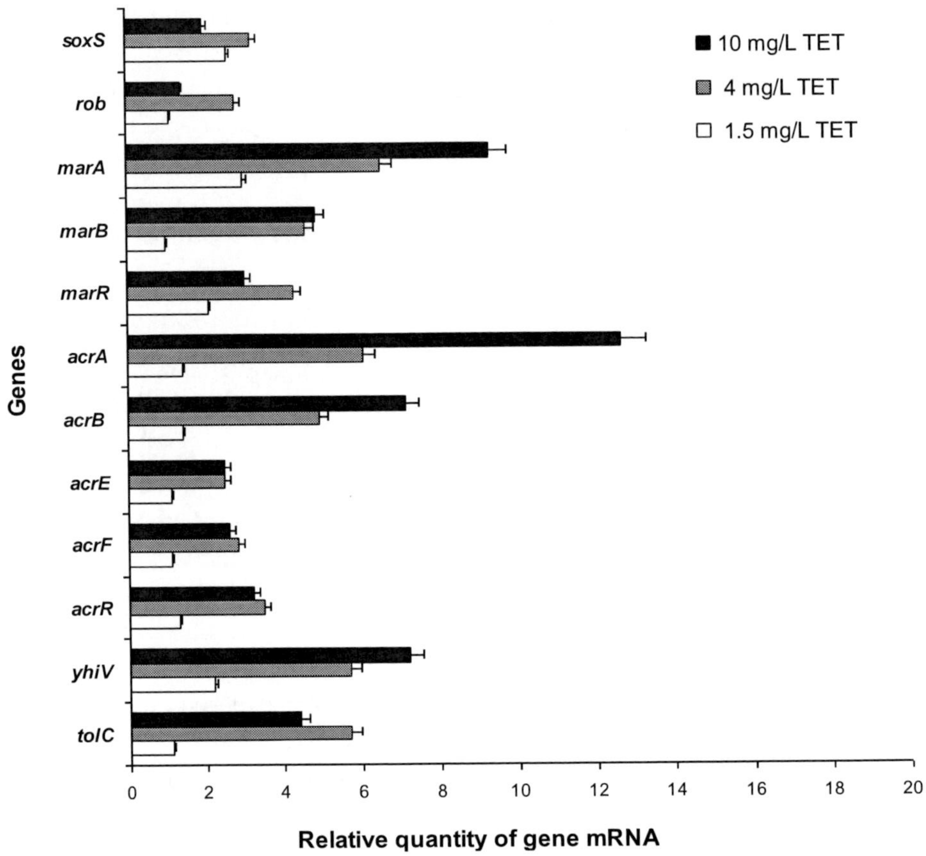

Figure 4. Relative expression of regulators and inner membrane transporter genes of *E. coli* AG100 gradually exposed to 1.5 mg/L, 4 and 10 mg/L of tetracycline (TET) compared to its parental non-induced strain.

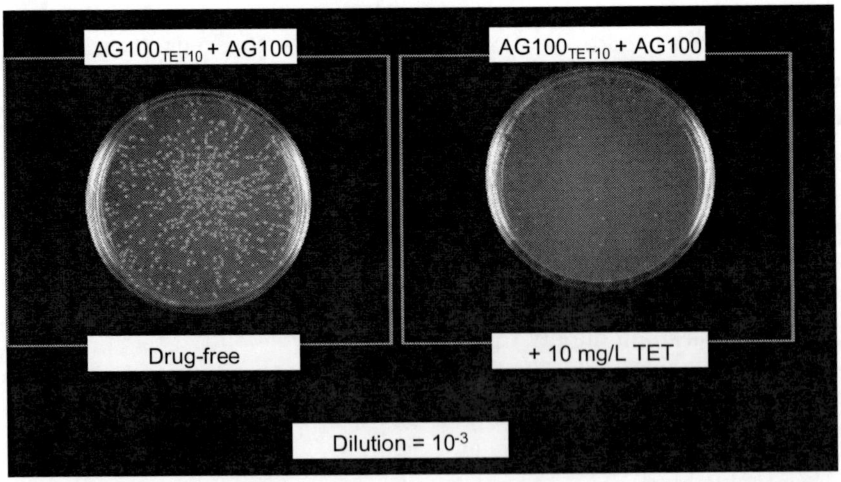

Figure 5. Survival fitness of $AG100_{TET10}$, that has been serially exposed to 10 mg/L of tetracycline. Plate on left is drug free and on right place contains 10 mg/L of tetracycline.

The question of whether the development of an extreme, non-reversible resistance phenotype to tetracycline caused a decrease of fitness was studied by inoculating 500 mL drug-free medium with equal numbers of the wild-type isogenic reference strain (AG100) and the strain that was now resistant to 120 mg/L of tetracycline (AG100$_{TET10}$), incubated at 37°C, and determination of cell number expressed as colony forming units (CFU) from both drug-free and tetracycline (10 mg/L) containing agar plates. As is shown by Figure 5, very few colonies detected on drug-free agar were of the highly tetracycline resistant strain. Indeed, the AG100$_{TET10}$ appears to pay a high fitness cost when it "decides" to reduce the available energy required to maintain a high efflux activity and embark on a rapid evolutionary pathway.

Evaluation of Intrinsic and Over-Expressed Efflux Pumps of Gram-Negative Bacteria

The recently developed semi-automated method that utilizes the common efflux pump fluorochrome substrate EB, affords the sensitivity for the characterization and assessment of the intrinsic efflux pump system of *E. coli* wild-type reference strain, as well as those that express an MDR phenotype [50, 64]. Laboratory methods used to evaluate an efflux pump system are best conducted as close to physiologically relevant conditions as possible, namely, conditions provided by the *in vivo* environment during infection of the human. Such conditions usually involve a temperature of 37°C, the presence of a metabolic energy source in the event that such a source is needed and suitable ionic conditions similar to the interstitial fluids of the infected host. EB must be at a concentration in the medium that does not yield a fluorescence signal, and yet, if and when it begins to be accumulated within the periplasmic space of the bacterium, the relative concentration much reach detectable levels that can be measured by an instrument on a real-time basis.

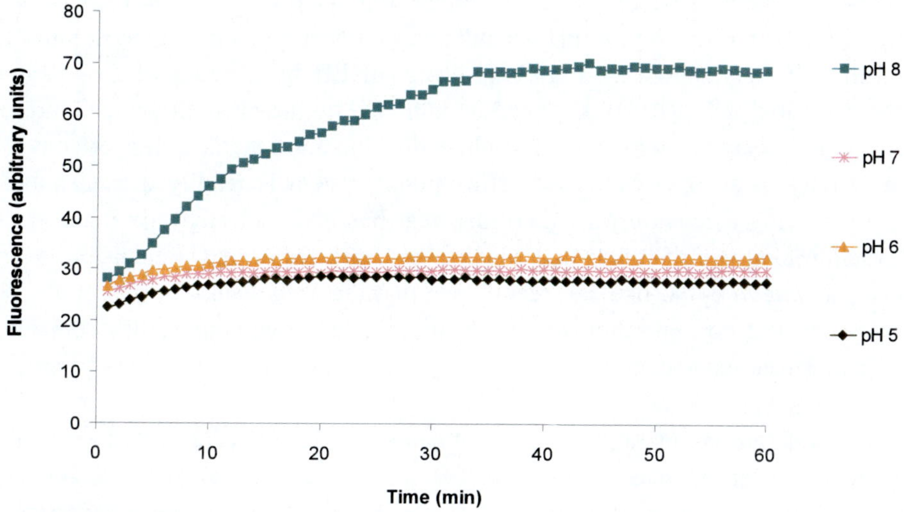

Figure 6. The effect of pH on the accumulation of EB used at 5 mg/L by *E. coli* AG100$_{TET}$ that over-expresses its AcrAB efflux pump.

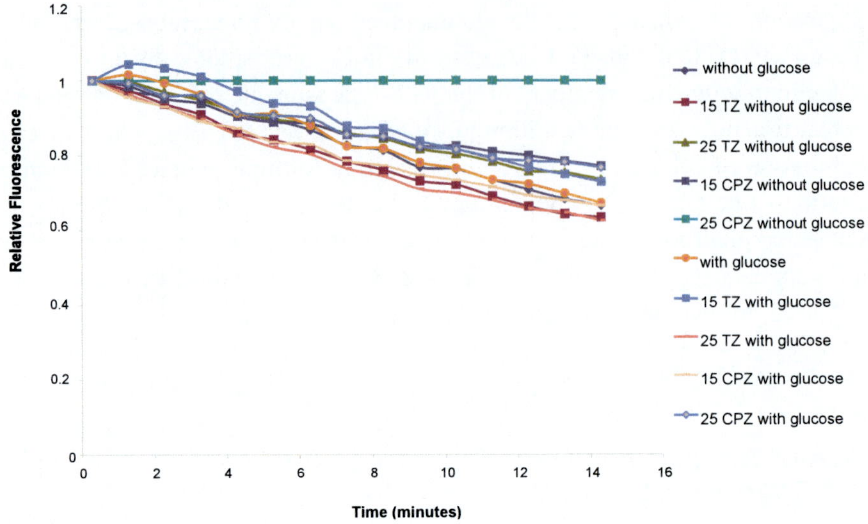

Figure 7. Demonstration of efflux of EB by *E. coli* AG100$_{TET}$ in the presence or absence of glucose at 0.4%.

Accumulation of EB is considered to be due to a concentration of EB that exceeds the efflux capacity of the pump or to the presence of an agent that inhibits the pump [50, 64]. As an example of the method, the *E. coli* tetracycline induced strain AG100$_{TET}$ is incubated at 37°C in a saline phosphate solution that is buffered at varying pH, containing glucose and increasing concentrations of EB. As shown by Figure 6, accumulation of EB by this over-expressing efflux pumps strain is minimal at low pH (5 to 7) compared to the accumulation observable at the higher pH of 8.

Efflux of EB and the physiological conditions that influence it are demonstrated by the following: cells are pre-loaded with EB under conditions that minimize efflux (temperature of 25°C; no energy source; presence of an EPI) and the accumulation of EB is followed on a real-time basis. When sufficient EB has accumulated in the presence of an EPI, the medium is replaced with EB-free medium at pH 7 containing an energy source (glucose) and efflux is followed at 37°C. As shown by Figure 7, efflux of EB by a strain of *E. coli* that over-expresses its efflux pump (AG100$_{TET}$) can be inhibited by the phenothiazine chlorpromazine in a concentration dependent manner. The phenothiazine thioridazine is less effective.

The activity of an over-expressed efflux pump system is readily demonstrated by the method. Employing a *Salmonella* Enteritidis, that has been selected and made resistant to ciprofloxacin (*Salmonella* 5408$_{cip}$) and which over-expresses *acrAB* some 6-fold over that of its parent *Salmonella* 5408, one can readily see that the *Salmonella* 5408$_{cip}$ strain begins to accumulate EB at a concentration of EB (5 mg/L) and above (Figure 8a) compared to its isogenic parent wherein accumulation of EB begins at lower concentrations (1 mg/L) (Figure 8b).

These results are comparable to those obtained by the EB-agar cartwheel method [64, 65], which show that whereas 1.0 mg/L of EB causes the colonies of the *Salmonella* 5408 strain to fluoresce, the *Salmonella* 5408$_{cip}$ does not fluoresce even with a concentration of EB of 2.5 mg/L (Figure 9).

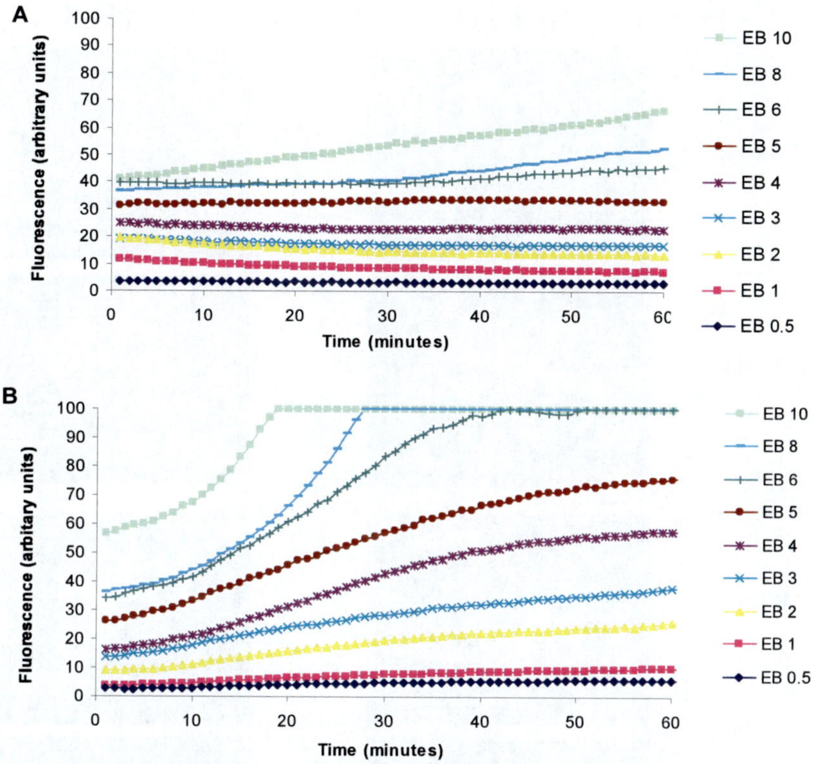

Figure 8. Determination of the highest concentration of EB that can be handled by Salmonella 5408cip (A) and Salmonella 5408 (B). The lines represent increasing concentrations of EB in mg/L.

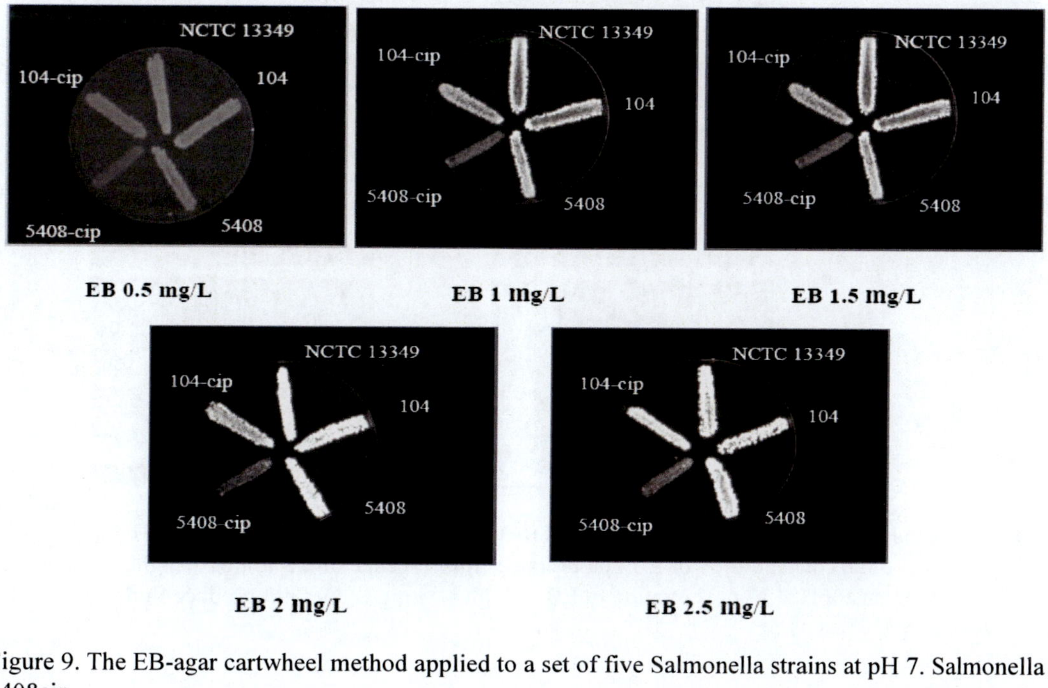

Figure 9. The EB-agar cartwheel method applied to a set of five Salmonella strains at pH 7. Salmonella 5408cip.

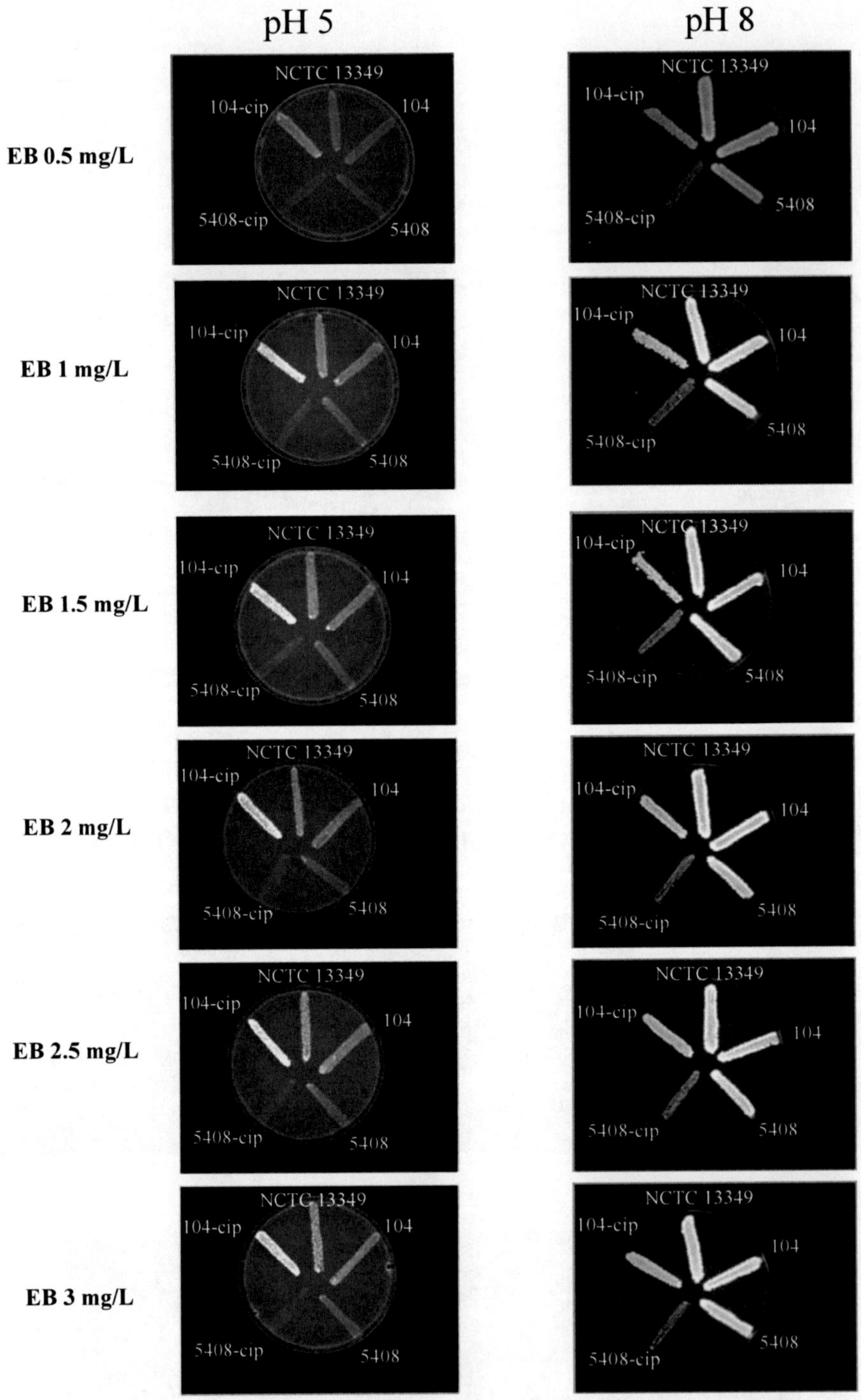

Figure 10. The EB-agar cartwheel method applied to a set of five *Salmonella* strains at pH 5 and 8. Note that at pH 5 the concentration of EB that produces fluorescence of the strains is higher than at pH 8. Moreover, even at pH 8, a concentration of EB as high as 3 mg/L does not produce fluorescence of the *Salmonella* 5408_{cip}.

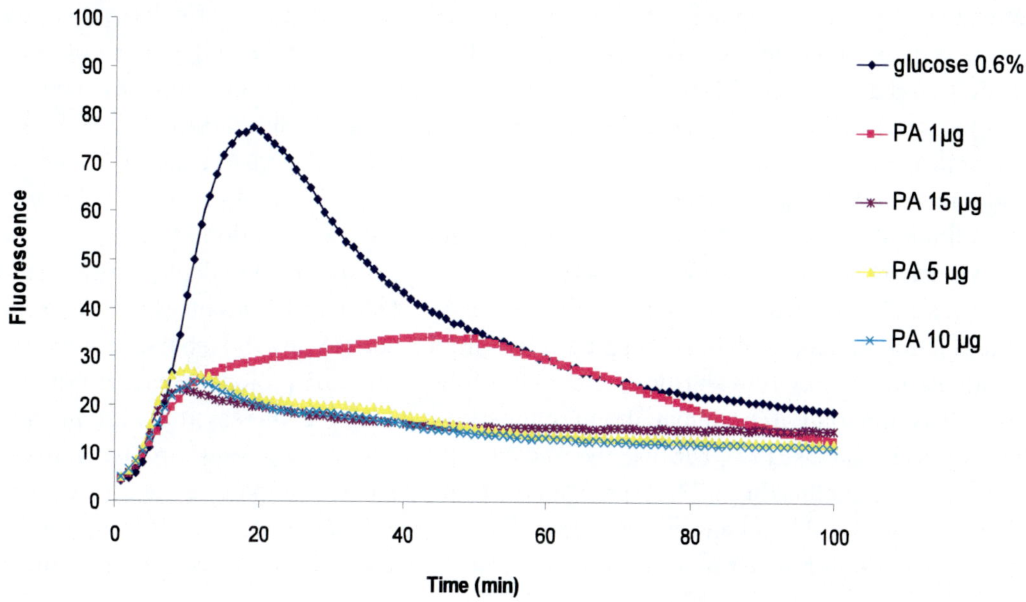

Figure 11. Accumulation of EB at 1 mg/L in the presence of thioridazine (TZ) at 50 mg/L by *Salmonella* 104 at pH 8. The addition of palmitic acid (PA) reduces the accumulation of EB.

The accumulation of EB by Gram-negative and Gram-positive bacteria, as previously discussed, is affected by pH; at low pH accumulation is minimal, at higher pH it is far greater. This observation can be reproduced using the EB-agar cartwheel method as shown by Figure 10. Note that at pH 5 the concentration that produces fluorescence of the colonies is always much higher than at pH 8. Also, at pH 8, a concentration of EB as high as 3 mg/L does not produce fluorescence of the *Salmonella* 5408_{cip}.

The permeability of *Salmonella* to antibiotics and other noxious agents and the bacterium response to these differs from that of *E. coli.*

The major differences include: i) the regulation of the main efflux pump of *Salmonella acrAB* which although very similar to that of *E. coli* [66] is also influenced by *ramA* a gene that is absent in *E. coli* [67, 68] ii) the regulation of permeability in *Salmonella* takes place as a consequence of the activation of *pmrA* by its cognate sensor kinase PmrB when the organism is cultured in medium at pH 5 [69] and the subsequent increase in the lipopolysaccharide deposition by the organism through the over-expression of genes that collectively result in the increased synthesis of Lipid A [70, 71]. That the pH of the medium is a major regulator of the permeability of *Salmonella* to an efflux pump substrate such as EB is clearly demonstrated by Figure 10.

The selection of the highest concentration at each pH that does not produce accumulation affords the opportunity to study additional conditions that may affect the concentrations of EB accumulated, such as the modulation of permeability to EB promoted by an EPI. As shown by Figure 11, the accumulation of EB by a *Salmonella* strain, in this case *Salmonella* 104, at pH 8 in the presence of 50 mg/L of the phenothiazine promotes rapid and substantial accumulation of EB. This step accumulation is soon followed by efflux. Because thioridazine inhibits ATPases and kinases [72-74], a metabolic source of protons would be required for activation of the efflux pump. Considering that *Salmonella* is primed for the activation of genes that are involved in the synthesis of Lipid A and increased deposition of the lipopolysaccharide layer [72-74], we considered the possibility that the source of energy that afforded the extrusion of EB as a consequence of exposure to thioridazine came from the metabolism of fatty acids. In *Salmonella* Enteritidis 104_{cip}, the *lpxC* gene is up-regulated (data not shown), resulting increased lipopolysaccharide synthesis. As shown by Figure 11, the addition of palmitic acid reduces thioridazine promoted accumulation of EB.

Although far from being understood, the above experiments demonstrate that for *Salmonella,* the status of permeability to a noxious agent such as EB involves a pH dependent efflux pump system which is supplemented in its activity by metabolic energy when conditions of the environment does not support the source of protons needed to drive the pump. It is important to note that although hydrolysis of ATP is increased at high pH due to the F_1F_0 ATP synthase [72], because the oxyreductase II as well as the F_1F_0 ATP synthase are inhibited by phenothiazines [73, 74] the source of protons needed to drive the efflux pump is removed. Because this organism is already primed by its PmrA/kinase PmrB to respond to a noxious agent by up-regulation of its lipopolysaccharide and Lipid A content, the source of protons needed to drive the efflux pump at pH 8 is assured.

Summary and Perspectives

The response of bacteria to a given antibiotic or other toxic agent that does not immediately kill them results in an adaptive response that secures their survival. This response may involve a number of distinct mechanisms, among which is the activation of genes that promote the appearance of transporters that extrude the agent prior to its reaching its target. These transporters extrude a large variety of chemically unrelated compounds and hence they bestow on the bacterium a MDR phenotype. The appearance of this MDR phenotype during therapy makes therapy problematic. Understanding the genetic and physiological properties of MDR efflux pumps is an absolute requirement if MDR bacterial infections are to be successfully managed. The material presented in this chapter is only the beginning for the evaluation and assessment of MDR efflux pumps. There is much to learn and methods that afford the needed understanding will eventually pave the way for the successful management of an MDR bacterial infection.

References

[1] Martins M., Dastidar S.G., Fanning S., Kristiansen J.E., Molnar J., Pagès J.M., Schelz Z., Spengler G., Viveiros M., Amaral L. (2008) Potential role of non-antibiotics (helper compounds) in the treatment of multidrug-resistant Gram-negative infections: mechanisms for their direct and indirect activities. *Int. J. Antimicrob. Agents* 31: 198-208.

[2] Poole K. (2007) Efflux pumps as antimicrobial resistance mechanisms. *Ann. Med.* 39: 162-176.

[3] Mahamoud A., Chevalier J., Davin-Regli A., Barbe J., Pagès J.M. (2006) Quinoline derivatives as promising inhibitors of antibiotic efflux pump in multidrug resistant *Enterobacter aerogenes* isolates. *Curr. Drug Targets* 7: 843-847.

[4] Piddock L.J. (2006). Clinically relevant chromosomally encoded multidrug resistance efflux pumps in bacteria. *Clin. Microbiol. Rev.* 19: 382-402.

[5] Pagès JM, Masi M, Barbe J. (2005) Inhibitors of efflux pumps in Gram-negative bacteria. *Trends Mol. Med.* 11: 382-389.

[6] Martins A., Couto I., Aagaard L., Martins M., Viveiros M., Kristiansen J.E., Amaral L. (2007) Prolonged exposure of methicillin-resistant *Staphylococcus aureus* (MRSA) COL strain to increasing concentrations of oxacillin results in a multidrug-resistant phenotype. *Int. J. Antimicrob. Agents* 29: 302-305.

[7] Viveiros M., Dupont M., Rodrigues L., Couto I., Davin-Regli A., Martins M., Pagès J.M., Amaral L. (2007) Antibiotic stress, genetic response and altered permeability of *E. coli*. *PLoS ONE* 2: e365.

[8] Viveiros M., Jesus A., Brito M., Leandro C., Martins M., Ordway D., Molnar A.M., Molnar J., Amaral L. (2005) Inducement and reversal of tetracycline resistance in *Escherichia coli* K-12 and expression of proton gradient-dependent multidrug efflux pump genes. *Antimicrob. Agents Chemother.* 49: 3578-3582.

[9] Viveiros M., Portugal I., Bettencourt R., Victor T.C., Jordaan A.M., Leandro C., Ordway D., Amaral L. (2002) Isoniazid-induced transient high-level resistance in *Mycobacterium tuberculosis*. *Antimicrob. Agents Chemother.* 46: 2804-2810.

[10] Couto I., Costa S.S., Viveiros M., Martins M., Amaral L. (2008) Efflux-mediated response of *Staphylococcus aureus* exposed to ethidium bromide. *J. Antimicrob. Chemother.* 62: 504-513.

[11] Kristiansen M.M., Leandro C., Ordway D., Martins M. Viveiros M., Pacheco T., Kristiansen J.E. and Amaral L. (2005) Thioridazine Reduces Resistance Of Methicillin Resistant *Staphylococcus aureus* By Inhibiting A Reserpine Sensitive Efflux Pump. *In Vivo* 20: 361-366.

[12] Kaatz G.W., Moudgal V.V., Seo S.M., Kristiansen J.E. (2003) Phenothiazines and thioxanthenes inhibit multidrug efflux pump activity in *Staphylococcus aureus*. *Antimicrob. Agents Chemother.* 47: 719-726.

[13] Lomovskaya O., Bostian K.A. (2006) Practical applications and feasibility of efflux pump inhibitors in the clinic – a vision for applied use. *Biochem. Pharmacol.* 71:910-918.

[14] Lomovskaya O., Watkins W.J. (2001) Efflux pumps: their role in antibacterial drug discovery. *Curr. Med. Chem.* 8:1699-1711.

[15] Kamicker B.J., Sweeney M.T., Kaczmarek F., Dib-Hajj F., Shang W., Crimin K., Duignan J. , Gootz T.D. (2008) Bacterial efflux pump inhibitors. *Methods Mol. Med.* 142: 187-204.

[16] German N., Kaatz G.W., Kerns R.J. (2008) Synthesis and evaluation of PSSRI-based inhibitors of *Staphylococcus aureus* multidrug efflux pumps. *Bioorg. Med. Chem. Lett.* 18: 1368-1373.

[17] Robertson G.T., Doyle T.B., Du Q., Duncan L., Mdluli K.E., Lynch A.S. (2007) A Novel indole compound that inhibits *Pseudomonas aeruginosa* growth by targeting MreB is a substrate for MexAB-OprM. *J. Bacteriol.* 189: 6870-6881.

[18] Ball A.R., Casadei G., Samosorn S., Bremner J.B., Ausubel F.M., Moy T.I., Lewis K. (2006) Conjugating berberine to a multidrug efflux pump inhibitor creates an effective antimicrobial. *A.C.S Chem. Biol.* 1:594-600.

[19] Pannek S., Higgins P.G., Steinke P., Jonas D., Akova M., Bohnert J.A., Seifert H., Kern W.V. (2006) Multidrug efflux inhibition in *Acinetobacter baumannii*: comparison between 1-(1-naphthylmethyl)-piperazine and phenyl-arginine-beta-naphthylamide. *J. Antimicrob. Chemother.* 57:970-974.

[20] Ramón-García S., Martín C., Aínsa J.A., De Rossi E. (2006) Characterization of tetracycline resistance mediated by the efflux pump Tap from *Mycobacterium fortuitum*. *J. Antimicrob. Chemother.* 57:252-259.

[21] Marquez B. (2005) Bacterial efflux systems and efflux pumps inhibitors. *Biochimie* 87: 1137-1147.

[22] Hendricks O., Butterworth T.S., Kristiansen J.E. (2003) The in-vitro antimicrobial effect of non-antibiotics and putative inhibitors of efflux pumps on *Pseudomonas aeruginosa* and *Staphylococcus aureus*. *Int. J. Antimicrob. Agents* 22: 262-264.

[23] Molnár J., Hevér A., Fakla I., Fischer J., Ocsovski I., Aszalós A. (1997) Inhibition of the transport function of membrane proteins by some substituted phenothiazines in *E. coli* and multidrug resistant tumor cells. *Anticancer Res.* 17: 481-486.

[24] Amaral L., Viveiros M., Kristiansen J.E. (2006) "Non-Antibiotics": alternative therapy for the management of MDRTB and MRSA in economically disadvantaged countries. *Curr. Drug Targets* 7: 887-891.

[25] Amaral L., Viveiros M., Molnar J. (2004) Antimicrobial activity of phenothiazines. *In Vivo* 18: 725-731.

[26] Amaral L., Viveiros M., Kristiansen J.E. (2001) Phenothiazines: potential alternatives for the management of antibiotic resistant infections of tuberculosis and malaria in developing countries. *Trop. Med. Int. Health* 6: 1016-1022.

[27] Amaral L., Kristiansen J.E., Viveiros M., Atouguia J. (2001) Activity of phenothiazines against antibiotic-resistant *Mycobacterium tuberculosis*: a review supporting further studies that may elucidate the potential use of thioridazine as anti-tuberculosis therapy. *J. Antimicrob. Chemother.* 47: 505-511.

[28] Amaral L., Kristiansen J.E. (2000) Phenothiazines: an alternative to conventional therapy for the initial management of suspected multidrug resistant tuberculosis. A call for studies. *Int. J. Antimicrob. Agents* 14: 173-176.

[29] Lorca G.L., Barabote R.D., Zlotopolski V., Tran C., Winnen B., Hvorup R.N., Stonestrom A.J., Nguyen E., Huang L.W., Kim D.S., Saier M.H. Jr. (2007) Transport capabilities of eleven gram-positive bacteria: comparative genomic analyses. *Biochim. Biophys. Acta* 1768: 1342-1366.

[30] Piddock L.J., Jin Y.F. (1999) Antimicrobial activity and accumulation of moxifloxacin in quinolone-susceptible bacteria. *J. Antimicrob. Chemother.* 43: 39-42.

[31] Muñoz-Bellido J.L., Alonzo Manzanares M., Martínez Andrés J.A., Guttiérrez Zufiaurre M.N., Ortiz G., Segovia Hernández M., García-Rodríguez JA. (1999) Efflux

pump-mediated quinolone resistance in *Staphylococcus aureus* strains wild type for *gyrA*, *gyrB*, *grlA*, and *norA*. *Antimicrob. Agents Chemother.* 43: 354-356.

[32] Jia B., Zhou T.Q., Huang A.L., Huang W.X. (2008) Role of TMS5: staphylococcal multidrug-efflux protein QacA. *Chin. Med. J. (Engl).* 121: 409-413.

[33] Smith K., Gemmell C.G., Hunter I.S. (2008) The association between biocide tolerance and the presence or absence of *qac* genes among hospital-acquired and community-acquired MRSA isolates. *J. Antimicrob. Chemother.* 61: 78-84.

[34] Sekiguchi J., Hama T., Fujino T., Araake M., Irie A., Saruta K., Konosaki H., Nishimura H., Kawano A., Kudo K., Kondo T., Sasazuki T., Kuratsuji T., Yoshikura H., Kirikae T. (2004) Detection of the antiseptic- and disinfectant-resistance genes *qacA*, *qacB*, and *qacC* in methicillin-resistant *Staphylococcus aureus* isolated in a Tokyo hospital. *Jpn. J. Infect. Dis.* 57: 288-291.

[35] Piddock L.J., Johnson M.M., Simjee S., Pumbwe L. (2002) Expression of efflux pump gene *pmrA* in fluoroquinolone-resistant and –susceptible clinical isolates of *Streptococcus pneumoniae*. *Antimicrob. Agents Chemother.* 46: 808-812.

[36] German N, Wei P, Kaatz GW, Kerns RJ. (2008) Synthesis and evaluation of fluoroquinolone derivatives as substrate-based inhibitors of bacterial efflux pumps. *Eur. J. Med. Chem.* 43: 2453-2463.

[37] Thota N., Koul S., Reddy M.V., Sangwan P.L., Khan I.A., Kumar A., Raja A.F., Andotra S.S., Qazi G.N. (2008) Citral derived amides as potent bacterial NorA efflux pump inhibitors. *Bioorg. Med. Chem.* 16: 6535-6543.

[38] Vidaillac C., Guillon J., Moreau S., Arpin C., Lagardère A., Larrouture S., Dallemagne P., Caignard D.H., Quentin C., Jarry C. (2007) Synthesis of new 4-[2-(alkylamino) ethylthio]pyrrolo[1,2-a]quinoxaline and 5-[2-(alkylamino) ethylthio]pyrrolo[1,2-a]thieno[3,2-e]pyrazine derivatives, as potential bacterial multidrug resistance pump inhibitors. *J. Enzyme. Inhib. Med. Chem.* 22: 620-631.

[39] Michalet S., Cartier G., David B., Mariotte A.M., Dijoux-franca M.G., Kaatz G.W., Stavri M., Gibbons S. (2007) N-caffeoylphenalkylamide derivatives as bacterial efflux pump inhibitors. *Bioorg. Med. Chem. Lett.* 17: 1755-1758.

[40] Vidaillac C., Guillon J., Arpin C., Forfar-Bares I., Ba B.B., Grellet J., Moreau S., Caignard D.H., Jarry C., Quentin C. (2007) Synthesis of omeprazole analogues and evaluation of these as potential inhibitors of the multidrug efflux pump NorA of *Staphylococcus aureus*. *Antimicrob. Agents Chemother.* 51: 831-838.

[41] Kaatz G.W., Seo S.M., Barriere S.L., Albrecht L.M., Rybak M.J. (1991) Development of resistance to fleroxacin during therapy of experimental methicillin-susceptible *Staphylococcus aureus* endocarditis. *Antimicrob. Agents Chemother.* 35: 1547-1550.

[42] Noguchi N., Okihara T., Namiki Y., Kumaki Y., Yamanaka Y., Koyama M., Wakasugi K., Sasatsu M. (2005) Susceptibility and resistance genes to fluoroquinolones in methicillin-resistant *Staphylococcus aureus* isolated in 2002. *Int. J. Antimicrob. Agents* 25: 374-379.

[43] Schmitz F.J., Fluit A.C., Brisse S., Verhoef J., Köhrer K., Milatovic D. (1999) Molecular epidemiology of quinolone resistance and comparative in vitro activities of new quinolones against European *Staphylococcus aureus* isolates. *FEMS Immunol. Med. Microbiol.* 26: 281-287.

[44] Ng E.Y., Trucksis M., Hooper D.C. (1994) Quinolone resistance mediated by *norA*: physiologic characterization and relationship to *flqB*, a quinolone resistance locus on the *Staphylococcus aureus* chromosome. *Antimicrob. Agents Chemother.* 38: 1345-1355.

[45] Kaatz G.W., Seo S.M. (1997) Mechanisms of fluoroquinolone resistance in genetically related strains of *Staphylococcus aureus*. *Antimicrob. Agents Chemother.* 41: 2733-2737.

[46] Muñoz Bellido J.L., Alonso Manzanares M.A., Yagüe Guirao G., Gutiérrez Zufiaurre M.N., Toldos M.C., Segovia Hernández M., Garcia-Rodríguez J.A. (1999) In vitro activities of 13 fluoroquinolones against *Staphylococcus aureus* isolates with characterized mutations in *gyrA*, *gyrB*, *grlA*, and *norA* and against wild-type isolates. *Antimicrob. Agents Chemother.* 43: 966-968.

[47] Kaatz G.W., Seo S.M. (1995) Inducible NorA-mediated multidrug resistance in *Staphylococcus aureus*. *Antimicrob. Agents Chemother.* 39: 2650-2655.

[48] Lee E.W., Chen J., Huda M.N., Kuroda T., Mizushima T., Tsuchiya T. (2003) Functional cloning and expression of *emeA*, and characterization of EmeA, a multidrug efflux pump from *Enterococcus faecalis*. *Biol. Pharm. Bull.* 26: 266-270.

[49] Spengler G., Martins A., Schelz Z., Rodrigues L., Aagaard L., Martins M., Costa S.S., Couto I., Viveiros M., Kristiansen J.E., Fanning S., Molnar J. and Amaral L. Characterisation of intrinsic efflux activity of *Enterococcus faecalis* ATCC29212 by a semi-automated ethidium bromide method. Accepted by *In Vivo*.

[50] Viveiros M., Martins A., Paixão L., Rodrigues L., Martins M., Couto I., Fähnrich E., Kern W.V., Amaral L. (2008) Demonstration of intrinsic efflux activity of *Escherichia coli* K-12 AG100 by an automated ethidium bromide method. *Int. J. Antimicrob. Agents* 31: 458-462.

[51] Lee E.W., Huda M.N., Kuroda T., Mizushima T., Tsuchiya T. (2003) EfrAB, an ABC multidrug efflux pump in *Enterococcus faecalis*. *Antimicrob. Agents Chemother.* 47: 3733-3738.

[52] Davidson A.L., Dassa E., Orelle C., Chen J. (2008) Structure, function, and evolution of bacterial ATP-binding cassette systems. *Microbiol. Mol. Biol. Rev.* 72: 317-364.

[53] Zakharov S.D., Li X., Red'ko T.P., Dilley R.A. (1996) Calcium binding to the subunit c of *E. coli* ATP-synthase and possible functional implications in energy coupling. *J. Bioenerg. Biomembr.* 28: 483-494.

[54] Thanassi D.G. and Hultgren S.J. (2000) Multiple pathways allow protein secretion across the bacterial outer membrane. *Curr. Opin. Cell Biol.* 12: 420-430.

[55] Borges-Walmsley M.I., McKeegan K.S., Walmsley A.R. (2003) Structure and function of efflux pumps that confer resistance to drugs. *Biochem. J.* 376: 313-338.

[56] Delepelaire P. (2004) Type I secretion in gram-negative bacteria. *Biochim. Biophys. Acta*; 1694: 149-161.

[57] Murakami S., Nakashima R., Yamashita E., Matsumoto T. and Yamaguchi A. (2006) Crystal structures of a multidrug transporter reveal a functionally rotating mechanism. *Nature* 443: 173-179.

[58] Akama H., Matsuura T., Kashiwagi S., Yoneyama H., Narita S., Tsukihara T., Nakagawa A. and Nakae T. (2004) Crystal structure of the membrane fusion protein,

MexA, of the multidrug transporter in *Pseudomonas aeruginosa*. *J. Biol. Chem.* 279: 25939-25942.

[59] Higgins M.K., Bokma E., Koronakis E., Hughes C., Koronakis V. (2004) Structure of the periplasmic component of a bacterial drug efflux pump. *Proc. Natl. Acad. Sci. U.S.A.* 101: 9994-9999.

[60] Fernandez-Recio J., Walas F., Federici L., Venkatesh Pratap J., Bavro V.N., Miguel R.N., Mizuguchi K. and Luisi B. (2004) A model of a transmembrane drug-efflux pump from Gram-negative bacteria. *FEBS Lett.* 578: 5-9.

[61] Lobedanz S., Bokma E., Symmons M.F., Koronakis E., Hughes C. and Koronakis V. (2007) A periplasmic coiled-coil interface underlying TolC recruitment and the assembly of bacterial drug efflux pumps. *Proc. Natl. Acad. Sci. U.S.A.* 104: 4612-4617.

[62] Pietras Z., Bavro V.N., Furnham N., Pellegrini-Calace M., Milner-White E.J. and Luisi B.F. (2008) Structure and mechanism of drug efflux machinery in Gram negative bacteria. *Curr. Drug Targets* 9: 719-728.

[63] Chopra I., O'Neill A.J., Miller K. (2003) The role of mutators in the emergence of antibiotic-resistant bacteria. *Drug Resist. Updat.* 6: 137-145.

[64] Viveiros M., Martins M., Martins A., Rodrigues L., Couto I., Fanning S. and Amaral L. (2008) New methods for the identification of efflux mediated MDR bacteria, genetic assessment of regulators and efflux pump constituents, characterization of efflux systems and screening for inhibitors of efflux pumps. *Curr. Drug Targets* 9: 760-778.

[65] Martins M., Santos B., Couto I., Viveiros M., Pages J.M., Molnar M., Cruz A. and Amaral L. (2006) Instrument free method for the demonstration and assessment of efflux pumps that cause bacterial resistance. *In Vivo* 20: 657-664.

[66] Mahamoud A., Chevalier J., Alibert-Franco S., Kern W.V., Pagès J.M. (2007) Antibiotic efflux pumps in Gram-negative bacteria: the inhibitor response strategy. *J. Antimicrob. Chemother.* 59: 1223-1229.

[67] Nikaido E., Yamaguchi A., Nishino K. (2008) AcrAB multidrug efflux pump regulation in *Salmonella enterica* serovar Typhimurium by RamA in response to environmental signals. *J. Biol. Chem.* 283: 24245-24253.

[68] Dowd S.E., Killinger-Mann K., Brashears M., Fralick J. (2008) Evaluation of gene expression in a single antibiotic exposure-derived isolate of *Salmonella enterica* typhimurium 14028 possessing resistance to multiple antibiotics. *Foodborne Pathog. Dis.* 5: 205-221.

[69] Perez J.C., Groisman E.A. (2007) Acid pH activation of the PmrA/PmrB two-component regulatory system of *Salmonella enterica*. *Mol. Microbiol.* 63: 283-293.

[70] Murata T., Tseng W., Guina T., Miller S.I., Nikaido H. (2007) PhoPQ-mediated regulation produces a more robust permeability barrier in the outer membrane of *Salmonella enterica* serovar typhimurium. *J. Bacteriol.* 189: 7213-7222.

[71] Gunn J.S. (2008) The Salmonella PmrAB regulon: lipopolysaccharide modifications, antimicrobial peptide resistance and more. *Trends Microbiol.* 16: 284-290.

[72] see: http://www.rpi.edu/dept/bcbp/molbiochem/MBWeb/mb1/part2/f1fo.htm for complete review of scheme.

[73] Teh J.S., Yano T., Rubin H. (2007) Type II NADH: menaquinone oxidoreductase of *Mycobacterium tuberculosis*. *Infect. Disord. Drug Targets* 7: 169-181.

[74] Tran S.L., Cook G.M. (2005) The F1Fo-ATP synthase of *Mycobacterium smegmatis* is essential for growth. *J. Bacteriol.* 187: 5023-5028.

In: Multiple Drug Resistance
Editors: A. Meszaros, G. Balogh, pp. 245-248
ISBN: 978-1-60741-595-4

Chapter XIII

Antimicrobial Resistance: Evolutionary Roots

Roberto Manfredi **[*]** ***and Leonardo Calza***
Department of Internal Medicine, Aging, and Nephrologic Diseases, Division of Infectious Diseases, " Alma Mater Studiorum" University of Bologna, S. Orsola-Malpighi Hospital, Bologna, Italy

Keywords: Antimicrobial resistance, spread, evolutionary perspective.

The extraordinary capacity of a number of bacterial organisms to develop resistance to antibiotic compounds remains a hot topic on the minds of doctors, hospital staff, reporters, and the community since several years. It is also heralded as a textbook example of "Darwinian evolution" continuously in action [1, 2]. As a consequence, these multiresistant bacteria are being studied also by "evolutionary" scientists, with the hope that they will reveal secrets or trace a pathway as to how molecules-to-man evolution could have happened [2, 3].

Basically, antibiotics are natural substances secreted by bacteria and fungi in order to kill other bacteria that are competing for limited nutrients; in fact, the majority of present antibiotics are synthetic derivatives of these natural products. Scientists are dismayed to discover that some bacteria have become resistant to antibiotics, mostly through various genomic (chromosomal-, plasmid-, or transposon-carried) mutations.

Changes in natural echosystems, including the release of large amounts of antimicrobial agents in the environment as happened in the last decades, might act on the population dynanmics of microorganisms too, including the selection of resistance determinants, with the visible consequences for human health, in terms of spread of multiresistant organisms in the community and especially in hospital facilities [3].

[*] Correspondence: Roberto Manfredi, MD. Associate Professor of Infectious Diseases, University of Bologna. c/o Infectious Diseases, S. Orsola Hospital. Via Massarenti 11. I-40138 Bologna, Italy. Telephone: +39-051-6363355. Telefax: +39-051-343500. E-mail: Roberto.manfredi@unibo.it

Hospitals have become a breeding ground for antibiotic resistant bacteria, and all microorganisms as whole. In these settings, bacteria proliferate in an "artificial" environment filled with sick people who have some underlying cause of immunodeficiency and concurrent diseases, and where antibiotics have eliminated competing bacteria that are not resistant to used compounds [3].

However, the history learns that bacteria which became resistant to modern antibiotics have even been found in the frozen bodies of people who died long before those antibiotics were discovered or synthesized [4].

As known, antibiotics were first discovered through a providential experiment conducted by Dr. Fleming in late 1920s. His work eventually led to the large-scale production of penicillin from the mold *Penicillium notatum* in the 1940s. Almost concurrently, as early as the late 1940s, resistant strains of penicillin-resistant bacteria began to appear [5]. Currently, it is estimated that over 70% of the different species of bacteria that cause hospital-acquired infections prove resistant to at least one of the antibiotics currently used to treat them [6].

Antibiotic resistance continues to expand for a very broad spectrum of reasons, including over-prescription of antibiotics by physicians, non-completion of prescribed antibiotic treatments by patients, self-prescription of antibiotics by patients themselves, use of antibiotics in animals as growth enhancers, increased international travel, and poor hospital hygiene [5].

In extreme synthesis, bacteria are known to develop antimicrobial resistance through two primary ways:

- By gene mutation, and
- By using a built-in design feature to swap DNA (called horizontal gene transfer); by this last way, bacteria have the possibility to transfer resistance genes among different species which share the same environment.

An antibiotic kills a bacterial cell by simply disrupting an essential structure, or by blocking a critical metabolic function [2]. Antibiotic resistance of bacteria also encompasses a loss of structural and/or functional systems. Anyway, on a general basis the evolutionary mechanisms require a gain of functional systems for bacteria, to evolve into more adaptive organism. For instance, an antibiotic may bind to a specific bacterial protein, so that this last protein cannot function properly. The normal protein is usually involved in copying the DNA, making proteins, or building the bacterial cell wall, all necessary mechanisms for bacteria, to grow and reproduce themselves. If the bacteria have a mutation in the DNA which encodes for one of those proteins, the compound cannot bind to the altered protein; as a direct consequence, the mutant bacteria survive and multiplicate. In the presence of antibiotics, the process of natural selection will occur, favoring the survival and reproduction of the mutant bacteria [2, 3]. Obviously, the mutant bacteria are better able to survive in the presence of the stated antibiotic(s), and will continue to cause illness in the patient, and to increase morbidity and mortality rates.

Although the mutant bacteria can survive well in the hospital environment, from an evolutionary point of view every change occurs at some cost. Actually, i.e. the altered protein is less efficient in performing its normal function, making the bacteria less fit in an specific environment, without the inducing antibiotics [2, 3]. Typically, the non-mutant bacteria are better able to compete for resources and reproduce faster than the mutant form. However, also adaptive mechanisms are activated by resistant microorganisms: the inhibition of some penicillin-binding proteins has been shown to elicit compensative responses in surviving colonies of *Pseudomonas aeruginosa* [7].

Bacteria can also become antibiotic-resistant by gaining mutated DNA from other bacteria. But this still is not an example of evolution in action. No new DNA is generated (a requirement for molecules-to-organism evolution), it is just DNA sequences moving around. However, this mechanism of exchanging DNA is necessary for bacteria to survive in extreme or rapidly changing environments like hospitals or nursing home facilities, or in experimental conditions [2, 8].

The mechanisms of bacterial mutations and natural selection aid microorganism populations in becoming resistant to antibiotics. However, mutation and natural selection also result in bacteria with defective proteins that have lost their normal functions. In general, the evolution process requires a gain of functional systems for bacteria to evolve [2, 3]. Mutation and natural selection, thought to be the driving forces of evolution, only lead to a loss of functional systems. Therefore, antibiotic resistance of bacteria is not an example of "evolution in action", but rather variation within a bacterial kind. It is also a testimony to the wonderful design "the destiny" gave to bacteria, master adapters and survivors in a sin-cursed world [2, 3].

Actually, evolutionary medicine is relevant also to family practice and family physician training, in a wide spectrum of perspectives [9]. Its incorporation into medical training and practice is underway, since its potential scientific burden may be supported by the generation of testable hypotheses and practical applications in relation to both disease pathogenesis, prevention, and treatment [1, 9].

References

[1] Alpert, JS. In Medicine, signs of evolution are ever-present. *Am. J. Med*, 2006, 119, 291.

[2] Gilmore, MS. The molecular basis of antibiotic resistance: where Newton meets Darwin. *Int. J. Med. Microbiol*, 2002, 292, 65.

[3] Martínez, JL. Antibiotics and antibiotic resistance genes in natural environments. *Science*, 2008, 321, 365-7.

[4] Bacterial antibiotic resistance: proof of evolution? www.apologeticspress.org/ articles/439.

[5] Antibiotic resistance: How did we get to this? flemingforum.org.uk/slides/antibiotic_ resistance.pdf.

[6] The problem of antimicrobial resistance, National Institute of Allergy and Infectious Diseases. www.niaid.nih.gov/factsheets/antimicro.htm/.

[7] Blázquez, J; Gómez- Gómez, JM; Oliver, A; Juan, C; Kapur, V; Martín, S. PBP3 inhibition elicits adaptive responses in *Pseudomonas aeruginosa*. *Mol. Microbiol*, 2006, 62, 84-9.

[8] Is natural selection the same thing as evolution? In "*The New Answers Book*", Ken Ham Ed., Master Books, *Green Forest, Arkansas*, 2006.

[9] Naugler, CT. Evolutionary medicine: update on the relevance to family practice. *Can. Fam. Physician*, 2008, 54, 1265-9.

Chapter Sources

Chapters 12 and 13 were also published in "Antibiotic Resistance: Causes and Risk Factors, Mechanisms and Alternatives", edited by Adriel R. Bonilla and Kaden P. Muniz, Nova Science Publishers. It was submitted for appropriate modifications in an effort to encourage wider dissemination of research.

Index

A

absorption, 101, 102, 104, 107, 121, 122
acceptor, 113
accuracy, 18, 20
acetaminophen, x, 99, 102, 127
acetylation, 178, 192
acid, x, 14, 19, 68, 69, 73, 76, 81, 83, 96, 99, 102, 105, 116, 117, 119, 127, 130, 131, 147, 149, 151, 155, 156, 157, 159, 160, 166, 169, 170, 172, 175, 176, 178, 180, 190, 192, 205, 215, 237, 238
acidic, xi, 131, 153
acidification, 37, 131, 147, 148, 149, 151
acidity, 132, 147, 148, 149
Acinetobacter, vii, viii, xiii, 31, 32, 33, 34, 35, 36, 37, 38, 39, 40, 41, 42, 43, 45, 46, 47, 48, 49, 50, 51, 52, 53, 54, 55, 56, 57, 58, 59, 60, 61, 62, 63, 75, 86, 90, 94, 154, 159, 163, 164, 165, 166, 170, 213, 214, 217, 240
acne, 171
actinomycetes, 75
activation, xiii, 3, 12, 121, 132, 133, 134, 156, 162, 220, 225, 237, 238, 243
activation energy, 133, 134
active site, 76
active transport, 67, 107, 157
acute, ix, 1, 2, 3, 4, 5, 6, 7, 9, 10, 11, 13, 14, 15, 16, 17, 18, 19, 20, 22, 23, 24, 25, 26, 27, 28, 29, 33, 50, 171, 197, 199, 211
acute leukemia, ix, 1, 2, 6, 14, 15, 16, 17, 19, 20, 22, 26, 29
acute lymphoblastic leukemia, ix, 1, 2, 3, 4, 5, 7, 9, 11, 13, 14, 22, 23, 24, 25, 26, 27, 28, 29
acute myeloblastic leukemia, 2
acute myelogenous leukemia, 27
acute myeloid leukaemia, 23, 26
acute myeloid leukemia, ix, 1, 3, 6, 7, 10, 14, 18, 23, 24, 25, 26, 27, 28, 211
acute renal failure, 171
acylation, 37
adaptation, 226, 231
adenocarcinoma, 148, 150, 205
adenosine, 148, 184
adenosine deaminase, 184
adhesion, 37, 174, 184
adjustment, 39, 112, 113
administration, xii, 9, 11, 39, 46, 55, 103, 104, 106, 107, 108, 109, 110, 127, 131, 162, 173, 177, 182, 195, 196, 199, 216
adolescents, 6, 11, 22
adrenal gland, 101
adriamycin, 131
adult, ix, 1, 5, 6, 7, 11, 12, 13, 18, 20, 23, 24, 25, 27, 28, 62, 101
adult population, 101
adult T-cell, 28
adulthood, 3, 4
adults, ix, 1, 2, 4, 7, 11, 12, 13, 14, 16, 22, 23, 26, 33, 59, 62, 100, 199, 201
aerobic, 32, 163
aerodigestive tract, 46
Afghanistan, 33, 50, 51, 159
agar, 233, 234, 235, 236, 237
age, 2, 4, 5, 7, 12, 21, 24, 27, 40, 47, 85, 106
agent, xiii, 4, 6, 17, 40, 42, 45, 47, 55, 56, 71, 81, 122, 131, 146, 165, 179, 183, 184, 189, 192, 193, 203, 210, 216, 225, 226, 228, 231, 234, 238

agents, x, xi, xiii, 6, 11, 16, 17, 19, 23, 32, 38, 39, 40, 42, 43, 45, 46, 54, 57, 66, 67, 68, 69, 71, 78, 80, 83, 85, 96, 99, 101, 130, 149, 151, 153, 162, 163, 165, 168, 170, 171, 173, 185, 188, 203, 204, 206, 209, 226, 237, 245
aging, 121
agricultural, 77, 168
agriculture, 154
aid, 26, 179, 217, 247
AIDS, 124
alanine, 175, 176, 188, 189
Albino, 188
alcohol, 47, 48
alcoholics, 48
alkaline, xi, 130, 131
alkalinity, 131
alkaloids, 150, 204, 210, 211
alkalosis, 130
alkylating agents, 20
alleles, 104
allergic reaction, 39
alternative, xii, 43, 45, 56, 61, 73, 81, 100, 112, 125, 130, 158, 167, 168, 170, 173, 179, 183, 240
alternative medicine, 100
alternatives, 175, 187, 240
Alzheimer's disease, 105, 123, 146
amide, 176
amiloride, 149
amino, 45, 74, 76, 81, 151, 168, 175, 176, 180, 205
amino acid, 74, 76, 81, 176, 180, 205
aminoglycosides, 34, 35, 36, 38, 41, 42, 44, 48, 71, 83, 97, 155, 157, 160, 215
AML, ix, 1, 3, 4, 5, 6, 7, 10, 12, 13, 14, 16, 18, 20, 23, 26, 27
amsacrine, 8, 10
Amsterdam, 163
anaerobes, 155
anesthetics, 151
aneuploidy, xiii, 219, 220, 221
angiogenesis, 146, 147
angiography, 33
animal models, 42, 170, 171, 197
animal studies, xii, 39, 45, 195, 196
animals, xii, 77, 78, 87, 89, 93, 94, 95, 164, 167, 170, 174, 178, 179, 181, 182, 183, 184, 200, 210, 246
antagonism, 126
antagonistic, x, 99, 105
antagonists, 157
anthrax, 181, 185
anti-apoptotic, 145
antibacterial, xii, 41, 45, 159, 166, 167, 173, 174, 175, 187, 190, 191, 193, 239
antibiotic, x, xi, xii, xiii, 31, 34, 36, 37, 41, 42, 45, 48, 54, 55, 57, 60, 65, 68, 69, 70, 71, 74, 76, 77, 78, 81, 82, 83, 84, 86, 87, 88, 89, 90, 92, 93, 94, 95, 96, 97, 153, 154, 155, 156, 157, 158, 159, 161, 162, 163, 164, 165, 167, 168, 173, 175, 182, 183, 184, 186, 188, 192, 193, 217, 225, 226, 227, 231, 238, 239, 240, 243, 245, 246, 247
antibody, 184, 192
anticancer, x, 17, 18, 99, 101, 129, 131, 132, 134, 145, 150, 211
anti-cancer, xii, 203, 204, 210
anticoagulant, 101
anticoagulants, x, 99, 101
antidepressant, 105, 121, 123
antidepressants, x, 99, 101, 123
antigen, 176, 193, 200, 201
anti-HIV, x, 99, 101, 191
antimetabolites, 9, 25
antimicrobial protein, 187
antimicrobial therapy, xi, 33, 45, 57, 61, 62, 153
antineoplastic, 152, 177, 192
antineoplastic agents, 152
antitumor, 122, 130, 146
anti-tumor, 177
antitumor agent, 130
anxiety, 116
apoptosis, 2, 6, 9, 16, 17, 19, 20, 21, 27, 130, 131, 147, 148, 149, 152, 211
apoptotic, 18
application, xiv, 226
arabinoside, 11
arginine, 240
Arkansas, 248
arrest, 223
ascites, 146, 150
Asia, 38, 54
aspiration, 46
aspirin, x, 99, 101
assessment, ix, xiv, 1, 11, 22, 26, 43, 54, 55, 60, 86, 92, 119, 226, 233, 238, 243
astrocytoma, 220, 222
asymmetry, 135, 143, 151, 152
Athens, 153
atmospheric pressure, 128

ATP, ix, xiii, 1, 2, 101, 120, 131, 204, 211, 219, 229, 238, 242, 244
ATPase, 131, 132, 145, 146, 151, 229
attachment, 172, 176, 178
Australia, 99
autolysis, 188
avoidance, 46, 112

B

BAC, 114, 115, 116, 117
bacilli, 31, 32, 48, 54, 57, 66, 163, 179, 181
bacillus, 185, 194, 196, 198
Bacillus, 171, 175, 180, 181, 187, 188, 190, 192, 193, 194
Bacillus subtilis, 188
bacteremia, 31, 42, 46, 47, 57, 58, 61, 62, 88, 90, 192
bacterial cells, 37, 70, 74, 155, 156, 171, 175
bacterial contamination, 186
bacterial infection, xii, xiv, 40, 54, 55, 56, 58, 154, 167, 171, 179, 180, 184, 185, 194, 226, 227, 238
bacterial strains, 69, 162, 168, 184, 226
bacteriocin, 184
bacteriocins, 191
bacteriolysis, xii, 167, 168, 169, 171, 174, 175, 179, 182, 189, 190
bacteriophage, 173, 184, 185, 186, 187, 188, 189, 190, 191, 192, 193
bacteriophages, 156, 158, 168, 171, 179, 180, 184, 185, 186, 189, 194
Bacteriophages, xii, 167, 168, 187
bacteriostatic, 40, 41, 66, 68, 81, 216
bacterium, xiii, 69, 156, 173, 179, 181, 182, 188, 213, 214, 216, 226, 231, 233, 237, 238
Badia, 60
barrier, xi, 32, 34, 44, 45, 101, 120, 133, 135, 136, 137, 154, 197, 210, 243
basic fibroblast growth factor, 147
B-cell, 7
B-CLL cells, 12
Belgium, 88
bending, 134, 135, 136
beta lactam, xi, 153
beta lactamase, xi, 153
Betel nut, 115, 127
bile, 101
binding, xiii, 2, 34, 36, 37, 38, 40, 41, 44, 53, 67, 68, 69, 93, 101, 103, 111, 120, 123, 126, 133, 148, 150, 156, 157, 160, 166, 176, 178, 179, 181, 204, 210, 211, 215, 219, 222, 242, 247
bioavailability, 104, 107, 115, 121, 124, 128, 142
biocontrol, 171
biofilm formation, 215
bioinformatics, 183
biological weapons, 181
biosynthesis, 19, 163, 169, 174
biotechnology, 96
biotic, 168
bleeding, 101, 106, 115, 127
blocks, 68
blood, 7, 32, 41, 44, 45, 85, 95, 101, 106, 111, 114, 116, 120, 124, 210
blood clot, 101
blood flow, 111
blood glucose, 210
blood pressure, 106, 210
blood-brain barrier, 32, 44, 45, 101, 120, 210
bloodstream, 50, 61, 89
body mass, 196, 197, 199
body mass index, 196, 197, 199
body weight, xii, 195, 199, 210
bolus, 108, 109
bone marrow, 6, 9, 21, 26
botulinum, 173
bovine, 181, 204
brain, 45, 101, 105, 120, 122, 123, 220
brain injury, 123
brainstem, 123
BRCA, 221
breast cancer, xii, xiii, 2, 148, 203, 204, 209, 211, 219, 221, 222
broad spectrum, xiii, 38, 68, 76, 91, 174, 203, 246
bronchoconstriction, 40
budding, 133, 134
Burkholderia, 76, 154
burn, 43, 63
bypass, 68, 136, 157

C

caffeine, 103, 110, 122
calcium channel blocker, 11
calorie, 199
Campylobacter jejuni, 170, 171
Canada, 33, 184
cancer, x, xi, xiii, 2, 3, 4, 14, 17, 22, 26, 27, 129, 130, 131, 132, 143, 144, 145, 146, 147, 148, 149, 150, 204, 211, 219, 220, 221, 222

cancer cells, xiii, 14, 17, 22, 130, 131, 132, 143, 145, 148, 149, 150, 219, 220, 221
cancer treatment, 204
candidates, xii, 113, 167, 168, 171
capsule, 37, 181
carbohydrate, 19, 192
carcinogens, 120
carcinoma, 103, 148, 222
caries, 180, 181, 193
carrier, 25
casein, 188
cassettes, 69, 70, 73, 87, 88, 90, 93, 96, 98, 158
catabolism, 3, 9, 228
catalase, 32, 188
catalysis, 220
catalytic activity, 128
catalytic properties, 190
catheterization, 80, 84
catheters, 33, 43, 45, 47, 55
cation, 142
cattle, 89, 90, 96, 158
causality, 196, 197
causation, 134
CCR, 10
CDC, 51, 66, 71, 80, 88
CDK2, 220
CDK4, 220
CDKs, 220
cDNA, 14, 19, 26, 103, 110, 120, 128, 177, 204
cell adhesion, 174
cell culture, 5, 23, 185
cell cycle, 2, 3, 16, 18, 21, 220, 221
cell death, 18, 132, 149, 174, 221
cell division, 130
cell growth, 19
cell line, xii, 140, 147, 148, 149, 203, 204, 208, 209, 211
cell lines, 140, 147, 148, 149, 211
cell membranes, 147, 151
cell metabolism, 130
cell surface, 169, 172
cementum, 180
Centers for Disease Control, 51, 63, 88
central nervous system, 2, 9, 56, 59, 118
cephalosporin, 82, 83, 84
cerebrospinal fluid, 59
CGT, 151
changing environment, 247
channel blocker, 11
channels, 34, 74
chemical weapons, 157
chemicals, ix, 113, 120, 204
chemoresistance, 148
chemotherapeutic agent, 16, 209
chemotherapeutic drugs, 16, 132, 145, 148, 149
chemotherapy, xiii, 2, 3, 4, 6, 9, 11, 13, 14, 16, 17, 18, 20, 27, 130, 145, 146, 147, 173, 177, 198, 201, 204, 210, 219, 220
chest, 40
chickens, 79, 92, 93, 98
childhood, 2, 3, 4, 5, 6, 7, 8, 9, 10, 12, 13, 16, 17, 19, 20, 22, 23, 24, 25, 26, 27, 28, 211
children, ix, 1, 2, 3, 4, 6, 7, 9, 11, 12, 13, 14, 17, 20, 23, 24, 25, 90, 91, 97, 171, 192
China, 98, 99, 164, 195, 203, 210
chlorpromazine, 228, 234
cholangiocarcinoma, 148
cholera, 172, 173
cholesterol, 196, 200
chromatography, 128
chromosomal abnormalities, 5, 25
chromosomal alterations, 73
chromosome, x, 7, 8, 9, 10, 24, 65, 69, 70, 91, 160, 214, 242
chromosomes, 5, 6, 8, 18, 21, 25, 69, 70, 158, 220
chronic lymphocytic leukemia, 12
chronic obstructive pulmonary disease, 47
cimetidine, 105
ciprofloxacin, 42, 78, 84, 88, 160, 168, 214, 217, 227, 234
cisplatin, 131, 147, 148, 150, 223
Cisplatin, 148
cisplatin resistance, 147, 148
cladribine, 12
classes, xi, 11, 34, 38, 42, 69, 71, 76, 79, 83, 84, 85, 153, 155, 160, 169, 210, 214, 216, 226
classical, 2, 20, 21, 107, 125, 134, 139, 157, 187
classification, 3, 14, 19, 20, 26, 28, 32, 94
clinical syndrome, 62
clinical trial, 100, 201
clonality, 48
clone, 160, 165, 220
cloning, 120, 183, 222, 242
clusters, 88, 160
CML, 3
CNS, 5, 44, 118, 120
coatings, 191
coding, 87, 97
cohort, 18, 21, 23, 42, 56, 61, 196

coil, 243
colitis, 39
colon, 101, 148, 149, 158, 204
colon cancer, 148, 149
colonisation, 84
colonization, 33, 37, 43, 45, 46, 47, 48, 50, 51, 63, 84, 92, 165, 171, 177, 179, 192, 193, 216
colonizers, 84
coma, 105, 106
combination therapy, 40, 58
commensals, 158
communication, 17, 19, 20, 77
communities, 70
community, x, 33, 47, 62, 65, 66, 77, 79, 80, 81, 86, 87, 88, 89, 93, 158, 164, 176, 241, 245
co-morbidities, 81
compaction, 68
competition, 155
complete remission, 6, 10, 18, 21
compliance, xi, 33, 77, 154, 162
complications, 199
components, 19, 68, 101, 102, 110, 112, 121, 128, 134, 170, 185, 203
composition, 94, 150, 186
compounds, xiii, 66, 74, 157, 163, 175, 214, 226, 238, 245, 246
concentration, 10, 25, 34, 35, 39, 74, 77, 104, 105, 106, 107, 108, 111, 112, 114, 116, 118, 119, 131, 142, 144, 151, 157, 177, 205, 206, 208, 210, 216, 228, 229, 231, 233, 234, 235, 236, 237
conflict, 51
confusion, 105, 116, 174, 175
coniferous, 211
conjugation, 70, 102, 107, 160
constraints, 135, 152
consumption, xi, 47, 153
contaminated food, 182
contamination, 32, 48, 63, 163, 172, 186, 194
contraceptives, x, 99, 101, 105, 106, 115, 127
control, ix, xii, 31, 32, 33, 35, 48, 49, 50, 51, 54, 55, 56, 59, 61, 63, 65, 82, 83, 89, 104, 147, 154, 163, 175, 178, 186, 191, 192, 195, 196, 197, 198, 199, 200, 205, 206, 207, 208, 209
control group, 208, 209
controlled studies, 81
controlled trials, xii, 195
conversion, xii, 173, 186, 187, 195, 198, 199, 202
correlation, ix, 1, 6, 7, 144, 150
correlations, 9, 90, 107
cortisol, 103
cost-effective, 183
costs, x, 60, 65, 81, 178
cough, 40
Coumadin, 101
coumarins, 101
cows, 174
CRC, 53
C-reactive protein, 199
critically ill, 41, 46, 50, 55, 58, 61, 165
cross-sectional, 196, 197
CRP, 2, 203
crystal structure, 113, 126, 151
CSF, 43, 45
C-terminal, 176
culture, 5, 23, 49, 144, 177, 180, 182, 185, 197, 198, 202
curing, 220
cyanide, 228
cycling, 163, 220
cyclins, 20, 220
cyclophosphamide, 9, 12, 192
cyclosporine, x, 11, 99, 101, 104, 106, 110, 112, 124
cyclosporine A, 118
cystic fibrosis, 55, 61
cytochrome, x, 99, 100, 101, 119, 120, 121, 122, 125, 126, 127, 128
cytogenetics, 2, 4, 16, 18, 26, 28
cytokine, 38, 200
cytokinesis, 220, 221
cytometry, xii, 9, 203, 205
cytoplasm, 139
cytoplasmic membrane, 67, 157, 170, 227
cytosine, 11
cytoskeleton, 20, 149
cytosol, 131, 132, 140, 147
cytosolic, xi, 130, 132, 142, 143, 144, 145, 146, 147
cytotoxic, 6, 11, 149, 206, 209, 211, 220, 221
cytotoxic agents, 6, 206, 209
cytotoxicity, xii, 10, 132, 149, 150, 203, 204, 209, 210, 223
cytotoxins, 204

D

Darwinian evolution, 245
de novo, 10

death, xiii, 18, 44, 68, 80, 132, 149, 174, 178, 198, 201, 219, 221
decolonization, 48
decontamination, 46, 63, 163, 171, 179
defense, 156, 163, 174, 177, 182, 196, 198, 199, 216
defenses, 37, 192
deficiency, 184, 196, 200
degradation, 164, 175, 176
degrading, 162, 175, 182, 190
dehydration, 134, 135, 140
delirium, 106, 114, 126
delivery, 93, 151
density, 138, 139, 140, 143, 144, 145, 182
dental caries, 181
dentistry, 187
dephosphorylation, 67
depolarization, 132
deposition, 237, 238
depression, 121, 126
deprivation, 196
derivatives, 11, 122, 150, 176, 226, 227, 239, 241, 245
dermatitis, 180
desiccation, 32
destruction, 68, 103, 181
detection, 52, 88, 96, 168, 179, 186, 193, 214
detoxification, 2
developed countries, 86, 100
developing countries, 77, 196, 240
dexamethasone, 7, 8, 11
diabetes, 47, 78, 196, 197, 200, 201
diabetic patients, 197, 201
diagnostic markers, 29
diaphoresis, 105
diarrhea, 39, 105
diarrhoea, xiii, 186, 213, 214, 216
diet, 121, 196, 200
dietary, 113, 121, 126, 199
differentiation, ix, 1, 148
diffusion, xi, xii, 79, 129, 133, 134, 135, 137, 139, 203, 204, 210, 216
diffusion time, 137
digestive tract, 48, 50, 63, 158
dimeric, 204
diphtheria, 173
disease-free survival, 9, 17
diseases, ix, x, xi, 1, 11, 129, 153, 155, 172, 179, 182, 216
disorder, 182
disposition, 211
distribution, 2, 4, 12, 13, 49, 70, 81, 85, 95, 101, 102, 121, 138, 174
disulfide, 122
diuretic, 106
diversity, 51, 89, 120, 158, 163, 179, 183
division, 41, 130
DNA, xi, 2, 3, 5, 9, 14, 15, 19, 20, 21, 26, 29, 32, 36, 68, 70, 71, 74, 88, 90, 97, 130, 151, 153, 156, 157, 158, 159, 160, 169, 171, 173, 180, 183, 192, 211, 216, 220, 221, 222, 246, 247
DNA damage, 68, 221
DNA repair, 2, 3, 19, 21
DNase, 84
doctors, 245
dopamine, 105, 126
dosage, 171, 173, 178
dosing, 39, 41, 60, 105, 106, 107
Down syndrome, 6
drug discovery, 16, 211, 239
drug efflux, 3, 104, 120, 210, 211, 227, 243
drug exposure, 3, 17
drug interaction, x, 5, 45, 99, 100, 102, 104, 105, 106, 107, 108, 109, 110, 111, 113, 117, 118, 119, 120, 122, 123, 125, 126, 127
drug metabolism, 2, 3, 103, 107, 120, 121, 125
drug resistance, ix, x, xi, xiii, 1, 2, 3, 4, 5, 6, 7, 8, 9, 10, 11, 12, 17, 18, 19, 20, 21, 22, 23, 24, 25, 27, 61, 65, 71, 77, 79, 81, 84, 87, 88, 90, 98, 130, 131, 133, 138, 142, 143, 144, 145, 153, 154, 155, 198, 211, 215, 219, 226
drug targets, 21, 156
drug therapy, 85
drug use, 139
drug-induced, 222
drug-related, 107
drug-resistant, 17, 24, 52, 54, 60, 66, 88, 150, 155, 166, 198
drugs, ix, x, xi, xii, xiii, 3, 5, 8, 10, 11, 13, 16, 17, 19, 25, 32, 42, 43, 44, 65, 66, 68, 77, 80, 81, 86, 99, 100, 101, 102, 103, 104, 105, 106, 107, 108, 109, 110, 111, 112, 113, 120, 121, 123, 125, 129, 131, 132, 133, 135, 136, 137, 138, 139, 140, 141, 142, 145, 148, 149, 150, 154, 155, 202, 203, 204, 208, 210, 215, 219, 220, 221, 242
duplication, 6, 90, 120
duration, 18, 40, 46, 82, 137, 162, 198

E

E. coli, x, xi, 65, 69, 70, 71, 73, 74, 75, 76, 78, 81, 82, 83, 153, 156, 157, 162, 170, 171, 174, 176, 183, 184, 185, 186, 187, 188, 190, 191, 192, 231, 232, 233, 234, 237, 239, 240, 242
ears, 174
Eastern Europe, 168
ecology, 164
economically disadvantaged, 240
EEG, 39
effluent, 77, 78, 88, 90
efflux transporter, 120, 211
efflux transporters, 120
egg, 187, 192
elderly, 6, 12, 105, 123
electrolytes, 142
electronic surveillance, 57
electrophoresis, 160, 193
elongation, 19, 68
emission, 205, 206
empyema, 47, 62
enantiomer, 101
encoding, xi, 52, 69, 71, 73, 88, 97, 104, 153, 156, 160, 165, 169, 187, 228
endocarditis, 47, 80, 180, 241
endocrine, 196
endocytosis, 133, 135, 137, 138, 139, 142, 145, 151
endonuclease, 149, 173
endothelial cell, 147
endotoxins, 170, 171, 173
energy, 133, 134, 135, 137, 140, 157, 197, 204, 227, 228, 230, 233, 234, 238, 242
enteritis, xiii, 180, 182, 213, 214
enterococci, 66, 80, 90, 93, 168, 184
environment, xi, 37, 48, 77, 78, 79, 92, 153, 156, 160, 178, 185, 233, 238, 245, 246
environmental conditions, 31
environmental contamination, 48, 63, 172
enzymatic, 35, 36, 158, 175, 178, 182, 189, 190
enzymatic activity, 35, 178
enzymes, xii, 2, 3, 9, 34, 35, 36, 37, 38, 51, 67, 71, 73, 74, 76, 88, 96, 102, 103, 106, 110, 113, 116, 119, 120, 121, 167, 174, 175, 176, 177, 178, 182, 183, 185, 189, 190, 192, 193, 194, 214, 229
epidemic, 33, 97, 160
epidemiology, xii, 32, 50, 51, 52, 53, 61, 62, 85, 89, 91, 92, 154, 165, 192, 196, 241
EPIs, 226, 228
epithelial cell, 37, 101, 177, 192
epitope, 192
erythrocyte, 151
Escherichia coli, 66, 79, 86, 87, 88, 89, 90, 91, 92, 93, 94, 95, 96, 97, 98, 154, 164, 170, 226, 231, 239, 242
esterase, 37, 176
estradiol, 115, 127
estrogen, 151
ethanol, 122
ethanol metabolism, 122
etiologic agent, 47
etiology, 145
etiopathogenesis, xi, 130, 146
eukaryotic cell, 68
Europe, 38, 41, 51, 54, 71, 77, 79, 80, 97, 154, 162
European Commission, 225
evolution, xi, 51, 86, 95, 153, 154, 156, 187, 193, 242, 245, 247, 248
excitation, 205, 206
excretion, 101, 102, 121
exocytosis, 135
experimental condition, 15, 247
exposure, 3, 17, 34, 41, 77, 79, 102, 104, 122, 155, 162, 178, 216, 226, 228, 231, 238, 239, 243
extraction, 14
extrapolation, 113, 125
extrusion, x, 129, 130, 131, 132, 133, 138, 144, 145, 149, 238
eyes, 62

F

fabrication, 14
factor analysis, 25
factorial, 202
faecal, 50, 79, 97
failure, 4, 16, 18, 20, 22, 28, 41, 46, 66, 71, 81, 82, 83, 104, 105, 131, 155, 171, 173, 186
familial, 96, 221
family, ix, 1, 68, 69, 71, 72, 73, 74, 75, 76, 78, 101, 120, 181, 211, 214, 220, 230, 247, 248
family physician, 247
farmers, 97
farms, 79, 94, 183
fatty acids, 238
FDA, 113, 170, 171

females, 128
fertilizer, 77, 79
fetal, 204
fetus, 210
fever, 43, 105, 180
fibroblast growth factor, 147
fibroblasts, 146
fibrosis, 55, 61
films, 191
fish, 89, 94, 170
fitness, 232, 233
flavonoids, 113, 126
floating, 92
flora, 78, 214
flow, xii, 9, 109, 111, 139, 203, 205
flow cytometry analysis, xii, 203
flow rate, 109, 111
fludarabine, 6, 12, 24
fluid, 59, 135, 151
fluidization, 151
fluorescence, 205, 206, 208, 209, 233, 236, 237
fluorogenic, 14
fluorometric, 103
fluoroquinolones, 36, 38, 42, 85, 156, 157, 160, 168, 214, 216, 227, 241, 242
flushing, 105
focusing, 17, 123
folate, 25, 157
food, 78, 87, 89, 91, 94, 95, 96, 123, 127, 157, 164, 170, 171, 174, 177, 179, 180, 181, 182, 184, 186, 196, 199
food intake, 199
food poisoning, 170, 180, 181, 182
food products, 172, 182, 186
food safety, 96, 171
France, 52
free radicals, 220
freeze-dried, 103
fruits, 171
FTC, 204, 205, 208
functional activation, 220
fungal, 174, 177
fungi, ix, 65, 66, 214, 245
Fusarium, 177
Fusarium oxysporum, 177
fusion, 7, 8, 24, 188, 230, 242

G

GABA, 105, 119, 123
GABAergic, 123
gas, 180
gas gangrene, 180
gastric, 46, 123, 216
gastrointestinal, 33, 104, 121, 125, 181
gastrointestinal tract, 33
gel, 160, 193
gender, 21, 106
gene, xi, 2, 4, 7, 8, 11, 14, 15, 16, 17, 18, 19, 20, 21, 22, 23, 24, 26, 27, 28, 29, 34, 36, 53, 69, 70, 71, 73, 74, 76, 86, 87, 88, 89, 90, 91, 93, 94, 96, 97, 98, 101, 120, 121, 153, 155, 156, 157, 158, 160, 161, 169, 170, 172, 173, 174, 180, 182, 183, 188, 189, 190, 191, 192, 211, 220, 221, 222, 223, 228, 231, 237, 238, 241, 243, 246
gene expression, 2, 4, 14, 15, 16, 17, 18, 19, 20, 21, 22, 23, 26, 27, 28, 29, 211, 222, 243
gene mapping, 120
gene therapy, 11
gene transfer, 157, 246
generation, 11, 71, 76, 78, 82, 145, 247
genetic abnormalities, 2, 10
genetic alteration, xiii, 18, 219
genetic factors, 105
genetic mutations, 157, 221
genetics, 96, 184, 188, 221
Geneva, 119, 199
genome, xi, 14, 15, 16, 92, 93, 153, 158, 169, 172, 183
genomes, 158, 187
genomic, 32, 88, 89, 113, 158, 173, 180, 187, 240, 245
genomics, 27, 187
genotype, 104
gentamicin, 74, 78, 83, 85, 88, 91, 97, 160, 214
Georgia, 168
Germany, 77, 92, 164, 203, 205
ginger, 117, 119, 127
gingivitis, 180, 181, 193
ginkgo biloba, 123, 126, 127, 128
ginseng, 101, 114, 119, 125, 126
glucocorticoids, 10, 25
glucose, 210, 228, 229, 234
glutamate, xi, 153
glutamate decarboxylase, xi, 153
glutamine, 205
glutathione, 119, 122
glycine, 189
glycolysis, 147

glycopeptides, 67, 71, 79, 81, 168
glycoprotein, xiii, 101, 152, 219
Glycoprotein, 2
glycoproteins, 120
glycoside, 175
glycosides, 45, 168
glycosyl, 176
glycosylated, 197
glycosylated hemoglobin, 197
gold, 43
gold standard, 43
gram negative, 31
gram-negative, 31, 36, 37, 38, 39, 40, 42, 45, 46, 50, 52, 54, 55, 56, 57, 58, 59, 60, 61, 66, 72, 75, 76, 81, 83, 87, 95, 96, 98, 154, 163, 170, 171, 173, 174, 175, 176, 178, 182, 188, 190, 192, 217, 227, 230, 237, 238, 239, 242, 243
gram-positive, 38, 66, 69, 72, 75, 87, 164, 168, 170, 171, 173, 174, 175, 176, 177, 178, 182, 191, 227, 228, 237, 240
granulocyte, 189
graph, 141
Greece, 153, 162, 165
ground water, 77
groups, 2, 4, 5, 14, 15, 16, 17, 18, 35, 76, 82, 103, 174, 176, 177, 179, 208, 209, 210
growth, 19, 32, 68, 77, 146, 147, 149, 157, 181, 182, 188, 192, 214, 222, 240, 244, 246
growth factor, 32, 147
gut, 92, 104, 108, 122, 216

H

half-life, 38, 41, 116, 119
handling, 113, 132, 139, 144, 145
hands, 50, 163
harm, 155
hazards, 156, 158
head trauma, 43
headache, 39, 115
health, ix, 31, 32, 33, 51, 65, 66, 93, 94, 96, 120, 123, 160, 179, 180, 184, 200, 245
heart, 106, 124
heavy smoking, 47
hematologic, 16
hematological, 216
hematopoietic, 16, 24
hematopoietic stem cell, 24
hemoglobin, 197
hemorrhage, 116
hemorrhages, 43
hepatocytes, 107, 110
herbal, x, 99, 100, 101, 102, 103, 104, 105, 106, 107, 108, 109, 110, 112, 113, 119, 121, 123, 124, 125, 128
herbal medicine, x, 99, 100, 101, 102, 119, 123
herbs, x, 99, 100, 101, 102, 103, 105, 106, 107, 108, 110, 112, 113, 114, 117, 121, 127
heterogeneity, 165, 197
heterogeneous, 7, 24, 32, 92, 113, 188
high risk, 2, 16, 18, 110
high-level, 35, 38, 52, 80, 86, 168, 226, 227, 231, 239
high-risk, 6, 16, 18, 23, 46
hip, 15
histone, 6, 20
HIV, ix, x, 65, 99, 101, 104, 112, 122, 177, 191, 198, 199, 201
HIV-1, 122
Holland, 185, 186
homeostasis, 147, 152
homology, 73, 120, 183
Hong Kong, 88, 89, 91, 195, 196
horizontal gene transfer, 157, 246
hormones, 200
hospital, x, 32, 33, 34, 38, 43, 46, 50, 51, 52, 60, 61, 62, 65, 66, 71, 77, 78, 79, 80, 81, 82, 83, 84, 86, 87, 89, 90, 91, 92, 93, 94, 95, 96, 98, 154, 158, 159, 160, 163, 165, 181, 200, 217, 241, 245, 246
hospital stays, 43
hospitalization, 45, 80, 84, 105
hospitalizations, 92
hospitalized, 74
hospitals, xi, 32, 33, 54, 61, 77, 78, 81, 86, 95, 96, 154, 160, 247
host, ix, xi, 37, 69, 70, 74, 75, 79, 91, 93, 153, 154, 169, 170, 172, 173, 174, 183, 185, 187, 192, 198, 233
household, 77, 93
households, 78
human, xii, xiii, 12, 17, 26, 33, 37, 42, 66, 73, 76, 77, 78, 84, 90, 92, 93, 94, 95, 96, 100, 101, 103, 107, 113, 119, 120, 121, 122, 123, 126, 127, 128, 131, 146, 147, 148, 149, 150, 154, 158, 164, 168, 171, 177, 178, 179, 180, 181, 182, 188, 190, 191, 192, 195, 196, 200, 204, 211, 219, 220, 221, 222, 223, 233, 245
human brain, 220
humanitarian, 198

humanity, 196
humans, x, 32, 33, 76, 87, 89, 93, 95, 96, 98, 99, 100, 101, 103, 110, 113, 114, 117, 121, 128, 164, 174, 181, 200
HUS, 171
hybridization, 14, 70
hydrazine, 103
hydro, 134
hydrogen, 113, 130, 142, 144, 145
hydrolases, xii, 167, 168, 174, 187
hydrolysis, 34, 76, 176, 204, 229, 238
hydrophilic, 134
hydrophilicity, 37
hydrophobic, 68, 113, 134, 135, 142, 210
hydrostatic pressure, 191, 192
hydroxyl, 176
hydroxylation, 104, 127
hygiene, ix, xi, 48, 153, 154, 163, 246
hyperactivity, 132
hypersensitivity, 39
hyphema, 114, 126
hypoglycemia, 116
hypothesis, xi, 130, 132, 154, 158, 222, 231
hypoxia, 147

I

icosahedral, 169
ICU, x, xiii, 50, 51, 63, 65, 85, 159, 160, 163, 164, 213, 216
identification, x, 16, 17, 28, 29, 32, 74, 76, 94, 99, 112, 113, 142, 158, 181, 183, 243
immune function, 168, 196, 200
immune response, 169, 178, 197, 201
immune system, 38, 173, 197
immunity, 171, 173, 186, 200
immunocompromised, 71, 84, 85, 92
immunodeficiency, 246
immunogenicity, 171, 175, 186
immunological, 197
immunology, 191
immunophenotype, 4, 7, 14, 16, 21, 24, 26
immunosuppressive, 211
immunotherapy, 6
implementation, 48, 163
in vitro, 5, 6, 7, 8, 10, 11, 12, 19, 23, 24, 25, 38, 42, 43, 54, 57, 58, 82, 86, 100, 103, 107, 110, 112, 113, 122, 125, 148, 151, 173, 177, 180, 211, 214, 217, 226, 241
in vivo, 5, 25, 37, 56, 100, 103, 107, 108, 110, 112, 113, 125, 147, 149, 173, 177, 178, 180, 233
inactivation, 68, 149, 156, 158, 159, 191, 221
inactive, 221
incidence, 4, 9, 45, 47, 80, 84, 85, 162, 200
incompatibility, 70
incubation, 140, 206, 221, 228
Indian, 87, 94, 97
indices, x, 99, 100, 101, 104, 112, 113
indole, 240
inducer, 103
induction, x, 4, 12, 16, 18, 75, 99, 101, 102, 107, 110, 114, 115, 116, 119, 122, 131, 154, 198, 211, 221, 223
induction chemotherapy, 18
industrial, 77, 90
infants, 4, 5, 7, 12, 33
Infants, 4, 6, 7
infection, xiv, 31, 33, 39, 41, 42, 43, 45, 46, 47, 48, 50, 53, 61, 63, 78, 79, 80, 81, 82, 83, 84, 85, 89, 92, 93, 154, 160, 162, 163, 170, 171, 172, 173, 184, 185, 188, 189, 192, 196, 199, 200, 216, 226, 233, 238
infections, ix, x, xi, xii, xiv, 31, 32, 33, 36, 37, 38, 39, 40, 41, 42, 43, 44, 46, 47, 49, 50, 51, 53, 54, 55, 56, 57, 58, 59, 60, 61, 62, 63, 65, 66, 69, 73, 74, 75, 76, 78, 80, 81, 82, 83, 84, 86, 91, 94, 96, 97, 98, 153, 154, 158, 162, 163, 165, 168, 170, 171, 172, 178, 180, 181, 182, 185, 186, 193, 215, 216, 217, 226, 227, 238, 240, 246
infectious, xi, 37, 66, 88, 153, 168, 171, 173, 183, 186, 189, 226
inflammation, 44, 45, 189
inflammatory, xii, 187, 195, 199
inflammatory response, xii, 195, 199
inflammatory responses, xii, 195, 199
influenza, ix, 65
ingestion, 126, 171
inhalation, 46, 181
inherited, 69, 221
inhibition, xii, 67, 68, 73, 101, 102, 103, 107, 108, 109, 110, 111, 113, 114, 115, 116, 119, 122, 124, 125, 131, 139, 146, 148, 203, 204, 205, 206, 208, 209, 211, 240, 247
inhibitor, 39, 40, 43, 76, 103, 105, 107, 108, 111, 116, 191, 192, 210, 220, 227, 240, 243

inhibitors, 6, 20, 103, 104, 105, 106, 112, 119, 122, 131, 145, 148, 150, 178, 192, 220, 226, 227, 239, 240, 241, 243
inhibitory, 104, 107, 108, 109, 110, 160, 187, 208, 226, 228
inhibitory effect, 104, 187
initiation, 68, 76, 130
injection, 169
injuries, 33
insects, 174
insertion, 133, 157, 158
insertion sequence, 157, 158
institutions, 34
insurance, 81
integrases, 89
integration, 91
intensive care unit, x, xi, xiii, 33, 40, 43, 46, 47, 49, 50, 58, 60, 63, 65, 97, 154, 160, 162, 163, 165, 166, 213
interaction, ix, x, 14, 15, 35, 99, 100, 102, 105, 106, 107, 108, 110, 112, 113, 114, 115, 116, 117, 119, 122, 123, 124, 125, 126, 137, 139, 140, 142, 145, 154, 164, 196
interactions, x, 5, 17, 22, 37, 99, 100, 101, 102, 104, 105, 106, 107, 110, 111, 112, 113, 118, 119, 120, 121, 122, 123, 125, 126, 133, 134, 152, 210
intercalation, 211
interface, 243
interfacial tension, 152
interference, xiii, 159, 205, 206, 219
interleukin, 18, 147
interstitial, 130, 230, 233
interval, 109, 110
intervention, 50, 196, 198
intestinal tract, 96
intestine, 101, 122, 210
intracerebral, 101, 127
intragastrically, 122
intramuscular, 170
intravascular, 47
intravenous, 39, 42, 43, 44, 45, 46, 55, 56, 59, 60, 107, 217
intravenously, 59, 169
intrinsic, 2, 12, 34, 35, 92, 108, 109, 134, 149, 155, 156, 227, 228, 233, 242
invasive, 43, 47, 58, 84
ion adsorption, 152
ion transport, 132, 148
ionic, 233
ionization, 128
ions, 142
Iraq, 50, 51, 159, 217
Ireland, 225
Irinotecan, 114
iron, 37, 53
isolation, xiii, 32, 40, 48, 50, 56, 84, 86, 161, 163, 181, 187, 213, 216
isoniazid, 201, 226
Isoquinoline, viii, 203
Italy, 160, 165, 213, 215, 217, 245

J

JAMA, 49, 93, 163
Jamaica, x, 65, 66, 71, 72, 79, 80, 82, 83, 85, 86, 87
Japan, 70, 71, 80, 88

K

K-12, 239, 242
karyotype, ix, 2, 7, 10, 13, 21
kidney, 41, 101, 106
killing, 81, 173, 177, 178, 179, 188, 191, 192, 221
kinase, 20, 147, 220, 237, 238
kinases, 220, 237
kinetic model, 107
kinetics, 133, 137, 138, 139, 142, 149
knockout, 121
Korea, 52, 91
Korean, 88

L

L1, 76
labeling, 14, 150, 152
laboratory method, 14
lactams, 34, 35, 67, 69, 71, 72, 81, 155, 162, 168
lactic acid, 157
lactic acid bacteria, 157
lactoferrin, 187
lactoglobulin, 191
lactones, 128
lactoperoxidase, 187
lambda, 192
Laos, 91
large-scale, 246
laryngoscope, 33

late-onset, 56, 61
Latin America, 38
law, 137, 139, 140, 141
leaks, 59
leptin, 196, 200
Lesion, 68
lesions, 169
lethargy, 115
leucine, 37
leukaemia, 23, 24, 25, 26, 28
leukemia, ix, 1, 2, 3, 4, 5, 6, 7, 9, 10, 11, 12, 13, 14, 18, 20, 22, 23, 24, 25, 26, 27, 28, 29, 147, 150, 205, 211
leukemia cells, 24, 28, 147
leukemias, ix, 1, 2, 3, 6, 14, 15, 16, 17, 19, 22, 26, 29, 145
leukemic, ix, xiii, 1, 2, 4, 5, 6, 10, 11, 16, 17, 21, 29, 143, 146, 149, 213, 214
leukemic cells, ix, 1, 5, 6, 10, 11, 16, 17, 21, 146
leukocytes, 177, 189
life cycle, 169, 170, 174
life-threatening, 40, 74, 100, 106, 154
ligand, 103, 230
ligands, 113
limitation, 81
limitations, 125, 130, 184
linear, 143, 196
links, 230
lipase, 84
lipid, 37, 53, 68, 133, 135, 142, 143, 144, 150, 151, 152, 162, 164, 166, 169, 175
lipids, 37, 133, 135, 142, 145, 150
lipophilic, xii, 203, 204, 210
lipopolysaccharide, 37, 39, 173, 176, 182, 237, 238, 243
lipopolysaccharides, 37, 166, 176
Lipoprotein, 188
Listeria monocytogenes, 170, 171, 175, 191
liver, 41, 47, 101, 103, 106, 107, 108, 110, 120, 122, 125, 128, 210
liver cirrhosis, 47
liver transplant, 125
liver transplantation, 125
livestock, 89, 184
location, 48, 70, 138
locus, 18, 162, 242
London, 96, 97, 211
longitudinal study, 89
Los Angeles, 186
loss of consciousness, 43
lovastatin, 149
low risk, 110
lower respiratory tract infection, 160
low-level, 80, 81, 156, 157
LPS, 37, 182
LSCs, ix, 1
lumen, 104, 210
lung, 3, 7, 8, 131, 140, 143, 146, 148, 150, 197, 201, 216, 221
lung cancer, 131, 221
lung disease, 201
lungs, 175, 191
lying, xiii, 219
lymphatic, 3
lymphoblast, 18
lymphocytes, 200
lymphoma, 192
lysine, 176
lysis, 169, 170, 171, 173, 174, 175, 182, 185, 188, 189
lysosomes, 131
lysozyme, 174, 177, 178, 179, 187, 188, 190, 191, 192

M

M1, 10, 180
machinery, 170, 243
macrophages, 177
magnesium, 162
magnetic resonance spectroscopy, 147
maintenance, 9, 19, 127, 132, 135
malaria, 240
males, 128
malignancy, 130
malignant, x, 129, 130, 131, 145, 146
malnutrition, 196, 197, 199, 200, 201
mammalian cells, 177, 220, 221
mammals, 174
management, xiv, 54, 55, 66, 198, 226, 238, 240
mania, 106
manic episode, 116
manipulation, 47, 199
manure, 77
MAO, 114, 116
marine environment, 88
marrow, 5, 6, 9, 21, 26
mask, 46, 142
mass spectrometry, 128
mastitis, 180

matrix, 14
maturation, 23
MDA, xii, 203, 204, 206, 208, 209
MDR, vii, viii, ix, x, xi, xii, xiii, 32, 39, 46, 51, 65, 66, 71, 78, 86, 129, 130, 131, 132, 133, 134, 136, 137, 138, 139, 140, 142, 144, 145, 147, 148, 149, 150, 154, 159, 160, 162, 163, 203, 204, 210, 214, 215, 216, 219, 226, 227, 230, 231, 233, 238, 243
measurement, 16, 147
measures, ix, xi, 33, 48, 81, 131, 153, 154, 163
meat, 170, 171, 191
mechanical properties, xi, 130, 133, 145
mechanical ventilation, 43, 45, 46, 47, 160
media, 32, 189, 231
median, 10, 12, 82
mediators, 200
medications, 105
medicine, 247, 248
membrane permeability, 39, 150, 151, 215
membranes, 37, 68, 133, 134, 151, 177, 178
men, 104, 200
meningeal inflammation, 44, 45
meningitis, 31, 39, 40, 42, 43, 44, 45, 47, 55, 56, 58, 59, 60, 62, 180, 217
mercury, 70
meta-analysis, 80, 88
metabolic, 23, 106, 107, 109, 110, 111, 113, 114, 118, 120, 124, 125, 155, 157, 196, 197, 200, 228, 233, 237, 238, 246
metabolic dysfunction, 196, 200
metabolic pathways, 23, 157
metabolism, 2, 3, 18, 19, 20, 101, 102, 103, 107, 111, 119, 120, 121, 122, 125, 126, 127, 130, 158, 197, 238
metabolite, 103, 110, 114
metabolites, 124, 210
metabolizing, 106, 113
metastasis, 16, 20, 21, 146, 147
metastatic, xiii, 130, 219
metastatic cancer, xiii, 219
methicillin-resistant, x, 50, 65, 80, 87, 88, 89, 91, 92, 93, 98, 157, 158, 181, 192, 193, 239, 241
Methotrexate, 9, 19, 25
metropolitan area, 80
mice, 37, 53, 101, 121, 122, 125, 170, 171, 173, 174, 177, 178, 180, 185, 187, 189, 191, 193, 196, 200, 210
microarray, ix, 1, 2, 7, 14, 15, 16, 17, 21, 22, 26, 231
microarray technology, 16
microbes, 174, 178, 183
microbial, 67, 68, 69, 158, 188, 189, 190, 192
microenvironment, 130
microflora, 171, 179
micrograms, 177
microinjection, 147
micronutrients, 198
microorganism, 45, 158, 247
microorganisms, xii, 37, 60, 66, 78, 167, 174, 245, 246, 247
microsomes, 103, 107, 110
microtubule, 221
microtubules, 221, 222
migration, 157
miliary tuberculosis, 197, 201
military, 33, 50, 51
milk, 33, 110, 112, 117, 118, 126, 174, 192
milligrams, 177
minimal residual disease, ix, 1, 2, 4, 16, 29
minimal residual disease (MRD), 16
Ministry of Education, 99
mitochondria, 164
mitochondrial, 2
mitosis, 221
Mitoxantrone, 205, 208, 209
mixing, 163
MLL, 6, 7, 13, 16, 21, 24
modeling, 147, 191
models, x, 42, 99, 107, 112, 149, 170, 171, 197, 230
modulation, 11, 25, 102, 104, 121, 149, 237
modulus, 134, 135, 136
moieties, 39
mold, 246
molecular biology, xi, 14, 16, 153, 190
molecular mass, 176
molecular mechanisms, 14, 16, 162
molecular weight, xi, 130, 152
molecules, 37, 113, 156, 169, 176, 184, 187, 215, 245, 247
monoclonal antibody, 53, 192
monocytes, 177
monosomy, 6
monotherapy, 2, 42, 45, 57, 58, 61
morbidity, x, xiii, 47, 65, 80, 198, 200, 213, 246
morphological, 169, 185
morphology, 14

mortality, x, xi, xii, xiii, 31, 40, 42, 43, 45, 47, 60, 62, 65, 80, 81, 82, 84, 85, 88, 93, 153, 162, 173, 195, 197, 198, 202, 213, 216, 219, 246
mortality rate, 31, 45, 47, 80, 82, 85, 162, 173, 246
mosaic, 156
mouse, 42, 57, 58, 103, 121, 148, 192
movement, xi, 129, 133, 135, 136, 139, 142
MRD, 6, 16
mRNA, 15, 17, 68
MRPs, 5
MRSA, x, 65, 66, 71, 72, 78, 79, 80, 81, 82, 87, 92, 93, 164, 181, 239, 240, 241
mucosa, 84
mucous membrane, 178, 192
mucous membranes, 178, 192
multidrug resistance, x, xii, 2, 4, 6, 7, 11, 12, 51, 61, 86, 88, 120, 129, 147, 148, 149, 150, 151, 152, 203, 211, 239, 241, 242
multidrug-resistant tuberculosis, 202
multiplication, 170, 185
mutant, 75, 173, 193, 246
mutation, 16, 74, 82, 155, 156, 157, 160, 171, 172, 173, 221, 228, 246, 247
mutations, 28, 34, 36, 53, 69, 73, 74, 104, 155, 156, 157, 164, 221, 227, 228, 231, 242, 245, 247
MYC, 13
mycobacteria, 71
Mycobacterium, 66, 75, 154, 196, 200, 226, 239, 240, 243, 244
myeloid, ix, 1, 3, 6, 7, 10, 14, 18, 20, 23, 24, 25, 26, 27, 28, 149, 211
myeloid cells, 149
myeloma, 211

N

Na^+, 131, 132, 146, 149, 227
N-acety, 36, 67, 97, 119, 128, 175, 176, 181, 188, 189, 193
NADH, 243
NAM, 178
nares, 78
nasal cavity, 179
nasopharynx, 178
National Academy of Sciences, 190, 191, 192, 193
natural, xi, xii, 71, 91, 153, 154, 155, 157, 171, 203, 204, 245, 246, 247, 248
natural environment, 247
natural selection, xi, 153, 154, 246, 247, 248
nausea, 39, 105
neonatal, 179
neoplastic, 130
nephrotoxicity, 39, 55, 58, 216
Netherlands, 79, 90, 163
network, 131, 170, 175, 176, 182
neurodegenerative diseases, 146
neuroendocrine, 196, 200
neurofilament, 222
neurotoxicity, 40
neutralization, 173
New England, 192
New Jersey, 211
New York, 88, 152, 163, 190, 192, 199
Newton, 247
Nielsen, 150, 151
nitrates, 32
nodulation, 41
non-infectious, 226
nontoxic, 183
norepinephrine, 105
norfloxacin, 227
normal, 10, 18, 21, 28, 41, 79, 101, 130, 131, 149, 179, 196, 221, 246, 247
North America, 38, 54, 80, 163
Northeast, 66
nosocomial pneumonia, 46, 55, 61, 98
nuclear, 103, 121, 222
nucleic acid, 14, 19, 68, 155, 156, 169, 170, 172, 183
nucleoside analogs, 6
nucleotide sequence, 98
nutrient, 196, 199
nutrients, 245
nutrition, xii, 32, 43, 195, 196, 197, 199
nylon, 14

O

obese, 196
obesity, xii, 195, 196, 200
obligate, 3
observations, 100, 131, 196, 228
ofloxacin, 42, 168, 227
oil, 103, 119
older adults, 26
oligomerization, 222
oligonucleotides, 14, 26

oligosaccharide, 37
omeprazole, 104, 123, 127, 241
oncogenes, 20
oncogenesis, 20, 21, 146
oncological, 177, 216
oncology, 1, 4, 23, 25, 28, 145
optimism, 183
oral, x, 46, 99, 101, 104, 105, 106, 107, 109, 114, 115, 116, 121, 122, 127, 177, 179, 181
oral cavity, 177, 180, 181
oral contraceptives, x, 99, 101, 105, 106, 127
organ, 107, 112, 124
organelles, 131
organic, 79
organism, ix, 32, 33, 34, 37, 41, 48, 71, 75, 84, 85, 171, 216, 226, 227, 231, 237, 238, 246, 247
osmotic, 151
osmotic pressure, 151
osteomyelitis, 33, 217
otitis externa, 78
otitis media, 189
outpatients, 80
ovary, 149
overproduction, 68
oxidation, 120
oxidative, 189
oxygen, 147

P

p53, xiii, 219, 221
Pacific, 38, 54, 220
paclitaxel, 131
pancreas, 101, 106
pancreatic, 101, 148
pancreatic cancer, 148
pan-European, 53, 94
paradoxical, 131
parasite, 214
parenteral, 39, 43, 46, 48
Paris, 49
paroxetine, 106
patents, 171, 183
pathogenesis, xii, 6, 133, 154, 175, 186, 247
pathogenic, xi, 75, 91, 153, 157, 158, 166, 168, 171, 173, 174, 177, 178, 181, 191, 192, 216
pathogens, x, xi, 31, 32, 38, 49, 54, 65, 66, 75, 86, 154, 155, 157, 158, 163, 164, 165, 168, 170, 171, 174, 175, 177, 178, 182, 186, 187, 192, 227
pathology, 189, 226
pathways, 2, 16, 17, 20, 21, 22, 23, 28, 148, 156, 189, 242
PCR, 26, 76, 87, 88, 96
pediatric, ix, 1, 2, 5, 6, 7, 8, 12, 16, 17, 18, 26, 27, 28, 216, 217
pediatric patients, 2, 17, 18, 216, 217
pelvic, 180
penalty, 135
penetrability, 32
penicillin, x, 34, 38, 44, 53, 65, 66, 67, 76, 79, 80, 83, 84, 155, 156, 157, 168, 177, 179, 188, 215, 246, 247
peptide, 68, 162, 166, 169, 175, 176, 243
peptide chain, 176
peptides, 73, 164, 166, 174, 177, 187, 189, 191
PER, 35, 52, 214
periodontal, 181
periodontal disease, 181
periplasm, 230
peritoneal, 33
peritonitis, 187
permeability, 34, 35, 39, 71, 74, 107, 133, 150, 151, 157, 159, 215, 227, 237, 238, 239, 243
permeation, 34, 137, 150
perturbation, 176
perturbations, 132
pets, 77, 78
P-glycoprotein, x, 7, 8, 99, 100, 101, 119, 120, 121, 122, 123, 129, 131, 132, 147, 149, 150, 151, 203, 211
pH, vii, xi, 104, 129, 130, 131, 132, 133, 142, 143, 144, 145, 146, 147, 148, 149, 152, 228, 229, 233, 234, 235, 236, 237, 238, 243
phage, xii, 92, 167, 168, 170, 171, 172, 173, 174, 175, 177, 179, 180, 181, 182, 183, 184, 185, 186, 187, 189, 190, 193, 194
phagocytic, 177
phagocytosis, 37
pharmaceutical, 90, 123, 204
pharmaceuticals, 174
pharmacodynamics, 119, 127
pharmacogenetics, 104, 120
pharmacogenomics, 16
pharmacokinetic, x, 2, 38, 41, 45, 59, 99, 101, 102, 105, 106, 107, 112, 113, 120, 124, 125, 173
pharmacokinetic parameters, 105

pharmacokinetics, 12, 101, 103, 104, 107, 119, 121, 123, 124, 125, 126, 127, 128
pharmacological, 100, 120, 149, 173, 211
pharmacology, 25
pharyngitis, 179
phenothiazines, 227, 228, 229, 238, 240
phenotype, ix, xi, xiii, 1, 130, 140, 144, 150, 153, 156, 226, 227, 230, 231, 233, 238, 239
phenotypes, xi, 34, 146, 153, 154, 226
phenotypic, 231
phenylbutyrate, 148
phenytoin, 105, 124
Philadelphia, 7, 8, 24
phlebitis, 39, 180
phosphate, 220, 234
phosphatidylcholine, 152
phosphatidylserine, 142, 151, 152
phospholipids, 135, 151
phosphoprotein, 222
phosphorus, 147
photosensitivity, 128
phylogenetic, 73
physical chemistry, 231
physical interaction, 133
physical properties, 37, 133, 137, 140
physicians, xiii, 216, 219, 220, 246
physics, 142
physiological, xiii, 19, 67, 120, 174, 183, 226, 228, 234, 238
physiology, 49, 192
pig, 94, 196
pigs, 73, 89, 158, 174, 200
pilot study, 185
placebo, 115
placenta, 210
plants, xii, 100, 167, 174, 183
plasma, 9, 33, 101, 104, 105, 106, 107, 110, 111, 112, 113, 116, 118, 124, 128, 132, 134, 138, 151, 176, 230
plasma levels, 110, 124
plasma membrane, 132, 134, 138, 151, 176, 230
plasma proteins, 111
plasmid, 35, 38, 39, 69, 70, 71, 73, 74, 79, 81, 86, 90, 91, 93, 94, 95, 96, 97, 98, 156, 162, 165, 181, 183, 215, 216, 245
plasmids, x, 36, 65, 69, 70, 73, 74, 75, 78, 87, 90, 92, 156, 158, 159, 162, 215
plastic, xi, 153
platelet, 101
platforms, 22
platinum, 10
play, ix, xi, 8, 36, 86, 101, 104, 133, 153, 175, 199, 210, 215, 221
ploidy, 25
pneumococcus, 189
pneumonia, 31, 38, 39, 40, 41, 42, 45, 46, 47, 49, 55, 56, 57, 58, 60, 61, 62, 71, 84, 94, 162, 165, 166, 179, 180, 189, 217
point mutation, 69
poisoning, 170, 171, 180, 181, 182, 211
Poland, 1, 86
politics, 200
polyelectrolytes, 189
polymer, 175
polymerase, 68, 97, 191
polymerase chain reaction, 97
polymerization, 67
polymers, 178
polymorphism, 106
polymorphisms, 119
polymorphonuclear, 177
polypeptide, 162
polypeptides, 172, 193
polysaccharide, 37, 182
polysaccharides, 37, 178
population, ix, 1, 22, 23, 33, 78, 87, 94, 96, 101, 139, 155, 172, 182, 184, 216, 245
pores, 170
Portugal, 192, 225, 239
positive correlation, 131
potatoes, 191
poultry, 33, 90, 97, 158, 185
poverty, 196, 199
power, 80, 139, 140, 141
prediction, 16, 20, 22, 27, 29, 106, 107, 111
predictors, 18, 202
predisposing factors, 89
Prednisolone, 19, 202
pre-existing, 40
preservatives, 174
pressure, 33, 78, 79, 84, 106, 128, 133, 151, 156, 163, 176, 184, 191, 192, 210, 231
prevention, 46, 48, 66, 146, 173, 183, 185, 193, 247
preventive, 187
probability, 133, 137, 138, 139, 140, 144
probable cause, 214
probe, 14, 17, 19, 20, 21, 70, 103, 104

production, 34, 35, 37, 38, 51, 53, 71, 78, 79, 81, 82, 83, 90, 147, 157, 162, 170, 171, 182, 200, 215, 246
progenitor cells, 23
prognosis, ix, xii, 1, 4, 6, 7, 8, 9, 10, 11, 12, 17, 19, 22, 25, 27, 28, 58, 84, 195
prognostic factors, ix, 1, 4, 17, 90, 163
prognostic value, 6, 7, 21, 197
proliferation, 19, 21, 130, 148, 177
promoter, 76, 190, 228
promoter region, 228
propagation, 157
prophylactic, 46
prophylaxis, 9, 46, 171, 179, 180, 185
propranolol, 105, 111, 124
Propranolol, 115
prostate, 222
prostate carcinoma, 222
protease inhibitors, 104, 112, 122
protection, 36, 37, 41, 156, 177, 178
protective genes, 157
protective role, 210
protein, xi, 2, 7, 8, 14, 19, 33, 36, 38, 41, 53, 69, 74, 97, 103, 111, 126, 129, 147, 148, 149, 150, 155, 156, 157, 162, 170, 173, 180, 185, 188, 189, 193, 196, 197, 199, 200, 204, 211, 222, 223, 230, 241, 242, 246
protein binding, 38, 111, 126
protein function, 222
protein synthesis, 41, 155
proteinases, 166
proteins, 2, 4, 11, 12, 16, 19, 34, 35, 38, 44, 53, 67, 68, 73, 75, 111, 120, 121, 149, 157, 159, 173, 174, 175, 176, 183, 187, 215, 222, 227, 240, 246, 247
proteomics, 26
protocols, 4, 5, 10, 12, 20, 46
proton pump inhibitors, 148
protons, 142, 228, 237, 238
Pseudomonas aeruginosa, 39, 51, 52, 54, 57, 58, 59, 61, 66, 71, 74, 83, 87, 88, 90, 91, 92, 94, 97, 154, 160, 161, 165, 166, 170, 177, 217, 240, 243, 247
PTA, 172
public, ix, 65, 66
pumps, xiii, 34, 35, 36, 41, 97, 159, 215, 226, 227, 228, 230, 231, 234, 238, 239, 240, 241, 242, 243
purification, 29, 188
purines, 68

Q

Quercetin, 117
quinine, 11

R

radiological, 201
radiotherapy, 3, 11
radius, 134, 135, 136, 137
random, xi, 10, 129, 137, 157
random walk, xi, 129, 137
range, 31, 46, 69, 70, 72, 74, 75, 81, 84, 85, 106, 157, 158, 160, 181, 204
rat, 91, 101, 105, 123, 177
rats, 103, 119, 121, 122, 128
RB1, 223
reactive oxygen species, 147
real-time basis, 233, 234
receptors, 105
recognition, 3, 37, 73, 190
recolonization, 178
recombination, 69, 73, 90
recovery, 51, 78, 84, 110
reductases, 73
refractory, ix, 2, 3, 4, 7, 10, 18
regional, 66
regression, 130, 143
regular, 48
regulation, 3, 21, 130, 147, 148, 156, 200, 237, 238, 243
regulations, 171
regulators, 231, 232, 243
rehabilitation, 33
rejection, 106, 112, 114, 124
relapse, xii, 2, 4, 5, 8, 12, 14, 16, 17, 18, 20, 21, 22, 26, 28, 29, 195, 198, 199, 201
relapses, ix, 1, 2, 21
relationship, 7, 9, 25, 73, 84, 92, 106, 130, 131, 133, 135, 140, 141, 142, 150, 196, 200, 202, 228, 230, 242
relationships, 96, 151, 152
relevance, 60, 119, 125, 189, 226, 248
remission, 4, 6, 10, 18, 21, 211
renal, 39, 40, 41, 47, 126, 127, 171
renal disease, 47
renal dysfunction, 40
renal failure, 39
repair, 2, 3, 19, 21, 156, 221

reparation, 121
replication, 68, 156, 172
repressor, 75
reproduction, 246
Reserpine, 239
reservoir, 33, 34, 63, 79, 87, 154, 178
reservoirs, 32, 77, 78
residual disease, ix, 1, 2, 4, 5, 6, 16, 29
residues, 78, 176, 227
resolution, 4, 163
resources, 199, 247
respiration, 210
respiratory, 33, 40, 41, 47, 83, 84, 94, 160, 168, 174, 177, 179, 192, 193, 197, 199, 214, 216
respiratory failure, 47, 197, 199
restriction enzyme, 97, 170
retardation, 182
retention, 131, 206, 208
retinoblastoma, 220, 222, 223
Retinoblastoma, 222
Reynolds, 148
rhabdomyolysis, 56, 105
rheumatic, 179, 180
rheumatic fever, 179, 180
ribosomal, 16, 19, 36, 41, 68, 74, 157
ribosome, 36, 68
rigidity, 115
risk, xii, 2, 4, 5, 6, 14, 16, 17, 18, 20, 23, 25, 27, 28, 38, 40, 43, 45, 46, 47, 60, 61, 62, 80, 82, 84, 85, 89, 92, 94, 97, 104, 110, 155, 160, 163, 166, 195, 196, 197, 198, 200, 201
risk factors, 4, 28, 40, 43, 47, 60, 61, 62, 82, 84, 85, 89, 92, 97, 198
risks, 77, 106, 113
RNA, 14, 19, 68, 169, 191
rods, 6, 32
Rome, 160
Royal Society, 191
ruminant, 188
Russia, 200

S

S phase, 220, 221
safety, 46, 61, 96, 100, 106, 112, 171, 183, 184, 187
saline, 234
saliva, 174
Salmonella, 70, 74, 75, 86, 87, 88, 89, 90, 95, 98, 154, 160, 170, 171, 180, 182, 191, 194, 234, 235, 236, 237, 238, 243
Salvia miltiorrhiza, 119
sample, 14, 79, 96, 198, 214
scaling, 107, 125, 136
Scandinavia, 79
Seattle, 171
seawater, 183
secretion, 37, 123, 242
sedation, 46
sedatives, x, 99, 101
seizures, 39
self-renewing, ix, 1
sensitivity, 8, 9, 16, 17, 19, 22, 24, 25, 27, 32, 148, 149, 174, 175, 191, 200, 214, 215, 223, 228, 233
separation, 174, 188, 193
sepsis, 83, 163, 178, 180, 192
septic shock, 38, 47
septicemia, 37, 189
sequelae, 189
sequencing, 188, 214, 228
series, 14, 28, 40, 41, 45, 46, 47, 53, 56, 57, 100, 114, 115, 116, 147, 170
serotonergic, 105
serotonin, 105, 106, 115, 116, 123
serotonin syndrome, 106, 123
sertraline, 105, 123
serum, 38, 45, 126, 204
severity, xii, 43, 47, 179, 195, 197, 201
sewage, 77, 78, 172
Shanghai, 98
sheep, 174
Shigella, 74, 75, 90, 97, 154, 187, 194
shock, 38, 47, 80, 179, 180
shortage, 162
shrimp, 183
side effects, 40, 173, 222, 226
signal transduction, 2, 21
signaling, 23
signals, 14, 208, 243
silicon, 14
simulation, 125, 151
single-drug, 85
sites, xii, 33, 48, 164, 176, 195
skin, 33, 50, 51, 78, 171, 174, 188, 197, 216
small intestine, 101, 170
smoking, 47
socioeconomic conditions, 196

sodium, 39, 42, 49, 59, 183
soil, 33, 77, 79, 95, 181, 191
solubility, 107
Soviet Union, 168
Spain, 31, 87, 129
species, x, xiii, 32, 33, 34, 38, 42, 49, 51, 57, 59, 60, 61, 65, 66, 69, 70, 88, 91, 100, 106, 147, 157, 162, 172, 174, 177, 179, 180, 181, 182, 187, 213, 214, 216, 246
specificity, 22, 168, 171, 172, 173, 192, 220
spectrophotometric, 206
spectrum, xiii, 33, 38, 43, 47, 52, 68, 71, 76, 86, 89, 90, 91, 92, 94, 95, 156, 160, 162, 168, 172, 174, 175, 177, 203, 204, 210, 214, 246, 247
spindle, 211
sporadic, 160
spore, 181, 193
sputum, xii, 71, 85, 195, 198, 199, 202, 214
stability, 38
stabilization, 33
staffing, 46
stages, x, 37, 99, 112, 113, 169
standards, 22
staphylococcal, x, 65, 79, 81, 91, 157, 175, 181, 183, 189, 193, 241
staphylococci, 75, 168, 175, 178, 191
Staphylococci, 157, 181
Staphylococcus aureus, 50, 66, 75, 79, 82, 87, 88, 89, 91, 92, 93, 96, 97, 98, 154, 158, 164, 170, 180, 181, 188, 189, 190, 191, 192, 193, 200, 226, 239, 240, 241, 242
stem cells, ix, 1, 4, 5, 23
sterilization, 196, 200
steroid, 2, 5, 7, 121
stimulus, 162
stomach, xi, 153
strategies, ix, x, xiii, 1, 6, 48, 65, 113, 169, 219
stratification, 5, 24, 27
strength, 169
streptococcal bacteria, 179
streptococci, 95, 175, 177, 178, 179, 180, 183, 186, 193
Streptomyces, 156
stress, 46, 231, 239
structural protein, 222
subgroups, 5, 10, 13, 21, 23, 174, 199
substances, 37, 77, 226, 245
substrates, x, 99, 101, 102, 103, 104, 110, 112, 119, 150, 204, 228
suffering, 198
sugars, 175
suicide, 103
sulfate, 39
sulfonamide, 94, 95, 97
sulfonamides, 96
supplements, 100, 124, 126, 127
supply, 73, 158
suppression, 130, 147, 162
suppressor, xiii, 219, 220, 221, 223
surface area, 139, 142
surface tension, 133, 134, 135, 136, 140, 142
surface water, 77, 96
surfactants, 150
surgery, 43, 198
surgical, 31, 40, 43, 44, 47, 60, 63, 80, 85, 89
surprise, 221
surveillance, 38, 48, 54, 57, 77, 80, 86, 177
survival, xiii, 6, 9, 12, 16, 17, 21, 28, 32, 42, 157, 170, 177, 185, 187, 219, 225, 238, 246
survival rate, 9, 170, 177
susceptibility, 38, 39, 41, 48, 52, 54, 57, 61, 71, 73, 79, 81, 86, 87, 88, 89, 92, 98, 160, 163, 168, 188, 214, 222, 223, 226, 231
Switzerland, 92, 94
symptoms, 37, 105, 115, 214
syndrome, 47, 71, 92, 105, 127, 171, 179, 180
synergistic, x, 42, 43, 58, 74, 99, 105, 185
synthesis, 19, 41, 67, 68, 130, 150, 155, 159, 162, 163, 220, 237, 238, 246
systems, 226, 227, 228, 240, 242, 243, 246, 247

T

T cell, 200
tacrolimus, x, 99, 101, 110, 127, 128
Taiwan, 62, 88, 217
Tamoxifen, 151
Tanzania, 198, 201, 202
targets, xi, 21, 34, 67, 86, 129, 156, 176, 181, 196, 221, 226, 231
taste, 171
taxanes, 204
Taxol, viii, xiii, 219, 220, 221, 222
taxonomic, 32
taxonomy, 32, 49
teaching, 50, 62, 80, 96, 200
teicoplanin, 67, 71, 79, 98, 155
TEM, 35, 76, 81, 86, 90, 92, 162, 214
temperature, 134, 150, 228, 233, 234
temporal, 160

tension, 133, 134, 135, 136, 140, 142, 152
testimony, 247
testosterone, 123
tetracycline, 36, 75, 78, 79, 83, 86, 89, 90, 91, 95, 96, 157, 170, 214, 226, 231, 232, 233, 234, 239, 240
tetracyclines, 11, 35, 36, 40, 41, 71, 75, 157, 215
Texas, 220
Thai, 50
Thailand, 94
therapeutic agents, xi, 85, 153, 171
therapeutic approaches, 32, 38
therapeutics, ix, xiii, 65, 134, 219, 221
therapy, ix, xii, xiii, 1, 2, 4, 5, 6, 7, 9, 11, 12, 14, 16, 17, 18, 20, 21, 28, 31, 33, 34, 36, 40, 41, 42, 44, 45, 46, 48, 57, 58, 59, 77, 81, 82, 85, 88, 90, 95, 113, 147, 167, 168, 170, 171, 172, 173, 175, 178, 184, 185, 186, 187, 190, 192, 198, 211, 215, 219, 220, 221, 226, 238, 240, 241
thiazide, 106
thioridazine, 228, 234, 237, 240
thiosulphate, 183
thioxanthenes, 239
third-generation cephalosporin, 33, 82, 88
Thomson, 54
threat, 54, 66, 164, 173
threshold level, 154
thymine, 73
tissue, ix, 1, 14, 37, 50, 81, 97, 151, 196, 216
TMP, 73
TNF, 19
Tokyo, 96, 241
tolerance, 79, 93, 241
Topoisomerase, 159
toxic, x, xiii, 17, 37, 39, 81, 99, 106, 112, 113, 120, 131, 171, 179, 180, 209, 215, 225, 226, 238
toxic shock syndrome, 179, 180
toxic substances, 226
toxicities, 105, 112, 113
toxicity, x, 37, 39, 40, 68, 99, 105, 112, 119, 121, 123, 171, 173, 175, 210
toxicological, 16, 127
toxin, 92, 172, 173, 187
toxins, 173, 214
tracheostomy, 33
traditional medicines, 119
traits, 156
transcription, 19, 20, 68, 76
transcription factor, 20
transcriptional, 27
transduction, 70
transfer, 68, 70, 89, 90, 96, 98, 134, 156, 157, 158, 159, 200, 216, 231, 246
transformation, 28, 70, 130, 146, 149, 156, 192
transgenic, 177, 191
transgenic mice, 177, 191
translation, 19, 68
translational, 76
translocation, 6, 7, 8, 18, 68, 135, 147, 149, 151
translocations, 5, 7, 10, 18
transmembrane, 132, 137, 139, 149, 151, 152, 204, 227, 230, 243
transmission, 32, 33, 48, 51, 69, 160, 163
transplant, 106, 124, 126, 127
transplant recipients, 126
transplantation, 24, 106, 124, 125
transport, 3, 9, 19, 67, 107, 120, 121, 132, 133, 145, 146, 148, 149, 150, 151, 157, 204, 227, 230, 240
transportation, 170
transposon, 36, 70, 76, 245
transposons, 36, 69, 70, 71, 75, 158, 159
trauma, 50, 51, 166
traumatic brain injury, 123
tremor, 105, 115
trial, 21, 26, 198, 199, 201, 202
triggers, 131
trisomy, 10, 18, 28
tuberculosis, xii, 66, 154, 155, 195, 196, 197, 198, 199, 200, 201, 202, 226, 239, 240, 243
tubular, 147
tumor, ix, xii, xiii, 1, 11, 17, 130, 131, 132, 145, 146, 147, 148, 149, 150, 151, 177, 203, 204, 211, 219, 220, 221, 223, 240
tumor cells, xii, 17, 145, 146, 148, 149, 150, 203, 204, 211, 240
tumor growth, 146, 149
tumorigenesis, 223
tumors, 16, 17, 149
tumour, 147, 149, 150, 203
turgor, 176
Turkey, 52, 94, 194
turnover, 137
tyrosine, 20, 147

U

ulcer, 46

underlying mechanisms, 102
undernutrition, xii, 195, 196
unification, 142
United Kingdom, 26, 51
United States, 2, 51, 54, 61, 88, 89, 92, 95, 97, 154, 171, 190, 191, 192, 193, 194, 200
United States Agency for International Development, 200
upper airways, xiii, 213, 216
upper respiratory infection, 193
upper respiratory tract, 168
urinary, 31, 38, 43, 81, 83, 103, 110, 172
urine, 174

V

vaccination, 185, 201
vacuum, xi, 129, 130, 132, 133
vaginitis, 168
validity, 140
valproic acid, 151
values, 8, 10, 110, 111, 134, 197, 208, 209, 214
Van der Waals radius, 136
vancomycin, 66, 67, 71, 74, 78, 79, 81, 88, 90, 92, 93, 98, 155, 157, 168, 170, 182, 187
variability, 37, 107
variables, 4, 22
variation, 199, 247
vascular endothelial growth factor, 147
vector, 69
vein, 222
ventilation, 46
ventilators, 33
verapamil, 11, 104, 122, 131, 146, 150, 151, 204, 206, 207, 208, 211, 228
vesicle, 134, 135, 136, 137, 151
veterinary medicine, 66, 76, 77
Vibrio cholerae, 70, 91, 93, 171, 186, 187
Victoria, 99
villus, 104
vinblastine, 131, 149, 151
virulence, 37, 81, 84, 88, 89, 90, 91, 93, 158, 164, 171, 173, 174, 187, 189
virus, 177, 189
viruses, ix, 65, 66, 156, 168, 170, 191
viscosity, 134, 135
vision, 239
vomiting, 115, 116

W

war, x, 33, 34, 50, 51, 65, 85
warfare, 178
warfarin, x, 99, 100, 101, 102, 105, 106, 112, 119, 125, 127
wastewater, 77
water, 33, 77, 79, 134, 157
watersheds, 79
weight gain, 198, 201
Weinberg, 146
West Indies, 65, 80, 82, 87, 94
western countries, 168
Western countries, 168, 170
white blood cell count, 7
WHO, 119, 164, 199
wild type, 241
wildlife, 79
women, 105
workers, 49, 79
World Health Organization, 100, 119, 199
wound infection, 31, 33, 47, 51
writing, 226

X

xenobiotic, 119
xenobiotics, 12, 102, 210
xerostomia, 187

Y

yeast, 146
yield, 42, 78, 177, 220, 226, 233
young adults, 22
young men, 200

Z

zinc, 191
zoonotic, 87